Pediatric Nurse Practitioner

Certification Review Guide

EDITOR

Virginia Layng Millonig, Ph.D, R.N., C.P.N.P.
Health Leadership Associates, Inc.
Potomac, Maryland

SECOND EDITION

Health Leadership Associates, Inc.
Potomac, Maryland

Family Nurse Practitioner Set
by
Health Leadership Associates, Inc.

**Adult Nurse Practitioner Certification
Review Guide**

**Pediatric Nurse Practitioner Certification
Review Guide**

**Women's Health Care Nurse Practitioner
Certification Review Guide**

Health Leadership Associates, Inc.

Production Manager:	Martha M. Pounsberry
Manuscript Editors:	Denise Colbert
Cover and Design:	Frances Weber, The Type House
Production:	Port City Press, Inc.

Second Edition

Copyright © 1994 by Health Leadership Associates, Inc.

Printed in the United States of America

Health Leadership Associates, Inc. ■ P.O. Box 59153 ■ Potomac, Maryland 20859

Library of Congress Cataloging-in-Publication Data

Pediatric nurse practitioner certification review guide / editor,
    Virginia Layng Millonig : contributing authors, Ellen Rudy Clore
    ... [et al.].—2nd ed.
       p.   cm.
    Includes bibliographical references and index.
    ISBN 1-878028-10-3
        1. Pediatric nursing—Outlines, syllabi, etc.   2. Examinations—
Study guides.   I. Millonig, Virginia Layng. II. Clore, Ellen Rudy
     [DNLM: 1. Pediatric Nursing—outlines.   WY 18 P37053 1994]
    RJ242.P43   1994
    610.73'62'076—dc20
    DNLM/DLC
    for Library of Congress   94-21935
                                                   CIP

10 9 8 7 6 5 4

Fourth printing January 1997

Contributing Authors

TEST TAKING STRATEGIES AND TECHNIQUES
Nancy Dickenson Hazard, M.S.N., C.P.N.P., F.A.A.N.
Executive Officer
Sigma Theta Tau International
Indianapolis, Indiana

GROWTH AND DEVELOPMENT
Lois A. Hancock, M.S.N., C.P.N.P.
Lecturer
Parent and Child Nursing
College of Nursing
University of Washington
Seattle, Washington

HEALTH MAINTENANCE AND PROMOTION
Margaret A. Hertzog, M.S.N., C.P.N.P.
Pediatric Nurse Practitioner
Pediatric Clinic
Sacred Heart Hospital
Allentown, Pennsylvania

ENDOCRINE DISORDERS
Jacalyn Peck Dougherty, M.S.N., C.P.N.P.
Former Assistant Professor
Primary Care of Infants, Children, Adolescents Program
School of Nursing
University of Colorado Health Sciences Center
Denver, Colorado

HEMATOLOGICAL/ONCOLOGICAL/IMMUNOLOGICAL DISORDERS
Jo-Anne Tierney, M.S.N., C.P.N.P.
Associate in Nursing
School of Nursing
Columbia University
New York, New York

DERMATOLOGICAL DISORDERS
Ellen Rudy Clore, M.S.N., C.P.N.P.
Assistant Professor
College of Nursing
University of Florida
Orlando, Florida

EYE, EAR, MOUTH DISORDERS
>Carole S. Stone, M.S.N., C.P.N.P.
>Assistant Professor
>Pediatric Nurse Practitioner Program
>School of Nursing
>The Catholic University of America
>Washington, D. C.

RESPIRATORY DISORDERS
>Carole S. Stone, M.S.N., C.P.N.P.
>Assistant Professor
>Pediatric Nurse Practitioner Program
>School of Nursing
>The Catholic University of America
>Washington, D. C.

CARDIOVASCULAR DISORDERS
>Carole S. Stone, M.S.N., C.P.N.P.
>Assistant Professor
>Pediatric Nurse Practitioner Program
>School of Nursing
>The Catholic University of America
>Washington, D. C.

NEUROLOGICAL DISORDERS
>Elizabeth Hawkins-Walsh, M.S.N., C.P.N.P.
>Assistant Professor
>Director
>Pediatric Nurse Practitioner Program
>School of Nursing
>The Catholic University of America
>Washington, D.C.

MUSCULOSKELETAL DISORDERS
>Elizabeth Hawkins-Walsh, M.S.N., C.P.N.P.
>Assistant Professor
>Director
>Pediatric Nurse Practitioner Program
>School of Nursing
>The Catholic University of America
>Washington, D.C.

GENITOURINARY/GYNECOLOGIC DISORDERS

Elizabeth Hawkins-Walsh, M.S.N., C.P.N.P.
Assistant Professor
Director
Pediatric Nurse Practitioner Program
School of Nursing
The Catholic University of America
Washington, D.C.

GASTROINTESTINAL DISORDERS

Elizabeth Hawkins-Walsh, M.S.N., C.P.N.P.
Assistant Professor
Director
Pediatric Nurse Practitioner Program
School of Nursing
The Catholic University of America
Washington, D.C.

TRENDS, PROFESSIONAL ISSUES, HEALTH POLICY

Marilyn Winterton Edmunds, Ph.D., C.R.N.P.
Associate Professor
Director, Gerontological Nurse Practitioner Program
School of Nursing
University of Maryland
Baltimore, Maryland

Debra Hardy Havens, B.S.N., R.N., F.N.P.
Vice President, Chief Executive Officer
Capitol Associates, Inc.
Washington, D. C.

HEALTH LEADERSHIP ASSOCIATES, INC.
POTOMAC, MARYLAND

Reviewers

Arlene Butz, Sc.D., C.P.N.P.
Assistant Professor
School of Nursing
Johns Hopkins University
Baltimore, Maryland

Linda K. Jonides, B.S., C.P.N.P.
Pediatric Nurse Practitioner
Private Practice
Ann Arbor, Michigan

Clare Marie Rodgers, M.S.N., C.P.N.P.
Pediatric Nurse Practitioner
Private Practice
Annapolis, Maryland

Agnes C. Tytko, M.S.N., RN,CS
Instructor
Coordinator Nurse Practitioner Program
Frances Payne Bolton School of Nursing
Case Western Reserve University
Cleveland, Ohio

Victoria A. Weill, M.S.N., C.P.N.P.
Lecturer
Primary Care/Young Family Program
School of Nursing
University of Pennsylvania
Philadelphia, Pennsylvania

Preface

The second edition of this book has been developed especially for pediatric and family nurse practitioners preparing to take Certification Examinations. The second edition differs substantially from the first edition in several respects. All sections have been expanded and updated. The number of questions has been increased and the bibliographies enhanced. The new additions to this edition are the chapters on endocrine and hematological/immunological/oncological disorders and the trends, professional issues, health policy chapter.

The purpose of the book is twofold. This book will assist individuals engaged in self study preparation for Certification Examinations, and may be used as a brief reference guide in the practice setting. It is also one of three books that comprises the "Family Nurse Practitioner Series," the others being the Adult Nurse Practitioner Certification Review Guide and the Ob-Gyn Nurse Practitioner Certification Review Guide.

The book has been organized to provide the reader with test taking strategies first. This is followed by the chapters on growth and development and health maintenance and promotion. The next 10 chapters address common disorders and provide succinct summaries of definitions, etiology, signs and symptoms, physical findings, differential diagnoses, diagnostic tests/findings and management/treatment. The final chapter addresses health policy, role, trends and professional issues for the nurse practitioner in the health care industry at large.

Following each chapter are test questions, which are intended to serve as an introduction to the testing arena. In addition a bibliography is included for those who need a more in depth discussion of the subject matter in each chapter. These references can serve as additional instructional material for the reader.

Many nurses preparing for certification examinations find that reviewing an extensive body of scientific knowledge requires a very difficult search of many sources that must be synthesized to provide a review base for the examination. This publication provides a succinct, yet comprehensive review of the core material.

The editor and contributing authors are certified nurse practitioners. They have designed this book to assist potential examinees to prepare for success in the certification examination process.

It is assumed that the reader of this review guide has completed a course of study in either a pediatric or family nurse practitioner program. The Pediatric Nurse Practitioner Certification Review Guide is not intended to be a basic learning tool.

Certification is a process that is gaining recognition both within and outside the profession. For the professional it is a means of gaining special recognition as a certified nurse practitioner which not only demonstrates a level of competency, but may also enhance professional opportunities and advancement. For the consumer, it means that a certified nurse has met certain predetermined standards set by the profession.

Acknowledgements

Appreciation is extended to the authors, reviewers and the many nurse practitioners throughout the country who have provided suggestions and directions in the development of the second edition of this Review Guide. And also, to the nurse practitioners who have found this review guide not only responsible for success in the certification process, but also as a useful tool in the clinical setting.

CONTENTS

Test Taking Strategies and Techniques

Nancy A. Dickenson Hazard

We all respond to testing situations in different ways. What separates the successful test taker from the unsuccessful one is knowing how to prepare for and take a test. Preparing yourself as a successful test taker is as important as studying for the test. Each person needs to assess and develop their own test taking strategies and skills. The primary goal of this chapter is to assist potential examinees in knowing how to study for and take a test.

STRATEGY #1 Know Yourself

When faced with an examination, do you feel threatened, experience butterflies or sweaty palms, have trouble keeping your mind focused on studying or on the test question? These common symptoms of test anxiety plague many of us, but can be used advantageously if understood and handled correctly (Divine & Kylen, 1979). Over the years of test taking, each of us have developed certain testing behaviors, some of which are beneficial, while others present obstacles to successful test taking. You can take control of the test taking situation by identifying the undesirable behaviors, maintaining the desirable ones and developing skills to improve test performance.

Technique #1: From the following descriptions of test taking personalities, find yourself (Table 1). Write down those characteristics which describe you even if they are from different personality types. Carefully review the problem list associated with your test taking personality characteristics. Write down the problems which are most troublesome. Then make a list of how you can remedy these problems from the improvement strategies list. Be sure to use these strategies as you prepare for and take examinations.

STRATEGY #2 Develop Your Thinking Skills

Understanding Thought Processes: In order to improve your thinking skills and subsequent test performance, it is best to understand the types of thinking as well as the techniques to enhance the thought process.

Everyone has their own learning style, but we all must proceed through the same process to think.

Thinking occurs on two levels—the lower level of memory and comprehension and the higher level of application and analysis (ABP, 1989). Memory is the ability to recall facts. Without adequate retrieval of facts, progression through the higher levels of thinking can not occur easily. Comprehension is the ability to understand memorized facts. To be effective, comprehension skills must allow the person to translate recalled information from one context to another. Application, or the process of using information to know why it occurs, is a higher form of learning. Effective application relies on the use of understood memorized facts to verify intended action. Analysis is the ability to use abstract or logical forms of thought to show relationships and to distinguish the cause and effect between the variables in a situation.

Table 1

Test Taker Profile

Type	Characteristics	Pitfalls	Improvement Strategies
The Rusher	• Rushes to complete the test before the studied facts are forgotten • Arrives at test site early and waits anxiously • Mumbles studied facts • Tense body posture • Accelerated pulse, respiration and neuromuscular excitement • Answers questions rapidly and is generally one of the first to complete • Experiences exhaustion once test is over	• Unable to read question and situation completely • At high risk for misreading, misinterpreting and mistakes • Difficult items heighten anxiety • Likely to make quick, not well-thought-out guesses	• Practice progressive relaxation techniques • Develop a study plan with sufficient time to review important content • Avoid cramming and last minute studying • Take practice tests focusing on slowing down and reading and answering each option carefully • Read instructions and questions slowly
The Turtle	• Moves slowly, methodically, deliberately through each question • Repeated rereading, underlining and checking • Takes 60 to 90 seconds per question versus an average of 45 to 60 seconds	• Last to finish; often does not complete the exam • Has to quickly complete questions in last part of exam, increasing errors • Has difficulty completing timed examinations	• Take practice tests focusing on time spent per item • Place watch in front of examination paper to keep track of time • Mark answer sheet for where one should be halfway through exam based on total number of questions and total amount of time for exam • Study concepts, not details • Attempt to answer each question as you progress through the exam

Table 1
Test Taker Profile

Type	Characteristics	Pitfalls	Improvement Strategies
The Personalizer	• Mature person who has personal knowledge and insight from life experiences	• Runs risk in relying on what has been learned through observation and experience since one may develop false understandings and stereotypes	• Focus on principles and standards that support nursing practice
		• Personal beliefs and experiences are frequently not the norm or standard tested	• Avoid making connections between patients in exam clinical situations and personal clinical experience
		• Has difficulty identifying expected standards measured by standardized examination	• Focus on generalities not experiences
The Squisher	• View exams as threat, rather than an expected event in education	• Procrastinates studying for exams	• Establish a plan of progressive, disciplined study
	• Preoccupied with grades and personal accomplishment	• Unable to study effectively since waits until last minute	• Use defined time frames for studying content and taking practice exams
	• Attempts to avoid responsibility and accountability associated with testing in order to reduce anxiety	• Increased anxiety over test since procrastinating in the study effort impairs ability to learn and perform	• Use relaxation techniques • Return to difficult items • Read carefully
The Philosopher	• Academically successful person who is well disciplined and structured in study habits	• Over analysis causes loss of sight of actual intent of question	• Focus on questions as they are written
	• Displays great intensity and concentration during exam	• Reads information into questions answering with their own added information rather than answering the actual intent of question	• Work on self confidence and not on question. Initial response is usually correct
	• Searches for questions hidden or unintended meaning		• Avoid multiple re-readings of questions
	• Experiences anxiety over not knowing everything		• Avoid adding own information and unintended meanings
			• Practice, practice, practice with sample tests
The Second Guesser	• Answers questions twice, first as an examinee, second as an examiner	• Altering an initial response frequently results in an incorrect answer	• Reread only the few items of which one is unsure. Avoid changing initial responses

Table 1
Test Taker Profile

Type	Characteristics	Pitfalls	Improvement Strategies
	• Believes second look will allow one to find and correct errors	• Frequently changes answers because the pattern of response appears incorrect (i.e. too many "true" or too many correct responses)	• Take exam carefully and progressively first time, allowing little or no time for rereading
			• Study facts
			• Avoid reading into the question
	• Frequently changes initial responses (i.e. grades own test)		
The Lawyer	• Attempts to place words or ideas into the question (leads the witness)	• Veers from the obvious answer and provides response from own point of view	• Focus on distinguishing what patient is saying in question and not on what is read into question
	• Occurs most frequently with psychosocial or communication questions which ask for the most appropriate response	• Reads a question, jumps to a conclusion then finds a response that leads to predetermined conclusion	• Avoid formulating responses aimed at obtaining certain information
			• Choose responses that allow patient to express feelings which encourage hope, not catastrophe, those which are intended to clarify, which identify feeling tone of patient or which avoid negating or confronting patient feelings
			• Carefully read entire question before selecting a response

From: "Making the grades as a test-taker," by N. Dickenson-Hazard, (1989) *Pediatric Nursing* 15, p.303. Adapted from: *Nurse's guide to successful test-taking*, by M. B. Sides and N. B. Cailles, 1989. Philadelphia: J. B. Lippincott, Co., pp 59-70, 199-203. Copyright 1989 by A. J. Jannetti, Inc. Reprinted by permission.

As related to testing situations, the thought process from memory to analysis occurs quite quickly. Some examination items are designed to test memory and comprehension while others test application and analysis. An example of a memory question is as follows:

A normal child is expected to walk by:

a) 6 months
b) 10 months
c) *14 months*
d) 18 months

To answer this question correctly, the individual has to retrieve a memorized fact. Understanding the fact, knowing why it is important or analyzing what should be done in this situation is not needed. An example of a question which tests comprehension is as follows:

> The mother of an otherwise healthy 11-month old boy voices concern that her son is not walking yet because her older daughter walked at this age. You should know that:
>
> a) Girls generally walk before boys
> b) *Her son should be walking by 14 months of age*
> c) The mother is demonstrating overanxious behaviour
> d) Her son is delayed developmentally

To answer this question correctly, an individual must retrieve the fact that walking well is not always achieved until 14 months of age, and understand that in this situation, a child of 11 months would not necessarily be expected to have achieved this developmental milestone.

In a higher level of thinking examination question, individuals must be able to recall a fact, understand that fact in the context of the question, apply this understanding to explaining why one answer is correct, after analyzing the answer choices as they relate to the situation (Sides & Cailles, 1989). An example of an application analysis question is as follows:

> After administering the Developmental Screening Test (Denver II), you note that an 18-month old boy is not walking. The child's mother is voicing concern about this. Your most apropriate action is to:
>
> a) Repeat the Denver II in 6 months
> b) *Consult with pediatrician*
> c) Reassure the mother that the child's not walking is normal at this age
> d) Recommend exercises to strengthen the lower extremities

To answer this question correctly, the individual must recall the fact at which age walking should be achieved; understand if it is normal or abnormal for an 18-months old child not to walk as depicted in this situation; apply this knowledge to each option, understanding why it may or may not be correct; and analyze each option for what action is most apropriate for this situation. Application/analysis questions require the examinee to use logical rationale, based on a well defined principle or fact. Problem solving ability becomes important as the examinee must think through each question option, deciding its relevance and importance to the situation of the question.

Building your thinking skills: Effective memorization is the cornerstone to learning and building thinking skills (Olney, 1989). We have all experienced "memory power outages" at some time, due in part to trying to memorize too much, too fast, too ineffectively. Developing skills to improve memorization is important to increasing the effectiveness of your thinking and subsequent test performance.

Technique #1: Quantity is NOT quality, so concentrate on learning important content. For example, it is important to know the various pharmacologic agents appropriate for the management of chronic obstructive pulmonary disease (COPD), not the specific dosages for each medication.

Technique #2: Memory from repetition, or saying something over and over again to remember it, usually fades. Developing memory skills which trigger retrieval of needed facts is more useful. Such skills are as follows:

Acronyms: These are mental crutches which facilitate recall. Some are already established such as PERRL (pupils equal, round, reactive to light), NOFTT for non-organic failure to thrive or SGA for small for gestational age. Developing your own acronyms can be particularly useful since they are your own word association arrangements in a singular word. Nonsense words or funny, unusual ones are often more useful since they attract your attention.

Acrostics: This mental tool arranges words into catchy phrases. The first letter of each word stands for something which is recalled as the phrase is said. Your own acrostics are most valuable in triggering recall of learned information since they are your individual situation associations. An example of an acrostic is as follows:

<u>M</u>om <u>C</u>arried <u>N</u>ell <u>E</u>very <u>P</u>lace <u>S</u>he <u>W</u>ent stands for the areas of assessment for a cast check: movement, color, numbness, edema, pulse, sensation and warmth.

ABCs: This technique facilitates information retrieval by using the alphabet as a crutch. Each letter stands for a symptom, which when put together creates a picture of the clinical presentation of the disease. The clinical picture of acute epiglottitis using the ABC technique is as follows:

    a) Aphonia
    b) Brassy cough
    c) Complaint of sore throat initially
    d) Dysphagia
    e) Expiratory and inspiratory stridor
    f) Forward leaning position

Imaging: This technique can be used in two ways. The first is to develop a nickname for a clinical problem which when said produces a mental picture. For example, the nickname "bloated blue baby" might be used to trigger visualization of an infant with a congenital heart defect who is cyanotic, edematous and having breathing difficulty. A second form of imaging is to visualize a specific patient while you are trying to understand or solve a clinical problem when studying or answering a question. For example, imagine a child with cerebral palsy. You are trying to understand the most appropiate feeding position for this child. In your mind, visualize the various positions of supine, prone and semi-prone, imaging what will happen to the child in each position.

Rhymes,   The absurd is easier to remember than the most common. Rhymes,
music   music or links can add absurdity and humor to learning and remembering
& links: (Olney, 1989). These retrieval tools are developed by the individual for specific content. For example, making up a rhyme about diabetes may be helpful in remembering the predominant female incidence, origin of disease, primary symptoms and management as illustrated by:

> There once was a girl
> > whose beta cells failed
> She grew quite thirsty
> > and her glucose levels sailed
> Her lack of insulin caused her to
> > increase her intake
> And her increased urinary output
> > was certainly not fake
> So she learned to watch her diet
> > and administer injections
> That kept her healthy, growing
> > and free of complications.

Setting content to music is sometimes useful to remembering. Melodies which are repetitious jog the memory by the ups and downs of the notes and the rhythm of the music.

Links connect key words from the content by using them in a story. An example given by Olney (1989) for remembering the parts of an eye is: IRIS watched a PUPIL through the LENS of a RED TIN telescope while eating CORN-EA on the cob.

Additional memory aids may also include the use of color or drawing for improving recall. Use different colored pens or paper to accentuate the material being learned. For example, highlight or make notes in blue for content about respiratory problems and in red for cardiovascular content. Drawing assists with visualizing content as well. This is particularly helpful for remembering the pathophysiology of the specific health problem.

The important thing to remember about remembering is to use good recall techniques.

Technique #3: Improving higher level thinking skills involves exercising the application and analysis of memorized fact. Small group review is particularly useful for enhancing these high level skills. It allows verbalization of thought processes and receipt of input about content and thought process from others (Sides and Cailles, 1989). Individuals not only hear how they think, but how others think as well. This interaction allows individuals to identify flaws in their thought process as well as to strengthen their positive points.

Taking practice tests are also helpful in developing application/analysis thinking skills. They permit the individual to analyze thinking patterns as well as the cause and effect relationships between the question and its options. The problem solving skills needed to answer application/analysis questions are tested, giving the individual more experience through practice (Dickenson-Hazard, 1990).

STRATEGY #3 Know The Content

Your ability to study is directly influenced by organization and concentration (Dickenson-Hazard, 1990). If effort is spent on both of these aspects of exam preparation, examination success can be increased.

Preparation for studying: Getting organized. Study habits are developed early in our education experiences. Some of our habits enhance learning while others do not. To increase study effectiveness, organization of study materials and time is essential. Organization decreases frustration, allows for easy resumption of study and increases concentrated study time.

Technique #1: Create your own study space. Select a study area that is yours alone, free from distractions, comfortable and well lighted. The ventilation and room temperature should be comfortable since a cold room makes it difficult to concentrate and a warm room makes you sleepy (Burkle & Marshak, 1989). All your study materials should be left in your study space. The basic premise of a study space is that it facilitates a mind set that you are there to study. When you interrupt study, it is best to leave your materials just as they are. Don't close books or put away notes as you will just have to relocate them, wasting your study time, when you do resume study.

Technique #2: Define and organize the content. From the test giver, secure an outline or the content parameters which are to be examined. If the test giver's outline is sketchy, develop a more detailed one for yourself using the recommended text as a guideline. Next, identify your available study resources: class notes, old exams, handouts, textbooks, review courses, or study groups. For national standardized exams, such as initial licensing or certification, it is best to identify one or two study resources which cover the content being tested and stick to them. Attempting to review all available resources is not only mind boggling, but increases anxiety and frustration as well. Make your selections and stay with them.

Technique #3: Conduct a content assessment. Using a simple rating scale of

> 1 = requires no review
> 2 = requires minimal review
> 3 = requires intensive review
> 4 = start from the beginning

Read through the content outline and rate each content area (Dickenson-Hazard, 1990). Table 2 provides a sample exam content assessment. Be honest with your assessment. It is far better to recognize your content weaknesses when you can study and remedy them, rather than wishing during the exam that you had studied more. Likewise with content strengths: if you know the material, don't waste time studying it.

Technique #4: Develop a study plan. Coordinate the content which needs to be studied with the time available (Sides and Cailles, 1989). Prioritize your study needs, starting with weak areas first. Allow for a general review at the end of the study plan. Lastly establish an overall goal for yourself; something that will motivate you when brought to mind.

Table 3 illustrates a study plan developed on the basis of the exam content assessment in Table 2. Conducting an assessment and developing a study plan should require no more than 50 minutes. It is a wise investment of time with potential payoffs of reduced study stress and exam success.

Table 2
Sample Content Assessment

Exam Content: Health Problems of Adolescents

Category: Provided by Test Giver   *Rating: Provided by Examinee*

I. Acne
    A. Pathophysiology 2
    B. Management 2
        1. General hygiene
        2. Medications
        3. Cleansing
        4. Expression of comedones
    C. Nursing Management 1
        1. Education
        2. Support
        3. Need for follow-up

II. Dysmenorrhea
    A. Etiology 4
    B. Pathophysiology 3
    C. Symptomatology 3
    D. Management 4
    E. Nursing Interventions 3

III. Infectious Mononucleosis
    A. Definition 1
    B. Pathophysiology 2
    C. Clinical Signs 1
    D. Diagnostic Tests 2
    E. Management 2
    F. Nursing Interventions 1

IV. Sports Injuries
    A. Types of Injuries 4
        1. Acute
        2. Chronic
    B. Management of Injuries 4
        1. Acute
        2. Chronic
    C. Injury prevention education 3
    D. Related health problems 4
        1. Nutrition
        2. Menstrual dysfunction
        3. Eating disorders
        4. Substance abuse
    E. Nursing Interventions 3

From "Study Smart" by N. Dickenson-Hazard, 1990, *Pediatric Nursing, 16*, p. 66 Copyright 1990 by A. J. Jannetti, Inc. Reprinted by permission.

Technique #5: Begin now and use your time wisely. The smart test taker begins the study process early (Olney, 1989). Sit down, conduct the content assessment and develop a study plan as soon as you know about the exam. DON'T PROCRASTINATE!

Getting Down To Business — The Actual Studying: There is no better way to prepare for an examination than individual study (Dickenson-Hazard, 1989). The responsibility to achieve the goal you set for this exam lies with you alone. The means you employ to achieve this goal do vary and should begin with identifying your peak study times and using techniques to maximize them.

Technique #1: Study in short bursts. Each of us have our own biologic clock which dictates when we are at our peak during the day. If you are a morning person, you are generally active and alert early in the day, slowing down and becoming drowsy by evening. If you are an evening person, you don't completely wake up until late morning and hit your peak in the afternoon and evening. Each person generally has several peaks during the day. It is best to study during those times when your alertness is at its peak (Dickenson-Hazard, 1990).

During our concentration peaks, there are mini peaks, or bursts of alertness (Olney, 1989). These alertness peaks of a concentration peak occur because levels of concentration are at their highest during the first part and last part of a study period. These bursts can vary from ten minutes to one hour depending on the extent of concentration. If studying is sustained for one hour there are only two mini peaks; one at the beginning and one at the end. There are eight mini peaks if that same hour is divided into four, 10-minute intervals. Hence it is more helpful to study in short bursts (Olney, 1989). More can be learned in less time.

Technique #2: Cramming can be useful. Since concentration ability is highly variable, some individuals can sustain their mini-peaks for 15, 20 or even 30 minutes at a time. Pushing your concentration beyond its peak is fruitless and verges on cramming, which in general is a poor study technique. There are, however, times when cramming, a short term memory tool, is useful. Short term memory generally is at its best in the morning. A quick review or cram of content in the morning can be useful the day of the exam (Olney, 1989). Most studying, however, is best accomplished in the afternoon or evening when long term memory functions at its peak.

Table 3
Sample Study Plan

Goal: Achieve a "B" on the adolescent health problem test.
Time Available: 2 Weeks

Objective	Activity	Date Accomplished
Master sports injury content	Read Chapter 26. Take notes on chapter content according to content outline	Feb. 5 & 6 1 hour
	Review class notes and combine with notes taken from text	Feb. 7 — 1 hour
	Review combined notes & sample test questions	Feb. 8 — 1 hour
Understand content on dysmenorrhea	Read Chapter 23. Take notes on chapter content according to content outline provided	Feb. 9 & 10 1 hour each day
	Review class notes and combine with text notes	Feb. 11 — 1 hour
	Review combined notes and sample test questions	Feb. 12 — 1 hour
Know material on infectious mononucleosis	Scan Chapter 27. Review class notes, supplementing class notes with text content	Feb. 13 — 1½ hours
Know material on acne	Scan Chapter 24. Review class notes supplementing class notes with text content	Feb. 15 — 1½ hours
Demonstrate under-standing of all material	Review with another person	Feb. 16 — 2 hours
	Review all notes	Feb. 18 — 2 hours
	Take sample test questions	Feb. 19 — 2 hours
Think positively	SMILE • Take frequent breaks • Reward myself after each study session	ON GOING

From "Study Smart" by N. Dickenson-Hazard, 1190, *Pediatric Nursing*, 16, p. 316. Copyright 1990 by A. J. Jannetti, Inc. Reprinted by permission.

Technique #3: Give your brain breaks. Regular times during study to rest and absorb the content is needed by the brain. The best approach to breaks is to plan them and give yourself a conscious break (Dickenson-Hazard, 1990). This approach eliminates the "day dreaming" or "wandering thought" approach to breaks that many of us use. It is better to get up, leave the study area and do something non-study related for longer breaks. For shorter breaks of five minutes or so, leave your desk, gaze out the window or do some stretching exercises. When your brain says to give it a rest, accommodate it! You'll learn more in less stress free time.

Technique #4: Study the correct content. It is easy for all of us to become bogged down in the detail of the content we are studying. However, it is best to focus on the major concepts or the "state of the art" content. Leave the details, the suppositions and the experience at the door of your study area. Concentrate on the major textbook facts and concepts which revolve around the subject matter being tested.

Technique #5: Fit your studying to the test type. The best way to prepare for an objective test is to study facts, particularly anything printed in italics. Memory enhancing techniques are particularly useful when preparing for an objective test. If preparing for an essay test, study generalities, examples and concepts. Application techniques are helpful when studying for this type of an exam (Burkle and Marshak, 1989).

Technique #6: Use your study plan wisely. Your study plan is meant to be a guide, not a rigid schedule. You should take your time with studying. Don't rush through the content just to remain on schedule. Occasionally study plans need revision. If you take more or less time than planned, readjust the plan for the time gained or lost. The plan can guide you, but you must go at your own pace.

Technique #7: Actively study. Being an active participant in study rather than trying to absorb the printed word is also helpful. Ways to be active include: taking notes on the content as you study; constructing questions then answering them; taking practice tests or; discussing the content with yourself. Also using your individual study quirks are encouraged. Some people stand, others walk around and some play background music. Whatever helps you to concentrate and study better, you should use.

Technique #8: Use study aids. While there is no substitute for individual studying, several resources, if available, are useful in facilitating learning. Review courses are an excellent means for organizing or summarizing your individual study. They generally provide the content parameters and the major concepts of the content which you need to know. Review courses also provide an opportunity to clarify not-well-understood content, as well as to review known material (Dickenson-Hazard, 1990). Study guides are useful for organizing study. They provide detail on the content which is important to the exam. Study groups are an excellent resource for summarizing and refining content. They provide an opportunity for thinking through your knowledge base, with the advantage of hearing another person's point of view. Each of these study aids increases understanding of content and when used correctly increase effectiveness of knowledge application.

Technique #9: Know when to quit. It is best to stop studying when your concentration ebbs. It is unproductive and frustrating to force yourself to study. It is far better to rest or unwind, then resume at a later point in the day. Avoid studying outside your A.M. or P.M. concentration peaks and focus your study energy on your right time of day or evening.

STRATEGY #4 Become Test-wise

Most nursing examinations are composed of multiple choice questions (MCQs). This type of question requires the examinee to select the best response(s) for a specific circumstance or condition. Successful test taking is dependent not only on content knowledge but on test taking skill as well. If you are unable to impart your knowledge through the vehicle used for its conveyance, i.e. the MCQ, your test taking success is in jeopardy.

Technique #1: Recognize the purpose of a test question. Most test questions are developed to examine knowledge at two separate levels: memory (or recall) and comprehension (or application). A memory question requires the examinee to recall facts from their knowledge base while an application question requires the examinee to use and apply the knowledge (ABP, 1989). Memory questions test recall while application questions test synthesis and problem solving skills. When taking a test you need to be aware of whether you are being asked a fact or to use that fact.

Technique #2: Recognize the components of a test question. Multiple choice questions may include the basic components of a background statement, a stem and a list of options. The background statement presents information which facilitates the examinee in answering the question. The stem asks or states the intent of the question. The options are 4 or 5 possible responses to the question. The correct option is called the keyed response and all other options are called distractors (ABP, 1989). Knowing the components of a test question helps you sift through the information presented and focus on the question's intent (see Table 4).

Table 4
Anatomy Of A Test Question

Background Statement:

A 20 year old woman brings her 3-week old infant to the clinic because she is concerned about the child's crying, especially at night, and the infant's constant feeding demands.

Stem: Which of the following histories would be most helpful in planning your management?

Options:
(A) Developmental
(B) Family
(C) Social
(D) *Dietary*
(E) Genetic

Technique #3: Identify the key word(s) in a test question. Key words are generally included in the stem of a test question, whereas key concepts or conditions appear in the background statement. You should pay particular attention to the key words in the stem and their impact on the intent of the question (See Table 5).

Table 5		
Test Question Key Words And Phrases		
First	Priority	True Statements
Best	Advice	Correct Statements
Most	Approach	Contributing to
Initial	Consideration	Of the following
Important	Management	Which of the following
Major	Expectation	Each of the following
Common	Intervention	
Least	Assessment	
Except	Contraindication	
Not	Evaluation	
Greatest	Counseling	
Earliest	Facilitative	
Useful	Indicative	
Leading	Suggestive	
Significant	Appropriate	
Immediate	Accurately	
Helpful	Likely	
Closely	Characteristics	

From "Anatomy of a test question" by N. Dickenson-Hazard, 1989, *Pediatric Nursing* 15, p. 395. Copyright 1989 by A. J. Jannetti, Inc. Reprinted by permission.

Technique #4: Recognize the item types. Basically two styles of MCQs are used for examinations. One requires the examinee to select the one best answer; the other requires selection of multiple correct answers. Among the one best answer styles there are three types. The A type requires the selection of the best response among those offered. The B type requires the examinee to match the options with the appropriate statement. C type items require the examinee to compare or contrast two related conditions. The X type asks the examinee to respond either true or false to each option (ABP, 1989). Table 6 illustrates these item types. **Most standardized tests, such as those used for nursing licensure and certification, are composed of four or five option-A type questions.**

Technique #5: Read the directions to the questions carefully. Since an examination may have several types of questions, it is imperative to read the directions carefully. If different item types are used on an exam, they are generally grouped together by type and marked clearly with directions. Be on the lookout for changing item types and be sure you understand how you are to answer before you begin reading the question.

Technique #6: Apply the basic rules of test taking. Examination candidates can avert many problems associated with test taking if they give thought to the mechanics of sitting down, reading the question and noting their answers. Timing yourself to avoid spending too much time on a question, returning to difficult questions, and not changing your answers are all techniques that can improve performance. Table 7 provides helpful hints for the basic rules of test-taking. Review these and apply them to the testing situation.

Technique #7: Practice, practice, practice. Taking practice tests can improve performance. While they can assist in evaluation of your knowledge, their primary benefit is to assist you with test taking skills. You should use them to evaluate your thinking process, your ability to read, understand and interpret questions, and your skills in completing the mechanics of the test.

Technique #8: Be prepared for exam day. It is important to familiarize yourself with the test site, the building, the parking and travel route prior to the exam day. If you must travel, arrive early to allow time for this familiarization. It is helpful to make a list of things you need on the exam day: pencils, admission card, watch and a few pieces of hard candy as a quick energy source. On exam day allow yourself plenty of time to arrive at the site. Wear comfortable clothes and have a good breakfast that morning. The night before the exam, go to bed at a reasonable hour; avoid last minute cramming; and avoid excessive drinking or eating (Sides & Cailles, 1989). The idea is to arrive on time at the test site, prepared and as rested as possible.

Table 6
Item Type Examples

A TYPE

Directions for One Best Choice Items: This item-type requires that you indicate the one best answer from the lettered alternatives offered for each item. After you have decided on the one BEST answer, completely blacken the corresponding lettered circle on the answer sheet.

#1   You have recommended that a 6-month old infant receive a DPT immunization. His mother reports that he had a tender red thigh for three days after his last shot and a hard knot that is still there. The infant should receive:

    a. No further DPT
    b. Adult dT
    c. Tetanus toxoid alone
    d. *The recommended DPT*
    e. DT

B TYPE

Directions: Each group of questions below consists of five lettered headings followed by a list of numbered words or statements. For each numbered word or statement, select the one lettered heading that is most closely associated with it and fill in the circle beneath the corresponding letter on the answer sheet. Each lettered heading may be selected once, more than once, or not at all.

#2 - #4 Blood test
    a. Direct Coombs test
    b. Direct serum bilirubin concentration
    c. Hemoglobin electrophoresis
    d. Heterophil antibody titer
    e. Osmotic fragility test

Important in the diagnosis of:
    2. Blood group incompatibility (A)
    3. Mononucleosis (D)
    4. Sickle cell disease (C)

C TYPE

Directions: Each set of lettered headings below is followed by a list of numbered words or phrases. For each numbered word or phrase fill in the circle on the answer sheet under A if the item is associated with (A) only, B if the item is associated with (B) only, C if the item is associated with both (A) and (B), D if the item is associated with neither (A) nor (B).

    (A) Diabetic acidosis
    (B) Insulin shock
    (C) Both
    (D) Neither

#5 - Elevated bicarbonate level in serum (D)
#6 - The duration of the condition before proper treatment is begun may influence the prognosis (C)
#7 - Deep breathing (A)
#8 - Coma (C)
#9 - Moist skin characteristic (B)

X TYPE

Directions: Each of the questions or incomplete statements below is followed by five suggested answers or completions. For EACH lettered alternative completely blacken one lettered circle in either column T or F on the answer sheet.

True statements about fractures in school aged children include:
    (A) Assessment of fractures is less difficult in children than adults
    (B) *The initial treatment for sprains and fractures is elevation and application of an ice pack*
    (C) After a plaster cast is applied, little care is necessary
    (D) *Fractures in children heal faster than fractures in adults*
    (E) *Clavicular fractures are generally benign*

Adapted from "Anatomy of a test question." by N. Dickenson-Hazard, 1989, *Pediatric Nursing* 15, p. 396. Copyright 1989 by A. J. Jannetti, Inc. Reprinted by permission.

Table 7

Basic Rules For Test Taking

Basic Rule	Helpful Hints
Use time wisely and effectively	Allow no more than 1 minute per question—If you can't answer question, make an intelligent guess

Know the parts of a question
    Background statement: Informational scenario
    Stem: Specific question or intent statement
	Select the option that best completes question or solves the problem
	Relate options to question and balance against each other
	Consider all options

Read question carefully	Understand stem first, then look for answer Underline key words in background information and stem (i.e. first, best, initial, early, most, appropriate, except, least, not).
Identify intent of item based on information given	Don't assume any information not given Don't read in or add any information not given Actively reason through question
Answer difficult questions by eliminating obviously incorrect options first	Select the best of the viable, options available using logical thought Re-read stem; select stongest option Skip difficult questions and return to them later or make an educated guess
Select responses guided by principles of communication	Choose therapeutic, respectful, communication enhancing options Avoid inappropriate, punitive responses
Know the principles of nursing practice	Select options that relate to common need or the population in general Select options that are correct without exception Select options which reflect nursing judgement
Know and use test-taking principles	Avoid changing answers without good reason Attempt every question Don't rely on flaws in test construction Be systematic and use problem-solving technique in answering questions

From "Making the grade as a test-taker" by N. Dickenson-Hazard, 1989. *Pediatric Nursing 15*, p. 304. Adapted from *How to take tests*. (pp 15-57) by J. Millman and W. Paul, 1969, New York: McGraw-Hill Co. and from *Nurses's guide to successful test taking*. (pp 43-53) by M. B. Sides and N. B. Cailles, 1989, Philadelphia: J. B. Lippincott Co. Copyright 1989 A. J. Jannetti, Inc. Adapted by permission.

STRATEGY #5 Psych Yourself Up: Taking tests is stressful

While a little stress can be productive, too much can incapacitate you in your studying and test taking (Divine & Kylen, 1979). Your attitude and approach to test-taking and studying can influence your outcomes. Psyching yourself up can have a positive affect and make examinations a non-anxiety laden experience (Dickenson-Hazard, 1990). The following techniques are based on the principles of successful test taking as presented by Sides & Cailles (1989). Incorporation of these techniques can improve response and performance in examination situations.

Technique #1: Adopt an "I can" attitude. Believing you can succeed is the key to success. Self belief inspires and gives you the power to achieve your goals. Without a success attitude, the road to your goal is much harder. We all stand an equal chance of success in this world. It is those who believe they can who achieve it. This "I can" attitude must permeate all your efforts in test taking from studying to improving your skills to actually writing the test.

Technique #2: Take control. By identifying your goal, deciding how to accomplish it and developing a plan for achieving it, you take control. Do not leave your success or failure to chance; control it through action and attitude.

Technique #3: Think positively. Examinations are generally based on a standard which is the same for all individuals. Everyone can potentially pass. Performance is influenced not only by knowledge and skill but attitude as well. Those individuals who regard an exam as an opportunity or challenge will be more successful.

Technique #4: Project a positive self-fulfilling prophecy. While preparing for an examination, project thoughts of the positive outcomes you will experience when you succeed. Self-talk is self-fulfilling. Expect success, not failure, of yourself.

Technique #5: Feel good about yourself. Without feeling a sense of positive self worth, passing an examination is difficult. Recognize your professional contributions and give yourself credit for your accomplishments. Think "I will pass," not "I suppose I can."

Technique #6: Know yourself. Focus exam preparation and test taking on your strengths. Try to alter your weaknesses instead of becoming hung up on them. If you tend to overanalyze, study and read test questions at face value. If you're a speed demon when taking a test, slow down and read more carefully.

Technique #7: Failure is a possibility. We all have failed at something at some point in our lives. Rather than dwelling on the failure, making excuses and believing you'll fail again, recognize your mistakes and remedy them. Failure is a time to begin again; use it as a motivator to do better. It is not the end of the world unless you allow it to be. It is best to deal with the failure and move on, otherwise it interferes with your success.

Technique #8: Persevere, persevere, persevere! Endurance must underlie all your efforts. Call forth those reserve energies when you've had all you think you can take. Rely upon yourself and your support systems to help you maintain a sense of direction and keep your goal in the forefront.

Technique #9: Motivation is muscle. Most individuals are motivated by fear or desire. The fear in an exam situation may be one of failure, the unknown or discovery of imperfection. Put your fear into perspective; realize you are not the only one with fear and that all have an equal opportunity for success. Develop strategies to reduce fear and use fear to your advantage by improving the imperfections. Desire is a powerful motivator and you should keep the rewards of your desire foremost in your mind. Whatever motivates you, use it to make you successful. Reward yourself during your exam preparation and once the exam has been completed. You alone hold the key to success; use what you have wisely.

This chapter has provided concepts, strategies and techniques for improving study and test taking skills. Your first task in improvement is to know yourself: how you study and how you take a test. You should use your strengths and remedy the weaknesses. Next you need to develop your thinking skills. Work on techniques to improve memory and reasoning. Now you need to organize your study and concentrate on using these new and used skills to be successful. Create a study space, develop a plan of action, then implement that plan during your periods of peak concentration. Before taking the exam be sure you understand the components of a test question, can identify key words and phrases and have practiced. Apply the test taking rules during the exam process. Finally, believe in yourself, your knowledge and your talent. Believing you can accomplish your goal facilitates the fact that you will.

Bibliography

American Board of Pediatrics, (1989). *Developing questions and critiques*. Unpublished material.

Burkle, C. A., & Marshak, D. (1989). *Study Program: Level 1*. Reston, Va: National Association of Secondary School Principals.

Dickenson-Hazard, N. (1989). Making the grade as a test taker. *Pediatric Nursing*, 15, 302-304.

Dickenson-Hazard, N. (1989). Anatomy of a test question. *Pediatric Nursing*, 15, 395-399.

Dickenson-Hazard, N. (1990). The psychology of successful test taking. *Pediatric Nursing*, 16, 66-67.

Dickenson-Hazard, N. (1990). Study smart. *Pediatric Nursing*, 16, 314-316.

Dickenson-Hazard, N. (1990). Study effectiveness: are you 10 a.m. or p.m. scholar? *Pediatric Nursing*, 16, 419-420.

Dickenson-Hazard, N. (1990). Develop your thinking skills for improved test taking. *Pediatric Nursing*, 16, 480-481.

Divine, J. H., & Kylen, D. W. (1979). *How to beat test anxiety*. New York: Barrons Educational Series.

Goroll, A., May, L., & Mulley, A (Eds.) (1988). *Primary care medicine* (2nd ed.). Philadelphia: J. B. Lippincott.

Hoekelman, R. A. (Ed.). (1992). *Primary pediatric care (2nd ed.)*. St. Louis: Mosby Year Book.

Millman, J., & Paul, W. (1969). *How to take tests*. New York: McGraw-Hill Book Co.

Olney, C. W. (1989). *Where there's a will, there's an A*. New Jersey: Chesterbrook Educational Publishers.

Sides, M., & Cailles, N. B. (1989). *Nurse's guide to successful test taking*. Philadelphia: J. B. Lippincott.

Whaley, L. F., & Wong, D. L. (1991). *Nursing care of infants and children* (4th ed.). St. Louis: Mosby Year Book.

Growth
and
Development

Lois A. Hancock

Data Gathering

- Process of Interviewing/Counseling
  1. Techniques
     a. Listening
        (1) Attend to both verbal and nonverbal cues
        (2) Paraphrase
        (3) Clarify by focusing discussion
        (4) Check perceptions with the client
     b. Leading
        (1) Use indirect or open questions to initiate a topic
        (2) Use direct questions to gather specific details
        (3) Focus if information seems vague
     c. Reflecting
        (1) Repeat idea in different words
        (2) Respond to a feeling
     d. Summarizing
        (1) Pull themes together and check your perceptions
     e. Confronting
        (1) Feed-back opinions
        (2) Promote self-confrontation
        (3) Facilitate more open expression of feelings
     f. Interpreting
        (1) Use interpretive questions to facilitate client awareness
        (2) Use metaphor to clarify an issue
     g. Informing
        (1) Give factual information
        (2) Give suggestions and opinions
  2. Interviewing clients of different ages

a. Preschool and young school-age

    (1)   Sit on floor or at child's level

    (2)   Use play and fantasy to facilitate comfort

    (3)   Allow sufficient time for responses

    (4)   Don't expect too much detail from child

b. Older schoolage and adolescents

    (1)   Separate from parents for part of interview

    (2)   Assure confidentiality

    (3)   Avoid confrontation

    (4)   Start with non-threatening topics

    (5)   Accept some silence

- Obtaining the History

   1. General guidelines

     a. Assure privacy

     b. Begin with open questions

     c. Use direct questions to obtain specifics

     d. Avoid giving reassurance or advice prematurely

   2. New patient history

     a. Demographic data

     b. Chief complaint (CC)

     c. Present problem or illness (HPI)

        (1)   Onset

        (2)   Course since onset

        (3)   Present description of the problem

           (a)   Quantity/quality

           (b)   Timing and duration

           (c)   Location

           (d)   Relieving and aggravating factors

           (e)   Significant positives and negatives

           (f)   Effect upon daily function and coping

(g) Treatments tried

   d. Past medical history

      (1) If child is under 2 years or has developmental problems include detailed pregnancy and birth data (see Health Maintenance and Promotion chapter)

   e. Family history (FH)

   f. Personal and social history

   g. Review of systems

3. Interval history

   a. Chief complaint

   b. Present problem

   c. Update past medical history from time of last history only

   d. Update personal and social history

   e. Review of systems since last history

4. Phone history (telephone triage)

   a. No visual cues available

   b. Focus on chief complaint and description of present problems

   c. Requires a triage decision

      (1) Manage over phone

      (2) Office visit

      (3) Refer to other provider

5. Sexual history

   a. Data fits in Past Medical History and Personal and Social History

   b. Include in visits for older school-age and adolescents

   c. Content

      (1) Development of secondary sexual characteristics

      (2) Onset of menses and present description

      (3) Sexual activity (both homo and hetero)

      (4) Use of contraceptives

      (5) Knowledge of and use of prevention for STDs and AIDS

        (6)   Satisfaction with decision to be sexually active

- Recording the history
    1. SOAP format
        a. Subjective—information given by client
        b. Objective observations and examination findings
        c. Assessment (diagnosis)
        d. Plan (management)
            (1) Teaching
            (2) Laboratory studies
            (3) Consultations or referrals
            (4) Medications
            (5) Diet or activity modifications
            (6) Follow-up visit schedule

- Physical Examination
    1. Modifications by age of client
        a. Young infant
            (1) Head to toe sequence or "opportunistic," i.e., auscultate heart and lung sounds while infant sleeping, and/or quiet
            (2) Keep on parent's lap when possible
            (3) Allow for a brief break if infant hungry or unduly stressed
        b. Older infant and toddler
            (1) Start with extremities, head last
            (2) Allow for exploration of instruments
            (3) Position self so child can see your actions
            (4) Allow child to sit on parent's lap or stay close to parent
            (5) Give choices when possible
        c. Older preschool and school-age
            (1) Can usually use head to toe sequence
            (2) Briefly explain all components
            (3) Answer questions factually and with age-appropriate vocabulary

      d. Adolescent (same as school-age, plus)

         (1) Recognize and discuss apprehension about pelvic examination

  2. Examination techniques

      a. Inspection

         (1) Gather data throughout visit

         (2) Validate findings with client

         (3) Use direct or tangential lighting, depending on data desired

      b. Palpation

         (1) Use palmar surface of fingers for most situations

         (2) Use ulnar surface of hand to detect vibration

         (3) Use dorsal surface of hand to estimate temperature

         (4) Always use light palpation before deep palpation

      c. Percussion

         (1) Tones (and examples)

            (a) Tympany (gastric bubble)

            (b) Hyperresonance (emphysematous lungs)

            (c) Resonance (healthy lungs)

            (d) Dullness (liver)

            (e) Flatness (muscle)

      d. Auscultation

         (1) Note intensity, pitch, duration and quality of sound

         (2) Identify individual sounds first

  3. Measurement of vital signs

      a. Temperature

         (1) Consider potential hazards in taking rectal temperature (most accurate method)

         (2) Tympanic membrane temperature measurement is quick and noninvasive; reliability problems

         (3) Child's temperature on several previous well visits is best

measure of "normal" for that child

b. Pulse

    (1) Norms (beats/min)

        (a) Newborn   120-170

        (b) 1 year   80-160

        (c) 3 years   80-120

        (d) 6 years   75-115

        (e) 10 years   70-110

c. Respirations

    (1) Norms (per minute)

        (a) Newborn   30-80

        (b) 1 year   20-40

        (c) 3 years   20-30

        (d) 6 years   16-20

        (e) 10 years   16-20

        (f) 17 years   12-20

4. Blood pressure

    a. Appropriate cuff size

        (1) Bladder width not more than 2/3 the length of the upper arm

        (2) Bladder length should cover 3/4 of the circumference of the arm

    b. Hypertension is average systolic and/or diastolic BP equal to or greater than the 95th percentile for age and sex on at least 3 occasions

        (1) Infant $S \geq 112$, $D \geq 74$

        (2) 3-5 years $S \geq 116$, $D \geq 76$

        (3) 6-9 years $S \geq 122$, $D \geq 78$

        (4) 10-12 years $S \geq 126$, $D \geq 82$

        (5) 13-15 years $S \geq 136$, $D \geq 86$

        (6) 16-18 years $S \geq 142$, $D \geq 92$

    c. Children who are taller or heavier for age have higher BP than smaller children of same age

- Laboratory
  1. Use of clinical laboratory tests
     a. Diagnosis vs monitor therapy
     b. Consider cost, pain, invasiveness vs. potential for data to be valid, reliable and contribute to accurate decision making
  2. Normal values
     a. Blood
        (1) Bilirubin (mg/dl)
            (a) At birth 1.5
            (b) Three to four days postnatal
                • Breastfed—7.3
                • Bottlefed—5.7
            (c) Older child
                • Total—less than 1.5
                • Direct—0.2-0.4
                • Indirect—0.4-0.8
        (2) Cholesterol (mg/100 ml)
            (a) Full-term newborn—45-167
            (b) Infant—70-190
            (c) Child—135-175
            (d) Adolescent—120-210
        (3) Iron—total (mg/dl)
            (a) Newborn—20-157
            (b) 6 wks-3 yrs—20-115
            (c) 3-9 yrs—20-141
            (d) 9-14 yrs—21-151
            (e) 14-16 yrs—20-181
        (4) Lead < 10 μg/dl whole blood—potential sources are lead-based paint, paint removal dust, industrial sources, contaminated soil, food, drinking water

(5)　CBC

	Newborn	1 month	1 year	8-12 years
Hb(gm/dl)	14-24	11-17	11-15	11.5-15.5
Hct (%)	54+10	35-50	36	35-45
WBC (1000/mm³)	9.4-34.0	5.0-19.5	6.0-17.0	4.5-13.5
RBC(mill/mm³)	4.1-7.5	4.2-5.2	4.1-5.1	4.5-5.4
Retic (%)	2-8	0-0.5	0.4-1.8	0.4-1.8
Plat	350,000	300,000	260,000	260,000
Lymphs (%)	20	56	53	31
Eosin. (mm³)	20-1000	150-1150	70-550	100-400
Monos (%)	10	7	6	7
MCV (μm³)	85-125	90	78	82
MCHC (%)	36	34	33	34

  b.　Urine

     (1)　ph

       (a)　Newborn 5.0-7.0

       (b)　Thereafter 4.8-7.8

     (2)　Specific gravity

       (a)　Newborn 1.001-1.020

       (b)　Thereafter 1.001-1.030

     (3)　Sugar—negative

     (4)　Protein—negative

  c.　Cerebrospinal fluid

	Preterm	Term	Child
Cell count (WBCX10⁶ cells/l)	0-25	0-22	0-7
(% polys)	57	61	0
Glucose (mg/dl)	24-63	34-119	40-80
Protein (mg/dl)	65-150	20-170	5-40
Pressure (mm H₂O)	< 200	< 200	< 200

- Screening Tests
  1. Vision screening
     a. Appropriate screening measures by age
        (1) Young infant
            (a) Identify risk factors
                - prenatal infections
                - congenital cyanotic heart disease
                - structural malformation
                - family history of vision problems
                - excessive O_2 in neonatal period
                - hearing problems
            (b) Pupillary response to light
            (c) Blink reflex
            (d) Ability to fix on and follow object
        (2) Older infant and toddler
            (a) Ability to fix on and follow object
            (b) Corneal light reflex test (Hirschberg)
            (c) Cover/uncover test
            (d) Red reflex (Bruchner) test
        (3) Preschool (same as toddler, plus)
            (a) Acuity tests (Pictures, HOVT, Sjogren hand, illiterate E)
            (b) Ishihara for color perception
        (4) School-age and adolescent
            (a) Far vision—Snellen alphabet chart
            (b) Near vision (Rosenbaum or Jaeger card)
     b. Normal acuity by age
        (1) 3 years 20/50
        (2) 4 years 20/40
        (3) 5 years 20/30
        (4) 6 years 20/20
  2. Hearing screening

a. Appropriate screening measures by age

    (1) Newborn

        (a) Identify high-risk factors
- affected family member
- bilirubin >20
- congenital CMV, Herpes, Rubella
- defects in ENT structure
- small at birth

        (b) Observation of responses to voices, loud noises

    (2) 4 to 24 months (above, plus)

        (a) Orienting to sound

        (b) Language development

    (3) 2 to 3 years (above, plus)

        (a) Play audiometry

    (4) Beyond 3 years

        (a) Pure tone audiometry

b. Interpretation of audiometry

    (1) 0-25 dB = normal

    (2) 26-40 dB = mild loss

    (3) 41-55 dB = moderate loss

3. Denver Developmental Screening Test revised (DDST-R) (Denver II)

a. Use for infant through 5½ years of age

b. Areas screened

    (1) Personal/social

    (2) Fine motor

    (3) Gross motor

    (4) Language

c. Interpretation: normal, suspect, or untestable

4. Denver Articulation Screening Exam (DASE)

a. Use for ages 2½ through 6 years

      b. Examiner pronounces word, child repeats

      c. Scoring: total correct sounds is the raw score

      d. Interpretation: chart on score sheet determines percentile rank and intelligibility

5. Early Language Milestone Scale (ELM)

      a. Use for ages 0 to 36 months

      b. Assesses language development

      c. Test screens expressive, receptive, visual language and intelligibility

6. Tuberculosis screening

      a. Two major types or tuberculin skin testing

          (1)   Multiple puncture tests (MPT)

               (a) Antigens either OT or PPD

               (b) Not as reliable as Mantoux

          (2)   Mantoux

               (a) PPD injected intracutaneously; examined for induration after 48 to 72 hours

               (b) Induration 15mm or greater considered positive in any person (AAP, 1994)

               (a) More reliable

      b. Host factors which can depress tuberculin reactions

          (1)   Age (very old or very young)

          (2)   Malnutrition

          (3)   Neoplastic disease

          (4)   Corticosteroids

          (5)   Presence of overwhelming illness of any type, including tuberculosis

          (6)   Immunization with an attenuated virus vaccine

Physical Growth and Development

■ General Parameters and Definitions

1. Newborn

a. "Preterm" designates newborn with gestational age of less than 37 weeks

b. Low birthweight infant (< 2500 gm)

    (1) AGA (appropriate for gestational age) refers to newborns who are preterm

    (2) SGA (small for gestational age) includes both preterm and term newborns

c. Average newborn

    (1) Weight between 6 to 12 lb; average weight 7½ lb (3.4 kg)

    (2) Approximately 10% of weight lost in first 3 to 4 days of life; greater in breast fed infants

    (3) Average length 20 inches (50 cm)

    (4) Average head circumference 13 to 14 inches (33.0 to 35.6 cm)

    (5) Chest circumference less than head by approximately 2 cm

2. Expected growth infants through school-age child

	Weight	Length/Height	Head Circumference
0-6 months	6-8 oz/wk (doubles birth wt by 5-7 months)	1 in/mo	½ in/mo
6-12 months	3-4 oz/wk (triples birth wt by 1 year)	½ in/mo	¼ in/mo
1-4 years	4½ to 6½ lb/year	3 in/yr	1 in/yr
5 years to adolescent	5 to 7 lb/year	2.5 in/yr	negligible growth spurt

3. Adolescent

a. Growth spurt average is 12 years for females; 14 years for males

b. Weight varies greatly after growth spurt

■ Use of Growth Charts

1. Use chart appropriate for child's ethnic background

2. Preterm infants

a. Use preterm growth chart

b. Use "corrected" age to plot measurement

3. Once an adolescent has started growth spurt, standard charts are

inaccurate

4. Use growth velocity chart for child whose gains seem inadequate

5. Interpretation

    a. Measurements that plot between the 10th to 90th percentile are considered normal

    b. Measurements that fall below the 5th percentile, consider

        (1) Failure to thrive

        (2) Short stature secondary to chromosomal or endocrine disorders

        (3) Familial short stature

    c. Weight measurement that plots above the 95th percentile

        (1) Plot weight for height to R/O obesity

    d. Need at least two measurements to determine a pattern

- Motor Development

1. Use Denver II or other standardized tool for screening

2. Gross motor milestones (mean age in months)

a. Roll prone to supine	3.6	SD 1.4
b. Roll supine to prone	4.8	SD 1.4
c. Sit tripod	5.3	SD 1.0
d. Sit unassisted	6.3	SD 1.2
e. Creep	6.7	SD 1.5
f. Crawl	7.8	SD 1.7
g. Pull to stand	8.1	SD 1.6
h. Cruise	8.8	SD 1.7
i. Walk	11.7	SD 1.9
j. Walk backwards	14.3	SD 2.4
k. Run	14.8	SD 2.7

3. Fine motor skills with pencil and paper

    a. Scribble in imitation—15 months

    b. Scribble spontaneously—18 months

     c. Imitate circle—30 months

     d. Copy square—4 years

     e. Copy triangle—5 years

     f. Copy horizontal diamond—6 years

     g. Copy cylinder—9 years

     h. Copy cube—12 years

■ Dental development

  1. Formation of teeth

     a. Deciduous teeth begin to develop at 4 months in utero

     b. Permanent teeth begin to develop at 3 to 4 months of age

  2. Eruption sequence—deciduous teeth (mean ages)

     a. Lower central incisors 6 months

     b. Lower lateral incisors 7 months

     c. Upper central incisors 7½ months

     d. Upper lateral incisors 9 months

     e. Lower first molars 12 months

     f. Upper first molars 14 months

     g. Lower cuspids 16 months

     h. Upper cuspids 18 months

     i. Lower second molars 20 months

     j. Upper second molars 24 months

  3. Eruption sequence—permanent teeth (mean ages)

     a. 6-7 years—upper and lower first molars;
              lower central incisors

     b. 7-8 years—upper central incisors;
              lower lateral incisors

     c. 8-9 years—upper lateral incisors

     d. 9-10 years—lower cuspids

     e. 10-11 years—upper first bicuspids

     f. 10-12 years—upper second bicuspids;

lower first bicuspids

    g. 11-12 years—upper cuspids;
                  lower second bicuspids

    h. 11-13 years—lower second molars

    i. 12-13 years—upper second molars

    j. 17-21 years—upper and lower third molars

   4. Variations in sequence of eruption are more significant than variation in timing

  ■ Sexual Development

    1. Puberty

	Females	*Males*
Beginning of puberty—average	10-11 years	11-12 years
Beginning of puberty—range	8-13 years	9½ to 14 years
Height spurt	9½ to 14½ years	10½ to 16 years
Peak height velocity	12-14 years; SD 0.88	14.6 years; SD 0.92
Initial pubertal event	Breast budding	Testicular growth
Precocious puberty	Breast development and/or pubic hair growth before age 8	Growth of testicles greater than 3 cm in diameter and/or pubic hair growth before age 9
Menarche	Range: 10-16½ years Mean: 12.6 years	
Nocturnal emissions		Mean: 14 years

    2. Tanner staging

Male	**Genital Development**
Stage 1	Pre-adolescent: Testes, scrotum and penis are about the same size and proportion as in early childhood
Stage 2	Scrotum and testes are enlarged. Skin of scrotum reddened and changed in texture. Little or no enlargement of penis is present at this stage
Stage 3	Penis is slightly enlarged, which occurs at first, mainly in length. Testes and scrotum are further enlarged
Stage 4	Increased size of penis with growth in both diameter and

development of glans. Testes and scrotum larger; scrotal skin darker than in earlier stages

Stage 5   Genitalia adult in size and shape

Female   **Breast Development**

Stage 1   Pre-adolescent: Elevation of papilla only

Stage 2   Breast bud stage: Elevation of breast and papilla as small mound. Enlargement of areola diameter

Stage 3   Further enlargement and elevation of breast and areola, with no separation of their contours

Stage 4   Projection of areola and papilla to form a secondary mound about the level of the breast

Stage 5   Mature stage: Projection of papilla only, due to recession of the areola to the general contour of the breast

Both Sexes   **Pubic Hair**

Stage 1   Pre-adolescent: The vellus over the pubes is not further developed than that over the abdominal wall; i.e., no pubic hair

Stage 2   Sparse growth of long, slightly pigmented, downy hair, straight or curled, chiefly at the base of the penis or along labia

Stage 3   Considerably darker, coarser and more curled. The hair spreads sparsely over the junction of the pubes

Stage 4   Hair now adult in type, but area covered is still considerably smaller than in adult. No spread to medial surface of thighs

Stage 5   Adult in quantity and type with distribution of the horizontal (or classically "feminine") pattern. Spreads to medial surface of thighs, but not up linea alba or elsewhere above the base of the inverse triangle

Stage 6   Spreads up linea alba

Interactive Growth and Development

- Developmental Theories
  1. Psychodynamic theories

	Freud	*Erikson*
Infant	oral	trust vs mistrust
Toddler	anal	autonomy vs shame and doubt
Preschooler	phallic	initiative vs guilt
School age	latency	industry vs inferiority
Adolescent	genital	identity vs role confusion

2. Piaget's levels of cognitive development

  a. Sensorimotor period—0 to 2 years

    (1) Thought dominated by physical manipulation of objects

    (2) By 8 months, infant begins to demonstrate goal-directed activity

    (3) By 12 months, infant begins to understand means-end relationships

    (4) By 24 months, child has beginning of symbolic representation

  b. Preoperational—2 to 7 years

    (1) Preconceptual (2-4 years)—uses representational thought to recall past, represent present, and anticipate future

    (2) Intuitive (2-7 years)—increased symbolic functioning

  c. Concrete operations—7 to 11 years

    (1) Mental reasoning processes assume logical approaches to solving concrete problems

  d. Formal operations—11 to 15 years

    (1) True logical thought and manipulation of abstract concepts emerge

3. Kohlberg's theory of moral development

  a. Preconventional (Premoral) Level

    (1) Step 0 (0-2 years): Naivete and egocentrism. Essentially no moral sensitivity; child does what pleases self

    (2) Stage 1 (2-3 years): Punishment and obedience orientation. Child essentially avoids punishment

   (3) Stage 2 (4-7 years): Naive instrumental hedonism. Child does what benefits self

  b. Conventional Level—follows external moral guidelines

   (1) Stage 3 (7-10 years): Good-boy orientation. Child avoids disapproval

   (2) Stage 4 (10-12 years): Law and order orientation. Child obeys law; "does one's duty", looks up to authority figures

  c. Postconventional-morality based on inner principles and reasoning

   (1) Stage 5 (13 years and up): Maintain respect of others; exceptions to rules in order to benefit an individual or group

   (2) Stage 6 (15 years and up): Implement personal principles regardless of legal sanction; great respect for life

   (3) Stage 7 (18 years and up): Live by external, universal principles; very few people reach this stage

■ Behaviorist Theory

 1. Focuses on behaviors that can be directly measured and observed, such as

  a. Physiological responses, e.g., blood values and brain waves

  b. Social behaviors

  c. Psychomotor skills

  d. Academic tasks

 2. All behavior is under the control of environmental contingencies

  a. Antecedent (stimulus or need) sets the occasion for behavior

  b. Consequences (contingencies) maintain the behaviors

 3. Key behaviorists

  a. J. B. Watson—father of "behavioral theory"

  b. B. F. Skinner—focused on systematically changing behavior

  c. Albert Bandura—social learning

■ Humanistic Theory

 1. Maslow's hierarchy of needs (from lowest to highest)

  a. Physiological

  b. Safety and security

   c. Love and belongingness

   d. Ego and esteem

   e. Self-actualization

    (1) Only about 1% of people fully actualize their potential

- Language Development
  1. Language is the best single measure of normal cognitive development in early childhood
  2. Expressive language milestones
     a. Coos 2 weeks to 3 months
     b. Babbles 4.5 to 8 months
     c. Dada/mama (indiscriminate) 5.5 to 10 months
     d. Da da/ma ma (discriminate) 7.5 months to 14 months
     e. First word 8 to 14 months
     f. Four to six words 12 to 18 months
     g. Mature jargon 15.5 to 23 months
     h. Two-word combinations 14 months to 23 months
     i. Fifty word vocabulary 18 months to 24 months
     j. Up to 425 word vocabulary, 75% of speech intelligible—30 months
     k. Sentences average 4 to 5 words, 95% of speech intelligible—42 months
     l. Defines ball, hat, stove, policeman; counts 5 objects—60 months
  3. Receptive language milestones
     a. Orients to voice—2 to 6 months
     b. Follows one-step command given with a gesture—8.5 to 12.5 months
     c. Follows one-step command given without a gesture—10.5 to 16.5 months
     d. Points to 5 body parts—12.5 to 20 months
     e. Distinguishes between one and many; understands "soon"—24 months
     f. Carries out 2- and some 3-item commands—36 months

     g. Can complete opposite analogies—48 months

     h. Understands "if", "because", "when"—60 months

4. Causes of delayed speech and language development

     a. Mental retardation

     b. Deafness

     c. Cerebral palsy

     d. Developmental disorders

     e. Infantile autism

     f. Severe malnutrition

     g. Emotional disturbances

5. Special situations

     a. Hearing children reared by deaf parents need to hear spoken language from others

     b. Children raised in bilingual homes will become proficient in both languages if both are equally used

         (1) Initial expressive language may be slightly late

     c. Twins or other siblings close in age may develop a "private" language understood only by them

6. Stuttering

     a. Repetition of whole words and phrases is normal for preschoolers

     b. Incidence of problematic stuttering: 4% of population; male to female ratio is 3.5:1; usually begins in preschool years

     c. Referral criteria

         (1) Prolongations and/or repetitions of first syllable of word with increased pitch toward end

         (2) Child avoids speaking or attempts to hide stuttering

         (3) Parent(s) greatly concerned

         (4) Stuttering present much of time

         (5) Present for more than 6 months

         (6) Visible struggle to get words out or trembling of mouth muscles

      d. Tips for parents

         (1) Model slower speech

         (2) Decrease stress in home

         (3) Do not correct or criticize child

         (4) Encourage child's strengths

   7. Speech/language screening tools

      a. Early Language Milestones Scale (ELM)— for 0 to 36 months

      b. Receptive—Expressive Emergent Language Scale (REEL)—for 0 to 36 months

      c. Clinical Linguistic and Auditory Milestone Tests (CLAMS)—for 0 to 36 months

      d. Fluharty Preschool Speech and Language Screening Test—for 2 to 6 years

      e. Goldberg's Speech and Language Screening Tool—for 3 to 12 years

Specific Normal Findings and Variations

■ Eyes

   1. History which indicates possible abnormalities

      a. Preterm

         (1) Resuscitated

         (2) Ventilator or O_2 used

         (3) Retrolental fibroplasia

      b. Infant

         (1) Failure to gaze at mother's face or other object

         (2) Mother uncertain if infant looks at her

         (3) Failure to blink in response to bright lights or threatening movements

      c. Young children

         (1) Excessive rubbing of eyes

         (2) Frequent hordeolum

         (3) Inability to reach for and pick up small objects

        (4)   Holds objects close to face

        (5)   Photophobia

   d. School-age

        (1)   Need to sit close to blackboard or TV

        (2)   Poor progress in school not explained by intellectual deficit

   e. Any age

        (1)   White area in the pupil visible in photographs (retinoblastoma)

        (2)   Excessive tearing; spills over lower eyelid

        (3)   Strabismus

2. Selected physical examination findings

   a. Position and placement: Inner canthal distance averages 2.5 cm., epicanthal folds present in Oriental children; palpebral fissures lie horizontally.

        (1)   Hypertelorism (wide set eyes) present in Down syndrome

        (2)   Epicanthal folds can be present in Down syndrome, renal agenesis, or glycogen storage disease

        (3)   Ptosis can be normal or indicate paralysis of oculomotor nerve

   b. Eyelids are normally the same color as surrounding skin

        (1)   "Stork Bite" marks (telangiectatic nevi) disappear by 12 months

        (2)   Blocked tear duct can cause inflammation of the lacrimal sac indicated by swelling, redness and purulent discharge

   c. "Allergic shiners" with discoloration and edema around the eyes usually indicative of allergies

   d. Conjunctiva is normally pink and glossy

        (1)   Redness can indicate bacterial or viral infection, allergy or irritation

        (2)   Excessive pallor indicates anemia

        (3)   Cobblestone appearance can indicate severe allergy

   e. Pupils and irises

(1) Unequal pupils (anisocoria) are usually congenital and normal, but if appear suddenly can indicate acute intracranial disease

(2) Constriction (miosis) or dilation (mydriasis) of pupils may occur with drug use

f. Normally, by 3 to 4 months, children can fixate on one visual field with both eyes simultaneously (binocularity)

(1) Assessment techniques to elicit strabismus

(a) Cover-uncover test

(b) Corneal light reflex test (Hirschberg)

(2) Intermittent alternating convergent strabismus is normal from 0 to 6 months of age

g. Ophthalmoscopic examination

(1) Red reflex should be elicited bilaterally in every newborn

(a) Absence of red reflex or an opacity in the lens may indicate cataracts

(2) In infants, the optic disc is pale and peripheral vessels not well developed

- Ears

1. History which indicates possible abnormalities

a. Prenatal exposure to maternal infection, irradiation or drug abuse

b. Birth weight less than 1500 g

c. Anoxia in neonatal period

d. Ototoxic antibiotic use

e. Cleft palate

f. Infections

(1) Meningitis

(2) Encephalitis

(3) Recurrent otitis media

g. Behaviors indicating hearing loss

(1) No reaction to loud or strange noises

(2) No babbling after 6 months of age

        (3) No communicative speech and reliance on gestures after 15 months of age

        (4) Inattention to children the same age

  2. Selected physical examination findings

    a. Position and placement

        (1) Low or obliquely set ears may indicate genitourinary or chromosomal abnormality or a multisystem syndrome.

    b. Pain

        (1) Pain produced by manipulation of auricle may indicate otitis externa

        (2) Pain and tenderness over mastoid process may indicate mastoiditis

- Nose/Sinuses

  1. History which indicates possible abnormalities

    a. Inability to move air through both nares

    b. Discharge

    c. Nasal flaring or narrowing on inspection

  2. Selected physical examination findings

    a. Flattened nose or bridge of nose (in other than Asian or African-American children) may indicate congenital anomalies

- Throat/Mouth

  1. History which indicates possible abnormalities

    a. Lack of, or excessive, fluoride supplementation or fluoridated water

    b. Infant or toddler who goes to sleep with bottle of milk or juice

    c. Thumbsucking or pacifier use beyond age 2

    d. Unusual sequence of tooth eruption

  2. Selected physical examination findings

    a. Lips

        (1) Cherry red color indicates acidosis

        (2) Drooping of one side of lips indicates facial nerve

impairment

    (3)   Fissures at corners of mouth can indicate riboflavin or niacin deficiency

  b. Teeth

    (1)   Mottling may indicate excessive fluoride intake

    (2)   Green or black staining can result from oral iron intake

  c. Adenoids not usually visible during gagging or saying "ah"

  d. Uvula rises and remains in midline when saying "ah"

    (1)   Deviation or absence of movement indicates involvement of glossopharyngeal or vagus nerves

  e. Voice

    (1)   Nasal quality indicates enlarged adenoids

    (2)   Hoarse cry indicates croup, cretinism or tetany

    (3)   Shrill, high-pitched cry may indicate increased intracranial pressure

- Face

  1. History which indicates possible abnormalities

    a. Difficult delivery, use of forceps

    b. Asymmetry of face when crying or speaking

    c. Facial features which are unusual or don't match family characteristics

    d. Drug or alcohol use during pregnancy

  2. Selected physical examination findings

    a. Asymmetry of nasolabial folds or drooping mouth indicates facial nerve impairment or Bell's palsy

    b. Child who demonstrates open mouth breathing and facial contortions may have allergic rhinitis

    c. Dysmorphic facial features are the hallmark of numerous syndromes and diagnoses should be pursued

- Head/Neck

  1. History which indicates possible abnormalities

    a. Difficult birth; use of forceps

    b. Unusual head shape or preferred position at rest

    c. Poor head control for age

    d. Lack of neonatal screening for hypothyroidism

2. Selected physical examination findings

    a. Fontanels

        (1) Posterior fontanel rarely palpable at birth; definitely closes by 2 months of age

        (2) Anterior fontanel should be no larger than 4 to 5 cm in diameter

        (3) Large anterior fontanel can indicate

            (a) Chronically increased intracranial pressure

            (b) Subdural hematoma

            (c) Rickets

            (d) Hypothyroidism

            (e) Osteogenesis imperfecta

        (4) Anterior fontanel closes between 9 to 18 months of age

    b. Large or unusual head size or shape

        (1) Hydrocephalus

        (2) Caput succedaneum—subcutaneous edema over the presenting part of the head at delivery; no specific treatment necessary; resolution usually occurs within 2 to 3 days

        (3) Cephalohematoma—subperiosteal collection of blood, bound by suture lines; often does not appear until several hours after birth and may increase over 24 hours; no specific treatment indicated

        (4) Premature or irregular closure of suture lines can cause unusual head shape

        (5) Preterm infants often have long narrow heads

        (6) Bossing (bulging) of the frontal area is associated with rickets and prematurity

    c. Head control

        (1) By 4 months of age, head should be held erect and in midline

(2) By 6 months of age, there should be no significant head lag when infant is pulled from supine to sitting position

d. Neck

(1) Pain and resistance to flexion may indicate meningeal irritation

(2) Torticollis can result from birth trauma, muscle spasm, viral infection or drug ingestion

(3) Unusual position of the trachea could indicate serious lung problem

(4) Mass in the neck

(a) Thyroglossal duct cyst

(b) Brachial cleft cyst

(c) Enlarged thyroid

(d) Enlarged lymph nodes

- Heart

1. Selected physical examination findings

a. Heart sounds and area of clearest auscultation

(1) S_1 — apex

(2) Split S_1 — tricuspid area

(3) S_2 — aortic and pulmonic areas

(4) Physiological splitting of S_2 — base

(5) S_3 — apex

(6) S_4 — apex

b. Functional (or innocent) murmurs are characterized by

(1) Usually grade I or II

(2) Medium pitch

(3) Blowing

(4) Brief

(5) No radiation (usually)

(6) Sounds heard best in second left intercostal space near left sternal border

        (7)   Sounds heard in a recumbent position which disappear when child sits or stands

        (8)   Murmur occurs in systole

        (9)   No cyanosis

        (10) Normal heart rate

   c. Murmurs in the newborn

        (1)   Transition from fetal to pulmonic circulation may take up to 48 hours

           (a)   Usually grade I or II

           (b)   Systolic

           (c)   Unaccompanied by other signs and symptoms

   d. Venous hums

        (1)   Usually of no clinical significance

        (2)   Heard in the neck or anterior portion of upper chest

   e. PMI (Point of Maximal Impulse)

        (1)   Children age 7 or younger—4th intercostal space

        (2)   Children over 7 years—5th intercostal space

        (3)   Lower, more lateral PMI may indicate cardiac enlargement

        (4)   Amplified PMI may indicate acute anemia, fever or anxiety

   f. Peripheral pulses are normally palpable, equal in intensity and rhythm

        (1)   Weak or absent femoral pulses may indicate coarctation of the aorta

■ Lungs

   1. History which indicates possible abnormalities

   a. Family history

        (1)   Tuberculosis

        (2)   Cystic fibrosis

        (3)   Allergy, asthma, atopic dermatitis

   b. Infants and young children

        (1)   Preterm with any respiratory complications

        (2)   Sudden onset of coughing or difficulty breathing

        (3)   Difficulty feeding

        (4)   Apnea episodes

    c. Older children and adolescents

        (1)   Smoking

        (2)   Cocaine use

  2. Selected physical examination findings

    a. Normal breath sounds

        (1)   Vesicular—low pitch, soft and short expirations; heard over most of lung fields

        (2)   Bronchovesicular—medium pitch, expiratory duration equals inspiratory duration; heard over main bronchus

        (3)   Bronchial/tracheal—high pitch, loud and long expirations; heard only over trachea

    b. Chest movement

        (1)   Children under 7 years are diaphragmatic (abdominal) breathers

        (2)   Girls over 7 years become thoracic breathers; boys continue to be abdominal breathers

        (3)   Retractions are more dramatic on younger children because of the lack of rigidity of the chest

    c. Chest structural abnormalities may compromise lung expansion

        (1)   Pectus carinatum—protuberant sternum

        (2)   Pectus excavatum—depressed sternum

■ Breasts

  1. History which indicates possible abnormalities

    a. Prepubertal breast enlargement in girls

    b. Gynecomastia in boys at any age

    c. Breast mass

    d. Galactorrhea not associated with childbearing

  2. Selected physical examination findings

a. Neonate may have gynecomastia and "witch's milk" which disappears within 2 weeks (or, at the latest, 3 months)

b. Gynecomastia in older male children may indicate

    (1) Obesity

    (2) Hormonal imbalance

    (3) Testicular or pituitary tumors

    (4) Medication with estrogens or steroids

c. Expect asymmetry in breast development in the adolescent female

d. Fibroadenoma is the most common breast mass in adolescent females

    (1) Characteristics

        (a) Single, unilateral mass

        (b) Round or discoid in shape

        (c) Firm in consistency

        (d) No retraction

        (e) Mobile

        (f) Nontender

        (g) No variation with menstrual cycle

■ Abdomen

1. History which indicates possible abnormalities

a. Birth weight under 1500 g puts infant at high risk for necrotizing enterocolitis

b. Failure to pass first meconium stool within 24 hours

c. Jaundice

d. Failure to grow or unexplained weight loss

e. Projectile vomiting or blood in emesis

f. Chronic diarrhea or constipation

g. Enlargement of the abdomen with or without pain

2. Selected physical examination findings

a. Prominent abdomen (pot-belly) is normal in infants and toddlers while standing; abdomen is flat when child is supine

b. Organ sizes

   (1) Liver span in infants and children

      (a) 6 months—2.4-2.8 cm

      (b) 24 months—3.5-3.6 cm

      (c) 4 years—4.3-4.4 cm

      (d) 8 years—5.1-5.6 cm

      (e) 10 years—5.5-6.1 cm

   (2) Liver edge may be palpable 1 to 3 cm below the right costal margin in infants and toddlers; in older children, lower edge should not extend below costal margin

   (3) Spleen tip may be palpated 1 to 2 cm below the left costal margin during *inspiration* in infants and young children

- Reproductive System

1. History which indicates possible abnormalities

  a. Discharge or bleeding from vagina or penis

  b. History, or suspicion, of sexual abuse

  c. Sexual intercourse without use of contraceptives

  d. Scrotal swelling with crying or bowel movement

  e. "Empty" scrotum vs retractable testes

  f. Unusual voiding pattern

2. Selected physical examination findings (see physical growth and development section for Tanner stages and sequence of pubertal development)

  a. Signs and symptoms of possible sexual abuse

    (1) Evidence of general physical abuse or neglect

    (2) Evidence of trauma or scarring in genital, anal or perianal areas

    (3) Changes in skin color or pigmentation in genital or anal area

    (4) Any sexually transmitted disease

    (5) Anorectal itching, bleeding, pain or poor sphincter tone

    (6) Rashes, sores or discharge in genital area

    b. Labial adhesions

        (1) R/O ambiguous genitalia

        (2) Adhesions of labia minora is most common in young infants

    c. Male genitalia

        (1) Phimosis—foreskin cannot be easily retracted in boy over 3 years old

        (2) Undescended testicle should be corrected by age 3

        (3) Hypospadias or epispadias should be referred

        (4) Large scrotum

            (a) Hydrocele

            (b) Spermatocele

            (c) Varicocele

            (d) Testicular tumor (common in adolescents and young men)

            (e) Indirect inguinal hernia

    d. Adolescent females

        (1) First gynecological examination can produce much anxiety

        (2) Choose appropriate speculum size

■ Musculoskeletal System

  1. History which indicates possible abnormalities

    a. Birth history

        (1) Large for gestational age

        (2) Abnormal presentation

        (3) Anoxia in perinatal period

    b. Delay in motor developmental milestones

    c. Unusual style of movement

    d. Leg pain

  2. Selected physical examination findings

    a. Specific examination maneuvers

        (1) Trendelenburg test to detect hip dislocation

(a) Lowering of iliac crest on side opposite weight-bearing leg shows defect in weight bearing hip

(2) Barlow-Ortolani test to detect hip dislocation or subluxation

(a) Palpable click, asymmetry or limited bilateral abduction are abnormal findings

(3) Allis sign to detect hip dislocation or shortened femur

(a) Unequal leg length is abnormal

(4) Gower's sign shows generalized muscle weakness; often indicative of muscular dystrophy

(a) Use of hands on legs to push self to standing is abnormal

b. Scoliosis (lateral curvature of the spine)

(1) Functional

(a) Child can voluntarily straighten spine

(b) Disappears when child recumbent

(2) Structural

(a) Persistent curvature

(b) Unequal height of shoulders and iliac crests when standing erect

(c) Asymmetric elevation of scapula when leaning forward

c. Developmental differences

(1) Longitudinal arch of foot can be obscured by fat pad until 3 years of age; child appears "flat footed"

(2) Bowleg (genu varum) gait is common until 18 months of age

(3) Knock knee (genu valgum) is common in children between 2 and 4 years of age

d. "Turned-in" foot may have different causes

(1) Femoral anteversion

(2) Tibial torsion

(3) Metatarsus adductus

■ Neurologic System

1. History which indicates possible abnormalities

      a. Delay or regression in developmental milestones

      b. Unusual behavior for age

      c. Headaches

      d. Seizures

      e. Clumsiness or progressive weakness

      f. Learning or school difficulties

  2. Selected physical examination findings

      a. Infant reflexes (automatisms)

Reflex	Appearance	Disappearance
Palmar grasp	birth	3 months
Plantar grasp	birth	8-10 months
Moro	birth	6 months
Stepping	birth to 8 weeks	varies
Tonic neck	2-3 months	6 months
Rooting	birth	4 months (except during sleep— up to 12 months)

      b. Use of Denver II or other general developmental screening tool will yield much data regarding age appropriate skills

      c. Babinski sign is normal up to age 2 years

      d. Age of disappearance of individual "soft signs" varies greatly

■ Dermatologic System

  1. History which indicates possible abnormalities

      a. Family history of atopic dermatitis, allergic skin disorders, familial hair loss or unusual pigmentation patterns

      b. Chronic or repeated acute episodes of skin lesions

      c. Frequent scratching or rubbing of body area

  2. Selected physical examination findings

      a. Birthmarks (nevi)

         (1) Salmon patch ("stork-bite")

            (a) Common on eyelids, naso-labial region or nape of neck

            (b) Disappears by 12 months

(2) Nevus flammeus (port-wine stain)

    (a) Enlarges as child grows

(3) Strawberry nevus (raised hemangioma)

    (a) Begins as circumscribed grayish white area; later becomes red and raised

    (b) Not always present at birth

    (c) Resolves spontaneously by 9 years of age

(4) Mongolian spot (hyperpigmented nevi)

    (a) Usually in sacral or gluteal areas

    (b) Generally seen in newborns of African, Asian or Latin descent

b. Common color changes in newborns

(1) Acrocyanosis—cyanosis of hands and feet

(2) Cutis marmorata—transient mottling when infant is exposed to decreased temperature

(3) Erythema toxicium—pink papular rash with vesicles superimposed on thorax, back, buttocks and abdomen

(4) Harlequin color change—as infant lies on side, lower half of body becomes pink and upper half is pale

c. Degree of dehydration can be estimated by length of time skin retains "tenting" after it is pinched

(1) < 2 seconds $= < 5\%$ loss of body weight

(2) 2 to 3 seconds $= 5$ to 8% loss of body weight

(3) 3 to 4 seconds $= 9$ to 10% loss of body weight

(4) > 4 seconds $= > 10\%$ loss of body weight

■ Lymph Nodes

1. History which indicates possible abnormalities

a. Recurrent infections, such as tonsillitis, adenoiditis, bacterial infections, oral candidiasis, chronic diarrhea

b. Poor growth; failure to thrive

c. Maternal HIV infection

d. Use of IV drugs

    e. Multiple and indiscriminate sexual contacts

  2. Selected physical examination findings

    a. Nodes enlarged due to infection are firm, warm, fluctuant, movable, and may be accompanied by redness of the overlying skin

    b. Children under age 2 frequently have enlarged lymph nodes which have no clinical significance

    c. "Shotty" nodes (e.g., under 0.5 cm in diameter and non-tender) can be present at any time in childhood and have no clinical significance

Anticipatory Guidance

- General Guidelines

  1. Ideally should be done before or at the very beginning of a stage of development or problem

  2. Provider and client should mutually discuss and decide on a plan

  3. Verbal coupled with written suggestions are more effective than either alone

  4. Limit topics to one or two per visit

- Play

  1. Stages (sequence) of play skill development

    a. Unoccupied (infancy)—auto-stimulation and random movements

    b. Solitary (young toddler)—engrossed, independent play with toys

    c. Onlooker behavior (early preschool)—observes peers; asks questions

    d. Parallel (preschool)—imitate each other and occasionally interact

    e. Associative (mid-preschool)—much borrowing and lending of toys

    f. Cooperative (late preschool)—highly organized activities centered around group goals

  2. Key points for parents

    a. Follow the child's lead

    b. Pace at the child's level

    c. Don't compete with the child

        d. Praise and encourage the child's ideas and creativity

        e. Use descriptive comments instead of asking questions

        f. Encourage problem solving

        g. Laugh and have fun

- Attachment
    1. Definition: The enduring and specific, affective bond that develops over time (beginning in utero and continuing through the first few months of life) between children and caregivers
    2. Age-specific indicators of secure attachment
        a. Early weeks—infant gives clear cues and caretaker accurately reads cues
        b. By 3 months—reciprocal vocal and affective exchanges
        c. By 3 to 5 months—baby has clear preference for primary caretaker
        d. Toddler—willingness to explore environment when caretaker is present
- Crying
    1. Definition: Crying is infant's way of communicating needs
    2. Normal patterns
        a. Less than 2 hours per day
        b. Incessant crying
        c. Peaks at about 6 weeks, then decreases
        d. Should decrease more as infant learns other ways to communicate
- Colic (Primary Excessive Crying)
    1. Definition: Poorly defined, incompletely understood state of excessive crying in otherwise healthy infants from age 2 to 3 weeks to 3 to 4 months
    2. Etiology is unknown. Colic is *not* caused by sensitivity or allergy to foods, acute disorders of the G.I. tract or "immaturity" of the CNS or G.I. tract
    3. Differential diagnosis
        a. Normal crying
        b. Secondary excessive crying—results from a physical problem

4. Management/Treatment/Nursing Considerations

   a. R/O physical problem by complete physical examination

   b. Acknowledge stress and difficulty of caring for infant

   c. Express optimism that this will end by 3 to 4 months

   d. Tips for parents:

      (1) Try soothing techniques such as rocking, walking, background music, decreased stimulation

      (2) Arrange for time away from infant

■ Infant Stimulation

   1. Definition: A program of multi-sensory stimulation aimed at facilitation of cognitive, physical and emotional development

   2. Target populations

      a. Infants with diagnosed developmental problems

      b. Infants at risk for lack of adequate environmental stimulation due to poverty, stress or parental barriers to interpreting infant cues

■ Separation Anxiety

   1. Definition

      a. Separation is the internal process and gradual awareness that the infant is an individual distinct from the primary caregiver

      b. Separation anxiety is a peak in the infant's concern about being separated from the primary caregiver which occurs between 9 to 18 months of age

   2. Tips for parents

      a. Recognize that bedtime, going to daycare, having a sitter at home are all separations

      b. Gradually introduce child to new situation/caretakers

      c. The child learns to accept separation through multiple, brief separations and reunions

      d. Games such as "peek-a-boo" and "hide-and-seek" may be helpful

■ Teething

   1. Eruption begins at about 6 months; new tooth erupts approximately every 2 months

2. Signs and Symptoms

   a. Local inflammation

   b. Local sensitivity

   c. Irritability

   d. Increased salivation

3. Myths: There is no scientific evidence that teething causes diarrhea, fever or other systemic illnesses

4. Comfort measures

   a. Hard rubber teething toy

   b. Chilled teething rings

   c. Wet wash cloth

5. Cautions

   a. Avoid liquid-filled teething rings

- Thumb Sucking

   1. Peaks between 18 to 21 months

   2. Tips for parents

      a. Ignore before age 4 unless child is not thriving

      b. At age 4 have dental evaluation to R/O malocclusion and speech evaluation if tongue thrust is suspected

- Sleep

   1. Common patterns by age

      a. The newborn sleeps from 10 to 23 hours per day; average is 16.5 hours

      b. The 2- to 4-month-old infant sleeps from 8 to 12 hours at night and takes 2 to 3 naps

      c. The 6- to 12-month-old infant sleeps 11 to 12 hours at night and takes 2 to 3 naps

      d. The 1- to 5-year-old sleeps 8 to 12 hours at night and gradually decreases from 2 naps to no nap

   2. Tips for parents

      a. Put the infant in crib when drowsy (not already asleep) so he learns to go to sleep in the crib

    b. Night feedings should be quiet, non-stimulating times

    c. Once night feedings stop, respond to night wakenings briefly and assure the child that he will go back to sleep

    d. Toddlers and preschoolers need ritual and consistency at bedtime

- Sleep Disturbances

    1. Nightmares start at about 3 years; the child generally wakens and remembers the dream

    2. Night terrors generally occur between 2 to 4 years; the child does not waken

    3. Tips for parents

        a. Quietly reassure child

        b. Let child fall asleep in own bed

- Toilet Training

    1. Most children are psychologically and physiologically ready between 18 to 30 months

    2. Majority of children achieve daytime bowel and bladder training simultaneously; average age is 28 months

    3. Bedwetting generally continues for about 1 year after daytime control is achieved

    4. Toilet training should not be started when family is unduly stressed, i.e., new baby, moving, holidays, divorce

    5. Tips for parents

        a. Praise all efforts

        b. Expect "accidents" to happen—don't punish the child

        c. If child is resistant, try again in a few weeks

        d. Follow the child's usual pattern of elimination

        e. Limit time on potty to 5 to 10 minutes

- Sibling Rivalry

    1. Can occur throughout childhood; is often most troublesome just after birth of new baby if older sibling is under 2 years

    2. Tips for parents

    a. Involve children in preparation for new baby

    b. Praise "big-kid" behaviors; ignore regression

    c. Provide special time for each child every day

    d. Stay out of minor sibling conflicts, but do discipline if aggression occurs

    e. Foster individual interests of each child and avoid comparing children

- Television

  1. There is a strong correlation between viewing aggression and the child's level of aggressive play

  2. TV fosters bad cognitive habits (i.e., rapid paced, superficial problem-solving) and obesity

  3. Tips for parents

     a. Limit TV time and types of programs watched

     b. Watch TV with the child and provide reality base, opportunity to discuss values, and stereotypes

     c. Set a good example in your own TV habits

- Exercise

  1. Limit TV, video game and other sedentary activities

  2. Children 6 and older should engage in light to moderate physical activity 4 to 7 times a week for 30 minutes

  3. Children 6 and older should engage in vigorous physical activity (i.e., sufficient to promote cardiorespiratory conditioning) for 20 minutes, 3 or more times per week

- Sports

  1. For 5- to 8-year-olds, sports participation should be noncompetitive and focused on learning rules, teamwork and having fun

  2. Older school-aged children and teenagers should have a preparticipation physical examination to identify conditions that could interfere with or be worsened by athletic participation

- Sex Education

  1. Sex education begins in infancy when caretakers label the genitals and accept genital exploration and masturbation as normal activities

2. By 5 years, children are curious about gender differences and "how babies are made" and their questions should be answered briefly and accurately

3. Components of sex education
   a. Anatomy and physiology
   b. Sexual activity
   c. Values clarification
   d. Decision making
   e. Contraception
   f. Prevention of STDs and AIDS

4. Sex education ideally comes from parents or parentally endorsed adult

■ Negativism

1. Normal developmental stage for children from 15 to 28 months as they develop a sense of autonomy

2. Expressed as "no," temper tantrums, breathholding

3. Tips for parents
   a. Offer choice of two acceptable objects or actions—allow independence when possible
   b. Ignore unacceptable behavior

■ Discipline/Limit Setting

1. Focus attention on prosocial behavior

2. Set age-appropriate limits and expectations

3. Give clear commands

4. Give commands only when necessary

5. Ignoring is the appropriate parental response for annoying or minor misbehavior (i.e., whining, temper tantrums)

6. Time out (T.O.)
   a. Use for aggressive, destructive or defiant behavior
   b. One minute of T.O. per year up to 5 years, then use 5 minutes

7. Removal of privileges is appropriate parental response for serious misbehavior of older school-age children and adolescents

    8.   Be consistent regarding expectations and parental responses

■ Lying/Cheating

    1.   Age parameter

        a. Preschoolers have difficulty separating fantasy from reality—they don't really "lie"

        b. School-age children lie to avoid trouble or gain an advantage

    2.   Appropriate response

        a. Confront the child in a positive way

        b. Try to understand the reason for the lie

        c. Follow through with age-appropriate discipline when needed

        d. Adults should model honesty

■ Substance Use

    1.   Differentiate between experimentation, regular use and dependence

    2.   Substance abuse prevention education should begin in primary grades

    3.   Content of substance use prevention program

        a. Hazards of individual substances

        b. How to resist peer pressure

        c. Decision making skills

        d. Values clarification

    4.   Signs of probable substance use

        a. Drop in school performance

        b. Personality change

        c. Mood swings

        d. Sleepiness or fatigue

        e. Depression

Impact of Infectious and Chemical Agents on Growth and Development

Acquired Immune Deficiency Syndrome (AIDS)

- Transmission
    1. Infants and young children
        a. Mother with HIV or AIDS during gestation or birth or via breast milk
        b. Sexual abuse
        c. Blood transfusion is an unlikely mode of transmission because of effective screening of blood for HIV
    2. Adolescents
        a. Sexual contact with persons infected with HIV
            (1) Homosexual or bisexual males
            (2) Multiple, indiscriminant sexual contacts
        b. IV drug use
        c. Received blood or blood products before March, 1985
        d. Hemophiliacs or sickle cell patients who receive frequent transfusions
- Effect on growth and development
    1. Poor gain in weight and height
    2. Small head circumference due to cortical atrophy and acquired microcephaly
    3. Mild to severe developmental lags

Cytomegalic Inclusion Disease (CMV)

- Transmission and Symptoms
    1. Perinatal transmission occurs in utero during delivery or post delivery via breast milk
    2. Transfusion of blood or blood products accounts for 10 to 30% incidence

- Effects on Growth and Development
  1. Intrauterine growth retardation
  2. Hepatosplenomegaly
  3. Mild to severe developmental delays due to microcephaly or hydrocephaly
  4. Sensorineural hearing loss
  5. Defective enamel of deciduous teeth resulting in higher rates of caries
- Presentations in the Newborn Period
  1. Ninety percent of infants with asymptomatic congenital CMV infection have no sequelae and only rarely have severe neurologic impairment
  2. Symptomatic infants with chorioretinitis microcephaly and intracranial calcifications will have severe intellectual and sensory deficits
  3. CMV acquired at delivery presents as an afebrile pneumonia in 50% of infants after an incubation period of 8 weeks

Chlamydia

- Transmission
  1. Infant most commonly infected on passage through a colonized or infected birth canal
     a. Fifty to 75% of infants colonized with *C. trachomatis* will develop conjunctivitis
        (1) Onset of symptoms is 5 to 14 days after birth
        (2) Clinical illness varies from mild mucoid discharge without significant conjunctival erythema to profuse discharge and edematous and friable conjunctivae
        (3) Untreated conjunctivitis will resolve in several weeks to months
        (4) Majority of infants will have normal visual acuity post infection
     b. Eleven to 29% will develop pneumonia
        (1) Onset of symptoms is 3 to 11 weeks after birth
        (2) Staccato cough is characteristic of *C. trachomatis* pneumonia
        (3) Preterm infants are at greater risk for requiring ventilatory

support

- Effects on Growth and Development
    1. Very small number of infants will have conjunctival scars which interfere with visual acuity
    2. Long-term pulmonary problems (asthma, chronic cough, abnormal pulmonary function tests) may impact rate of growth and development
- Treatment
    1. Conjunctivitis and pneumonia—erythromycin (50 mg/kg/24 hr) for 14 days
    2. Oral sulfonamides after immediate neonatal period for infants who do not tolerate erythromycin (AAP, 1994)
- Prevention
    1. Identification and treatment of pregnant women colonized with *C. trachomatis* and their sexual partners
    2. Erythromycin ophthalmic ointment shortly after birth—effectiveness questionable

Fetal alcohol syndrome (FAS)

- Etiology—alcohol intake by pregnant woman
- Presentation in the Newborn Period
    1. Irritable infant
    2. Poor suck
    3. Small for gestational age and microcephaly
    4. Typical FAS facial features
        a. Short palpebral fissures
        b. Hypoplastic philtrum (vertical ridge in upper lip)
        c. Narrow upper lip
- Effects on Growth and Development
    1. Cardiac defects
    2. Borderline to severe mental retardation
    3. Fine motor delays or deficits
    4. Unusual facial appearance may result in emotional difficulties

Gonococcal Infection

- Transmission
    1. At birth during passage through infected birth canal
    2. After birth from infected mother or in nursery from other infected infants
    3. After newborn period and before puberty, sexual abuse should be considered
- Presentation in the Newborn Period
    1. Conjunctivitis 2 to 5 days after birth
        a. Generally bilateral
        b. Purulent drainage
        c. Severe lid edema with marked chemosis
- Effects on Growth and Development
    1. Severe loss of visual acuity secondary to ulceration and scarring of cornea
    2. Loss of eye secondary to perforation in untreated cases
- Treatment
    1. Hospitalization/isolation
    2. IV or IM Ceftriaxone—25-50 mg/kg/day for 7 to 10 days
    3. Frequent saline irrigation of eyes
- Prevention
    1. Ophthalmic prophylaxis immediately after birth
        a. 1% silver nitrate
        b. 0.5% erythromycin ointment
        c. 1% tetracycline ointment
    2. If mother has untreated gonococcal infection at time of birth, infant should receive a single IM dose of Ceftriaxone
    3. Diagnosis and treatment of infected pregnant women

Hepatitis B

- Transmission

1. Transplacental transmission

2. During delivery as infant comes in contact with maternal secretions

3. Household contacts with children or adults who are infected or are chronic carriers

- Presentation in the Newborn Period

  1. Generally asymptomatic with only mild elevation of transaminase levels

- Effects on Growth and Development

  1. Slowed growth and development secondary to chronic hepatitis and/or cirrhosis

  2. At great risk of developing hepatocellular carcinoma as a young adult

- Treatment

  1. Infants born to HB_sA_g-positive women should receive

     a. HBIG (hepatitis B immune globulin) 0.5 mL, within 12 hours of birth AND

     b. Hepatitis B vaccine concurrently at different sites

     c. Subsequent doses should be given at 1 and 6 months of age (AAP, 1994)

- Prevention

  1. Diagnosis and treatment of pregnant women

  2. Immunization of all children with hepatitis B vaccine started in 1992 (See health maintenance chapter for dose and schedule)

Herpes Simplex Virus (HSV)

- Transmission

  1. Intrauterine period

  2. At delivery especially if mother has primary HSV infection

  3. During postpartum period from labial and cutaneous herpetic lesions

- Presentation in the newborn period

  1. Intrauterine HSV infection characterized by

     a. Cutaneous scars or vesicles

     b. Seizures

      c. Microcephaly, hydrencephaly

      d. Intracranial calcifications

      e. Microphthalmia

      f. Hepatosplenomegaly

      g. Chorioretinitis

  2. Neonatal HSV acquired at birth

      a. Disseminated disease with or without evidence of CNS, skin, eye and mouth involvement

      b. CNS disease (encephalitis) with or without skin, eye and mouth involvement

      c. Localized infection of skin, eye and mouth without visceral organ or CNS involvement

- Treatment

  1. Acyclovir—30 mg/kg/day in 3 divided doses is preferred drug for 14 days

  2. Vidarabine—15 to 30 mg/kg over 12 hours-24 hours for 21 days

  3. If ocular involvement present, use either 1% to 2% trifluridine or 3% vidarabine topical ophthalmic preparations

- Prevention

  1. Identification of HSV infected pregnant women and delivery by C-section within 4-6 hours of rupture of membranes

  2. Contact isolation of infant in hospital

Rubella

- Transmission

  1. Transplacental transmission occurs first trimester, early second trimester in the pregnant woman

  2. Incidence of anomalies—highest in weeks 1 to 4 of gestation (61%) and decreases progressively; weeks 5 to 8 (26%), weeks 9 to 12 (8%), and weeks 21 to 40, fewer than 1%

- Effects on Fetus

  1. Spontaneous abortion

  2. Stillbirth

3. Intrauterine growth retardation

4. Major organ defects (especially if maternal infection is before 12 weeks gestation)

- Presentation in the Newborn Period

  1. Hepatosplenomegaly

  2. Thrombocytopenia

  3. Adenopathy

  4. Meningoencephalitis

  5. Interstitial pneumonia

  6. Myocarditis (uncommon)

  7. "Blueberry Muffin" rash

- Effects on Growth and Development

  1. Sensorineural hearing loss; deafness in 50% of children

  2. Cardiac anomalies

  3. Cataracts, microphthalmia, retinitis

  4. CNS signs: microcephaly, seizures, severe mental retardation

  5. Growth retardation

- Prevention

  1. Universal immunization of all children at 15 months and at 10 to 11 years of age

  2. Rubella antibody studies on any pregnant woman of unknown immune status exposed to rubella

  3. Immune globulin 20 ml given in a single IM dose to pregnant woman within 72 hours of exposure may prevent or decrease effects on fetus

  4. Discuss termination of pregnancy if exposure occurs during first 12 weeks of pregnancy

Syphilis

- Transmission

  1. Transplacental—transmission any time during pregnancy

  2. At delivery through contact with a genital lesion

  3. Through sexual abuse

- Effects on Fetus
    1. Spontaneous abortion, stillbirth, perinatal death
    2. Premature delivery
    3. Intrauterine growth retardation
- Presentation in the Newborn Period
    1. Small for gestational age
    2. Hepatosplenomegaly
    3. Lymphadenopathy
        a. Epitrochlear node involvement is characteristic
    4. Thrombocytopenia with petechia and purpura
    5. Mucocutaneous manifestations ("snuffles")
    6. Maculopapular vesicular or bullous rashes
- Effects on growth and development
    1. Skeletal abnormalities
    2. Poor growth
    3. Visual impairment
    4. Dental deformities
    5. CNS involvement can result in mental retardation, seizure disorder, hydrocephalus or cranial nerve palsies
- Treatment
    1. Treatment at birth is required if
        a. Infant is symptomatic
        b. Maternal treatment was inadequate, unknown
        c. Mother was treated with drugs other than penicillin
        d. Mother was treated within 4 weeks of delivery
        e. Adequate follow-up care of infant is uncertain
    2. Symptomatic infants or infants with abnormal CSF results
        a. Aqueous crystalline penicillin G, 100,000 to 150,000 U/kg/day IV every 8 to 12 hours for 10 to 14 days *OR*
        b. Aqueous procaine penicillin G, 50,000 U/kg/d IM for 10 days

3. Asymptomatic infants with normal CSF may be treated with a single dose of 50,000 U/kg of benzathine penicillin G IM

- Prevention
  1. Prenatal screening and penicillin treatment of infected women and their sexual partners

Toxoplasmosis

- Transmission
  1. Transplacental transmission from mother to fetus
     a. Most severe outcomes for infants occur when maternal infection occurs in first trimester
  2. Direct contact with infected cat feces or ingestion of undercooked infected meat
- Effects on Fetus
  1. Stillbirth—severely affected
- Effects in the Neonatal Period
  1. Most infants asymptomatic at birth
  2. Sequelae include mental retardation, learning disabilities, impaired vision, or blindness
- Treatment
  1. Refer for treatment with pyrimethamine and sulfonamides
- Prevention
  1. Treatment of infected pregnant women with spiramycin (has been used in Europe)
  2. Pregnant women and young children should
     a. Cook meat to "well done" stage
     b. Wash hands after handling uncooked meat
     c. Avoid cat feces
     d. Avoid contact with cat litter boxes
     e. Use gloves when gardening

Impact of Genetic Factors on

Growth and Development

Trisomy 18 (Edward's Syndrome)

- Definition: A syndrome of multiple malformations due to presence of an extra number 18 chromosome
- Etiology/Incidence
    1. Nondisjunction (80%) or translocation (10%) of chromosome 18
    2. Advanced maternal age is a contributing factor
    3. Frequency of occurrence is 1 in 8,000 births
- Clinical Findings
    1. Small for gestational age
    2. Severe developmental retardation
    3. Failure to thrive
    4. Seizures and hydrocephaly
    5. High rate of congenital heart defects
    6. High rate of hernias
    7. Distinctive facial appearance
        a. Prominent occiput
        b. Narrow bifrontal diameter of face
        c. Low set malformed ears
        d. Short palpebral fissures
        e. Microphthalmia
        f. Microcephaly
- Management/Treatment
    1. Less than 10% of infants survive beyond 12 months; 50% die by 2 months of age; therapy is supportive
    2. Counseling and support to parents who must deal with loss of infant and decisions about future pregnancies

Down Syndrome (Trisomy 21)

- Definition: A syndrome of multiple malformations, characteristic physical appearance and mental retardation

- Etiology/Incidence
    1. Trisomy or translocation of chromosome 21
    2. Greater risk in women over age 35
    3. Most common chromosomal abnormality of a generalized syndrome
- Clinical Findings
    1. Mental retardation from mild to severe
    2. Atlantoaxial instability
    3. Congenital heart defects in 33 to 50% of cases
    4. Altered immune function—more susceptible to illness
    5. Distinctive facial appearance
        a. Microcephaly with flat occiput
        b. Oblique palpebral fissures (upward, outward slant)
        c. Inner epicanthal folds
        d. Flat profile
        e. Protruding tongue; high arched palate, hypoplastic mandible
- Management/Treatment
    1. Genetic counseling for parents
    2. Prompt referral for surgical correction of congenital anomalies
    3. Enrollment in an early intervention program
    4. Careful monitoring of growth, development, sensory function
    5. Titers to monitor immune status because these children do not develop immunity in an expected way
    6. Support and respite for parents
    7. Special education placement

Fragile X Syndrome

- Definition: An inherited condition that is commonly believed to occur only in males; various degrees of mental retardation, with certain physical and/or behavioral traits are usually present
- Etiology/Incidence
    1. Fragile site or break in the X chromosome; abnormal gene or genes

on the lower end of long arm of the X chromosome

2. Males are usually more severely affected; estimated to affect 1 in every 1000 to 2000 liveborn males

3. Incidence in females is increasing; females can also be carriers

4. Thought to be most common inherited form of mental retardation

- Clinical Findings

1. No typical facial appearance, but may have a long narrow face and prominent ears

2. Mild to profound mental retardation

3. Hyperactivity and poor attention span; autistic-like behaviors

4. Poor social skills

- Management/Treatment

1. Chromosome analysis and diagnosis of other family members with Fragile X

2. Medication to control hyperactivity and attentional problems

3. Appropriate school placement and monitoring

4. Support and referral to National Fragile X Foundation

Turner Syndrome (XO Karotype)

- Definition: A form of abnormal gonadal development characterized by short stature, phenotypic stigmata, and ovarian failure (Avery & First, 1994)

- Etiology/Incidence

1. Partial or complete deletion of one X chromosome

2. Incidence is 1:2000 to 1:5000 female births

- Clinical Findings

1. Many females with Turner Syndrome have minimal dysmorphic features and are not diagnosed early in life

2. Classic finding is lymphedema of hands and feet in neonatal period

3. As girl matures, other findings become more evident

   a. Short stature

   b. Broad chest with widely spaced nipples

   c. Webbed posterior neck

    d. Low posterior hairline

    e. Amenorrhea

■ Management/Treatment

1. Screening for hypertension, hearing loss and renal abnormalities which are common in this syndrome

2. Counseling regarding inability to have children

3. Support for girl who is sensitive about her appearance

4. Estrogen and androgen therapy to enhance growth

Klinefelter Syndrome (XXY Karotype)

■ Definition: Syndrome characterized by abnormality of the sex chromosomes

■ Etiology/Incidence

1. Two or more X chromosomes and one or more Y chromosomes

2. Occurs in 1:1000 male births

3. Associated with advanced maternal age

■ Clinical Findings

1. Tall, slim build through childhood

2. Hypogenitalism; sterile, male secondary sex characteristics may be deficient

■ Management/Treatment

1. Testosterone replacement therapy

2. Gynecomastia may require surgery

Tay-Sachs Disease

■ Detention: An autosomal recessive disorder

■ Etiology/Incidence

1. Abnormality in enzyme activity

2. Persons of Eastern-European Jewish ancestry have a carrier rate of 1:27

■ Clinical Findings

1. Affected children are usually normal at birth

2. Symptoms develop between 6 and 12 months of age

a. Hypotonia

b. Psychomotor retardation

c. Exaggerated startle response to noise

3. Steady progression of CNS degeneration with spasticity and blindness after one year of age

4. Death occurs between 2nd and 4th years

- Management/Treatment

1. Screening and genetic counseling of all persons of Eastern European Jewish ancestry

2. Supportive care to child

3. Support and respite for parents caring for and mourning loss of child

Questions

1. All of the following are appropriate interview strategies for a preschooler, except
   a. Use play to facilitate comfort
   b. Separate from parents for part of interview
   c. Allow sufficient time for responses
   d. Sit at the child's level

2. Which of the following interview techniques will be least productive when working with an adolescent client?
   a. Reflecting
   b. Summarizing
   c. Informing
   d. Confronting

3. When recording a client's history, the review of systems is included in which part of the chart note?
   a. Objective
   b. Subjective
   c. Plan
   d. Assessment

4. Allowing exploration of instruments, starting the PE with examination of the extremities and positioning yourself so the client can see your actions are modifications you might make in doing a PE on which age client?
   a. Young infant
   b. Toddler
   c. Older schoolager
   d. Adolescent

5. When percussing the abdomen, you would expect to hear which tone over the liver?
   a. Tympany
   b. Flatness
   c. Resonance
   d. Dullness

6. When examining a 12-month-old, you would expect vital signs to be?
   a. P= 80   R=16   BP 114/76
   b. P=120   R=42   BP 120/78
   c. P=100   R=30   BP 94/68
   d. P=130   R=18   BP 100/84

7. A normal total bilirubin level is

    a. Less than 1.5 mg/dl
    b. Less than 2.0 mg/dl
    c. Less than 2.5 mg/dl
    d. Less than 2.8 mg/dl

8. Risk factors for visual impairment in the young infant include all of these, except

    a. Congenital cyanotic heart disease
    b. Hearing problem
    c. Increased bilirubin in the newborn period
    d. Prenatal infections

9. Which of these is an appropriate instrument to test visual acuity in a 4-year-old child?

    a. Ishihara
    b. Hirschberg
    c. Sjogren hand
    d. Rosenbaum

10. Pure tone audiometry is an appropriate screening measure for hearing acuity after what age?

    a. 3 years
    b. 4 years
    c. 5 years
    d. 6 years

11. Responses to 30 to 35 dB when using pure tone audiometry are interpreted as

    a. Normal hearing
    b. Mild hearing loss
    c. Moderate hearing loss
    d. Severe hearing loss

12. The most accurate results for Tuberculosis screening is obtained with the

    a. Tine test
    b. Old Tuberculin (Mono-Vac)
    c. Mantoux test
    d. PPD

13. "Preterm" is the correct term for a newborn who

    a. Weighs under 2500 gm
    b. Has a gestational age of less than 37 weeks
    c. Is SGA

d. Is less than 19 inches in length

14. A weight increase of 3-4 oz per week and length increase of 1/2 inch per month is typical for a child of what age?

    a. 4 months
    b. 9 months
    c. 15 months
    d. 36 months

15. Which of these statements about use of growth charts is true?

    a. Once an adolescent has started the pubertal growth spurt, standard growth charts are inaccurate
    b. Standard growth charts should be used until age 18
    c. Preterm infant's growth can be accurately plotted on a standard growth chart after 3 months of age
    d. Weight measurements that plot above the 90th percentile indicate obesity

16. Which of these fine motor skills is typically first to develop?

    a. Copy a triangle
    b. Copy a square
    c. Imitate a circle
    d. Copy a diamond

17. Which are the first deciduous teeth to emerge?

    a. Upper cuspids
    b. Lower lateral incisors
    c. Upper central incisors
    d. Lower central incisors

18. Permanent teeth begin to develop and thus could be damaged at

    a. 32 weeks gestation
    b. 3-4 months of age
    c. 9-12 months of age
    d. 15-18 months of age

19. A 14-year-old girl comes to see you because she has not started her menstrual periods yet. You note that she has breast buds and some axillary and pubic hair growth. Your plan for this visit includes

    a. A laboratory workup for delayed puberty
    b. Radiographs for bone age
    c. Reassurance that her development is within normal limits
    d. Chromosome analysis to R/O Turner's Syndrome

20. Freud's phallic stage corresponds to which of Erikson's tasks?

a. Industry vs. inferiority
b. Identity vs. role confusion
c. Trust vs. mistrust
d. Initiative vs. guilt

21. According to Kohlberg's theory of moral development, a child of what age is cognitively able to accept external moral guidelines such as laws and regulations to maintain social order?

a. 4-5 years
b. 7-8 years
c. 10-12 years
d. 13-15 years

22. Which of the following would Maslow identify as the need just below self-actualization?

a. Ego and esteem
b. Safety and security
c. Love and belongingness
d. Physiological

23. Ability to follow a one-step command given without a gesture and using 4 to 6 individual words are skills you would expect of what age child?

a. 8 months
b. 10 months
c. 14 months
d. 20 months

24 The parents of 4-year-old David are concerned about his stuttering. Which of the following would lead you to refer David for language evaluation at this time?

a. Stuttering present for past 4 months
b. His age
c. Stuttering present whenever child is excited
d. Child avoids speaking

25. Which of the following is not an appropriate screening tool for language development in a four- year-old?

a. Ishihara test
b. Early Language Milestones Scale
c. Fluharty Preschool Speech and Language Screening Test
d. Goldberg's Speech and Language Screening Tool

26. Children with Down Syndrome typically have wide set eyes. The appropriate term for this is

a. Hypertelorism
b. Ptosis
c. Anisocoria
d. Hordeolum

27. As you are examining the eyes of a 12-year-old, you note miosis of her pupils. You may want to ask her about

a. Allergies
b. Her intake of iron-rich foods
c. Drug use
d. Recent eye infection

28. Which of these behaviors could indicate a moderate to severe hearing loss?

a. Use of gestures rather than expressed language after 12 months of age
b. No babbling after 6 months of age
c. No reaction to strangers at 4 months of age
d. No communicative speech after 12 months of age

29. Cherry red lips are an indication of

a. Acidosis
b. Riboflavin deficiency
c. Low fluoride intake
d. Niacin deficiency

30. If you observe greenish stains on a child's teeth, you would want to ask about?

a. Fluoride dosage
b. Tetracycline taken by mother while pregnant
c. Iron therapy
d. Recent tonsillitis

31. During your exam of a 2-month-old child, you note that the anterior fontanel is 7 cm in diameter. Your differential would include all of the following, except

a. Hypothyroidism
b. Subdural hematoma
c. Rickets
d. Within normal limits

32. At what age would you expect to see no significant head lag when an infant is pulled from a supine to a sitting position?

a. Over 2 months of age
b. Over 4 months of age
c. Over 6 months of age
d. Over 8 months of age

33. A split S_2 is best heard in which auscultatory area?

    a. Aortic
    b. Pulmonic
    c. Base
    d. Tricuspid

34. A particularly loud PMI could indicate

    a. Acute anemia
    b. Cardia enlargement
    c. Aortic regurgitation
    d. None of the above

35. At what age do you expect to see girls convert from diaphragmatic (or abdominal) to more thoracic movement with respirations?

    a. 2 years
    b. 7 years
    c. 11 years
    d. 14 years

36. Gynecomastia in older school-age boys can be a symptom of

    a. Obesity
    b. Testicular or pituitary tumors
    c. Steroid use
    d. All of the above

37. A 16-year-old young woman reports a breast mass that she noticed 2 months ago. Which of these findings is not characteristic of a fibroadenoma?

    a. There is a similar, though smaller mass in the other breast
    b. The mass is mobile and non tender
    c. The mass is firm in consistency
    d. No variation with menstrual cycle

38. Which of the following is a normal finding in a 2-year-old?

    a. Bluish tint in the umbilical area
    b. Visible peristaltic waves when child is supine
    c. "Pot-belly" appearance when standing
    d. Liver edge palpable 4 cm below right costal margin

39. Tenderness elicited during palpation of the lower abdominal quadrants would suggest

    a. Splenic enlargement
    b. Gastroenteritis

c. Hepatitis
d. None of the above

40. When you see a 4-month-old infant with a large scrotum, you would want to include all of the following in your differential, except

a. Hydrocele
b. Indirect inguinal hernia
c. Varicocele
d. Testicular tumor

41. The type of hernia which affects females more often than males and is more common on the right than left side is

a. Indirect inguinal hernia
b. Direct inguinal hernia
c. Femoral hernia
d. None of the above

42. Which of the following is not an examination technique used to detect hip dislocation?

a. Allis
b. Trendelenburg
c. Gower's sign
d. Barlow maneuver

43. Functional scoliosis is characterized by

a. Disappearance when the child is recumbent
b. Unequal height of shoulders and iliac crest when child is standing
c. Asymmetric elevation of scapula when child leans forward
d. Persistent curvature

44. Which of these primitive reflexes would you expect to see in an 8 month old infant?

a. Moro
b. Tonic neck
c. Palmar grasp
d. Plantar grasp

45. The parents of a 6-month-old are concerned about a "stork bite" (salmon patch) on their child's face. You tell them that a birthmark of this type

a. Tends to enlarge as the child grows
b. Usually gets darker as the child grows
c. Usually disappears by 12 months
d. Will require laser light treatments

46. A neonate with a pink papular rash with superimposed vesicles on chest, back,

buttocks and abdomen; no fever and no change in appetite, most probably has

a. Cutis marmorata
b. Erythema toxicum
c. Harlequin rash
d. Milia

47. On physical examination of a 12-month-old you note non tender mobile 0.3 to 0.4 cm diameter cervical lymph nodes. The most likely diagnosis in your differential is

a. Possible HIV infection
b. Acute tonsilar infection
c. Cytomegalovirus infection
d. Normal lymph nodes

48. Which of these infections cannot be acquired by the fetus in utero?

a. Hepatitis B
b. *Chlamydia trachomatis*
c. Cytomegalic inclusion disease
d. Herpes simplex virus

49. Infants who acquire cytomegalic inclusion disease (CMV) at birth

a. Typically present as an afebrile pneumonia about 8 weeks after birth
b. Very often have severe neurologic sequelae
c. Typically present as conjunctivitis about 2 weeks after birth
d. None of the above

50. A staccato cough is a characteristic finding in pneumonia caused by

a. Toxoplasmosis
b. Cytomegalovirus
c. *Chlamydia trachomatis*
d. None of the above

51. A 4-day-old infant presents with purulent eye drainage and marked eyelid edema which began in the past 24 hours. The most likely cause is

a. Chlamydia conjunctivitis
b. Gonococcal conjunctivitis
c. Delayed reaction to silver nitrate prophylaxis
d. None of the above

52. A newborn infant whose mother tests positive for HB_sA_g, should receive

a. Hepatitis B vaccine
b. Hepatitis B immune globulin
c. Both of the above

d. Neither of the above

53. Epitrochlear lymphadenopathy is characteristic of which of these congenital conditions?

   a. Toxoplasmosis
   b. Gonorrhea
   c. Syphilis
   d. Rubella

54. Exposure to which of these maternal infections results in more severe symptoms if the exposure is in the first rather than the third trimester?

   a. Toxoplasmosis
   b. Rubella
   c. Both of the above
   d. Neither of the above

55. Advanced maternal age increases the risk of which of these conditions?

   a. Trisomy 18
   b. Down Syndrome
   c. Both of the above
   d. Neither of the above

56. Fewer than 10% of infants with this chromosomal disorder will survive more than 12 months

   a. Klinefelter Syndrome
   b. Fragile X Syndrome
   c. Tay Sachs Disease
   d. Trisomy 18

57. You are seeing a 6-year-old boy who is hyperactive, has a poor attention span, seems to lack age appropriate social skills and is not able to do first grade school work. Of the following the most likely diagnosis is

   a. Trisomy 18
   b. Down Syndrome
   c. Klinefelter Syndrome
   d. Fragile X Syndrome

58. You have a new client in your practice, a 13-year-old girl with Turner Syndrome. You might expect to find all of the following, except

   a. School failure
   b. Short stature
   c. No pubertal changes
   d. Hypertension

59. A couple of Eastern European Jewish ancestry are planning to have a child. You would recommend genetic testing and counseling regarding

    a. Tay-Sachs Disease
    b. Trisomy 18
    c. Trisomy 21
    d. Fragile X Syndrome

60. Cooperative play is first seen in which age children?

    a. Toddlers
    b. Young preschoolers
    c. Older preschoolers
    d. Third graders

61. You have been asked to speak to a group of parents of children ages 3 to 6 about play, and how parents can participate in their child's play. You would plan to include all of these points, except

    a. Praise and encourage the child's creativity
    b. Don't compete with the child
    c. Follow the child's lead
    d. Correct the child's errors in describing the real world

62. If you are assessing the attachment between a young mother and her infant, you would look for which of these behaviors by 5 to 6 months of age?

    a. Reciprocal vocal and affective exchanges between mother and infant
    b. Baby has clear preference for mother
    c. Baby gives clear cues
    d. Mother notices baby's distress when placed on scale

63. In talking to the parents of a 2-month-old about colic you would include all of the following, except

    a. Colic is common in infants of this age
    b. Colic usually stops by 3 to 4 months
    c. Colic is caused by allergy to formula
    d. Medications to control colic are not usually needed

64. Teething can cause all of the following signs and symptoms, except

    a. Irritability
    b. High fever
    c. Increased salivation
    d. Local inflammation

65. The father of a 4-year-old calls you because his son is having nightmares. The boy

is afraid to go to sleep in his own bed and insists on sleeping with the father. The father is not comfortable with the arrangement but doesn't know how to manage the situation. You would want to include all of the following in your discussion with the father, except

a. Nightmares are common at this age
b. A small light in the boy's room may be reassuring to him
c. When he has a nightmare, go into his room and reassure him that you are close
d. Turn the room light on and read to him for 15 to 20 minutes to help him forget the nightmare

66. A parent is concerned because their 32-month-old boy is not toilet trained and all the other children his age at the daycare are successfully using the toilet. You would want to tell this mother

a. All children are different, and this boy is still within the range of normal for not being toilet trained
b. This boy should be seen by a urologist
c. This boy should be put on a potty chair or the toilet for 15 minutes after every meal
d. None of the above

67. A mother of a 5-year-old asks you about the pros and cons of TV viewing for her child. You would include all of the following in your discussion with her, except

a. TV can foster superficial problem solving
b. Viewing aggression on TV or videos can lead to increased use of aggression by the child
c. Extended TV watching can foster obesity
d. Don't limit the amount of time spent watching TV, but do control the types of programs watched

68. "Time out" is an appropriate discipline measure for a 5-year-old child when he

a. Whines for more than 5 minutes
b. Hits a playmate
c. Ignores a command to pick up his coat
d. All of the above

69. A key distinction between caput succedaneum and cephalohematoma

a. Cephalohematomas don't cross the suture line
b. Linear skull fractures occur with 25% of babies with caput succedaneum
c. Caput succedaneum is usually not apparent immediately after birth
d. Cephalohematomas result from pressure on the presenting part during a vertex delivery

Answer key

1. b	26. a	51. b
2. d	27. c	52. c
3. b	28. b	53. c
4. b	29. a	54. c
5. d	30. c	55. c
6. c	31. d	56. d
7. a	32. c	57. d
8. c	33. c	58. a
9. c	34. a	59. a
10. a	35. b	60. c
11. b	36. d	61. d
12. c	37. a	62. b
13. b	38. c	63. c
14. b	39. b	64. b
15. a	40. d	65. c
16. c	41. c	66. a
17. d	42. c	67. d
18. b	43. a	68. b
19. c	44. d	69. a
20. d	45. c	
21. c	46. b	
22. a	47. d	
23. c	48. b	
24. d	49. a	
25. b	50. c	

Bibliography

American Academy of Pediatrics (1994). *1994 Red Book: Report of the Committee on Infectious Disease* (23rd ed.), Elk Grove Village, IL: American Academy of Pediatrics.

Avery, M. E., & First, L. R. (1994). *Pediatric Medicine* (2nd ed.), Baltimore, MD: Williams & Wilkins.

Behrman, R., & Vaughan, V. (Eds.). (1992). *Nelson textbook of pediatrics* (14th ed.). Philadelphia: W. B. Saunders.

Bergen, K. S. (1991). *The developing person through childhood and adolescense* (3rd ed.). New York: Worth.

Edelman, C., & Mandle, C. (Eds.) (1993). *Health promotion throughout the lifespan* (3rd ed.). St. Louis: C.V. Mosby.

Jackson, P. L., & Vessey, J. A. (1992). *Primary care of the child with a chronic condition*. St. Louis: Mosby Year Book.

Jarvis, C. (1992). *Physical examination and health assessment*. Philadelphia: W. B. Saunders.

Levine, M., Carey, W., & Crocker, A. (1992). *Developmental-behavioral pediatrics* (2nd ed.). Philadelphia: W. B. Saunders.

Oski, F. (Ed.). (1994). *Principles and practice of pediatrics*. Philadelphia: J. B. Lippincott.

Schuster, C., & Ashburn, S. (1992). *The process of human development: A holistic life span approach*. New York: J. B. Lippincott.

Webster-Stratton, C. (1992). *The incredible years: A trouble shooting guide for parents of children aged 3-8*. Toronto: Umbrella Press.

Health Maintenance and Promotion

Margaret A. Hertzog

Health Maintenance

One of the primary functions of the pediatric nurse practitioner is health maintenance and promotion. A sound knowledge of growth and development and an understanding of the number of disorders that can affect children and adolescents provides the foundation of practice.

Health is a complex phenomenon. According to the World Health Organization (WHO), it is "a state of complete physical, mental, and social well-being and not merely the absence of disease." In order to provide a holistic approach to child care, the importance of developing a relationship early in the child-rearing process cannot be overemphasized. It is therefore appropriate to begin this chapter with the prenatal visit. The basic premise of the prenatal visit is to provide an opportunity to introduce yourself to the potential parents, provide the groundwork for what may become a long term relationship with the parent(s), and provide an opportunity for exploration of parental feelings and concerns. It ultimately builds the infrastructure for comprehensive child care.

Prenatal Visit

- Prospective Parenting Interview
  1. Physiological data
  2. Psychological data
     a. Readiness for parenthood
     b. Prenatal classes, childbirth preparation
     c. Sibling preparation, if applicable
     d. Choice of infant feeding (breast/bottle)
     e. Circumcision, if applicable
     f. Special concerns of prospective parents
     g. Use of tobacco, alcohol, drugs
     h. Genetic testing
  3. Sociological Data
     a. Family type—extended, single parent, nuclear, etc.
     b. Introduction of pets to infant, number of pets and type, safety around children

- Plan or Information Needed
    1. Reasons to seek attention from health care provider
    2. How, where to reach care when needed; available hours
    3. Frequency of scheduled visits
    4. Fees, if applicable; family's financial situation; health care, eligibility for assistance
    5. Language barriers; need for transportation
- Anticipatory Guidance/Plan of Care
    1. Options of birthing arrangements; rooming-in
    2. Infant equipment needed
    3. General infant care
    4. Safety factors
    5. Psychological adjustments

Parent/Infant Visit—Newborn Examination

- Initial History
    1. Family History: Maternal/Paternal
        a. Review of systems (ROS)
        b. Social/emotional
            (1) History of mental illness
            (2) Separation, divorce, single parent
            (3) Substance abuse
    2. General Health of Mother
        a. Mother's age and gestation at first prenatal visit; regularity of visits
        b. History of maternal infection—prenatal
        c. Substance abuse, tobacco use
        d. History of chronic disease
        e. Medications during pregnancy
        f. Weight gain; nutritional status
        g. Number of weeks of gestation

       h. Number of living children

3. Labor and Delivery

    a. Length of labor

    b. Medications used; Anesthesia

    c. Type of facility—birthing center, hospital, other

    d. Type of delivery—spontaneous, C-Section (explanation needed if yes)

    e. Blood type, including Rh factor

4. Infant's Status at Delivery

    a. Identification verified

    b. Term, preterm (number of weeks)

    c. Determination of gestational age (Ballard/Dubowitz)

    d. Apgar scores

    e. Oxygen required

    f. Blood Type, Rh Factor; other values

    g. Length, weight, head circumference

    h. Physical examination results—note any abnormal findings

    i. Correct date of birth

5. Nursery course; presence of jaundice; type of treatments

6. Medications; immunizations given, e.g., Hepatitis B vaccine (See Tables 1 and 2 and chapter on Growth and Development)

7. Length of stay at facility

8. Circumcision/cord condition

9. Infant's Social History

    a. Name of infant properly recorded

    b. Infant's caretaker

    c. Number of adults in home; any smokers

    d. Number of children; infant's place in family

    e. Infant equipment available for infant's care

    f. Number of pets; type, e.g., discuss safety and introduction of infant to pets

   g. Infant's sleeping arrangements

■ Common Questions/Concerns of Parent

   1. Initial weight loss, appearance of infant (cephalohematomas, molding)

   2. Rashes, skin markings—telangiectasis, cafe-au-lait, hemangiomas

   3. Infant's habits—feeding, stooling, sleeping, development, normal crying

   4. Breast engorgement, vaginal discharge—female infant

■ Objective Data

   1. Verify identification of mother, infant

   2. Parent/infant interaction

      a. Eye contact

      b. Holding; response to crying

   3. Behavioral—consolability, self-quieting

   4. Physical examination

      a. Weight, length, head circumference percentiles

      b. Visually alert; fix, follow

      c. Orient to sound

      d. Gestational Age (Ballard, Dubowitz)

      e. HEENT

         (1) Anterior fontanelle, posterior fontanelle (note any molding, craniosynostosis, cephalohematomas, asymmetry)

         (2) Presence of red reflex

         (3) Patency of nares; note any unusual findings in mouth

      f. Auscultation of lungs

      g. Cardiac evaluation, femoral, brachial, pulses

      h. Abdomen—number of blood vessels (two umbilical arteries and one umbilical vein); cord appearance, condition of stump

      i. Genitourinary—circumcision; prominence of labia; number of testicles and position; hypospadias

      j. Skeletal—hips, feet, range of motion; note any crepitus; positive

Ortolani/Barlow; note presence of equinovarus

    k. Neurological

        (1)   Root/suck

        (2)   Gag reflex

        (3)   Moro

        (4)   Head lag

        (5)   Plantar/palmar

        (6)   Stepping

5. Laboratory—Hereditary/Metabolic Screening—thyroid, PKU, MSUD hemoglobinopathies, galactosemia hemoglobiinopathies (according to state law)

- Anticipatory Guidance/Plan of Care

1. Reinforce infant care; cord care, circumcision care

2. Emphasize individuality of infant, positive aspects

3. Discuss feedings, amounts, time at breast

4. Reinforce instructions on when to seek medical advice—fever, vomiting, diarrhea, jaundice, feeding problems

5. Reinforce safety factors from earlier visits, car seat use

6. Episodes of crying; symptoms of colic

Health Maintenance: Infancy (1 Week to 1 Year)

- Interim Visit 1 Week to 1 Year

1. Subjective Information

    a. Feeding—amounts, time at breast, name of formula

    b. Elimination—frequency, color, consistency

    c. Number of saturated diapers

    d. Sleep

    e. Development

    f. Concerns of parent, caregiver

    g. Interval history; emergency care; illness, medications used

- Objective Data

1. Age; height, weight, head circumference percentiles; vital signs

2. Vision and hearing screening (can be subjective, by history)

3. Physical examination

4. Developmental assessment; Denver Developmental Screening, or equivalent and results

5. Laboratory

   a. Urinalysis at 6 months unless indicated otherwise

   b. Hematocrit or hemoglobin between 6 and 9 months or if indicated otherwise

- Anticipatory Guidance/Plan of Care

   1. Immunizations (See Tables 1, 2, 3)

   2. Counseling

      a. Side effects of immunizations; the National Childhood Vaccine Injury Act of 1986 requires all health care providers who administer vaccines to report occurrences of certain adverse events stipulated in the Act (see Table 4 "Reportable Events Following Immunization")

      b. Medications prescribed

      c. Nutrition—amounts, diet progress

      d. Parenting aspects related to subjective, objective data and developmental level of infant

      e. Safety; appropriate for developmental age

      f. Referrals to other nurse practitioners, physicians, clinics, community resources as needed

      g. Schedule for next visit

Table 1
Recommended Schedule for Immunization of Healthy Infants and Children[a]

Recommended Age[b]	Immunization(s)[c]	Comments
Birth	HBV[d]	
1-2 mo	HBV[d]	
2 mo	DTP, Hib,[e] OPV	DTP and OPV can be initiated as early as 4 wk after birth in areas of high endemicity or during outbreaks
4 mo	DTP, Hib,[e] OPV	2-mo interval (minimum of 6 wk) recommended for OPV
6 mo	DTP, (Hib[e,f])	
6-18 mo	HBV,[d] OPV	
12-15 mo	Hib,[e] MMR	MMR should be given at 12 mo of age in high-risk areas. If indicated, tuberculin testing may be done at the same visit
15-18 mo	DTaP or DTP	The 4th dose of diphtheria-tetanus-pertussis vaccine should be given 6 to 12 mo after the third dose of DTP and may be given as early as 12 mo of age, provided that the interval between doses 3 and 4 is at least 6 mo and DTP is given. DTaP is not currently licensed for use in children younger than 15 mo
4-6 y	DTaP or DTP, OPV	DTaP or DTP and OPV should be given at or before school entry. DTP or DTaP should not be given at or after the 7th birthday
11-12 y	MMR	MMR should be given at entry to middle school or junior high school unless 2 doses were given after the 1st birthday
14-16 y	Td	Repeat every 10 y throughout life

[a] Table is not completely consistent with all package inserts. For products used, also consult manufacturer's package insert for instructions on storage, handling, dosage, and administration. Biologics prepared by different manufacturers may vary, and package inserts of the same manufacturer may change from time to time. Therefore, the physician should be aware of the contents of the current package insert.

[b] These recommended ages should not be construed as absolute. For example, 2 mo can be 6 to 10 wk. However, MMR usually should not be given to children younger than 12 mo. if measles vaccination is indicated, monovalent measles vaccine is recommended, and MMR should be given subsequently, at 12-15 mo.

[c] Vaccine abbreviations: HBV = Hepatitis B virus vaccine; DTP = diphtheria and tetanus toxoids and pertussis vaccine; DTaP = diphtheria and tetanus toxoids and acellular pertussis vaccine; Hib = *Haemophilus influenzae* type b conjugate vaccine; OPV = oral poliovirus vaccine (containing attenuated poliovirus types 1, 2, and 3); MMR = live measles, mumps, and rubella viruses vaccine; Td = adult tetanus toxoid (full dose) and diphtheria toxoid (reduced dose), for children ≥ 7 y and adults.

[d] See Table 2. An acceptable alternative to minimize the number of visits for immunizing infants of HBsAg-negative mothers is to administer dose 1 at 0-2 mo, dose 2 at 4 mo, and dose 3 at 6 to 18 mo.

[e] See Table 3.

[f] (Hib: dose 3 of Hib is not indicated if the product for doses 1 and 2 was PedvaxHIB [PRP-OMP], available from Merck & Co., West Point, PA)

NOTE: From American Academy of Pediatrics. [Active and Passsive Immunization]. In: Peter G, ed. *1994 Red Book: Report of the Committee on Infectious Diseases.* 23rd ed. Elk Grove Village, IL: American Academy of Pediatrics; 1994: [p. 23]. Reprinted by permission.

Table 2
Recommended Schedules of Hepatitis B Vaccination for Infants Born to HBsAg-Negative Mothers.*
(These guidelines may not apply to preterm infants.)

Hepatitis B vaccine	Timing †
Dose 1	Birth (i.e., preferably before hospital discharge) to 2 mo of age
Dose 2	1 to 2 mo after dose 1
Dose 3	6 to 18 mo of age ‡

* Hepatitis B vaccine can be given concurrently with other vaccines, including DTP, *Haemophilus influenzae* type b conjugate, MMR, and/or oral poliovirus vaccine.

† See p. 231 of AAP "Red Book" for further explanation of possible variations in the schedule.

‡ Infants in populations with high rates of childhood infections should complete the 3-dose series by 6 to 9 mo of age (see p. 231 of AAP "Red Book").

NOTE: From American Academy of Pediatrics. [Summaries of Infectious Diseases]. In: Peter G, ed. 1994 Red Book: Report of the Committee on Infectious Diseases. 23rd ed. Elk Grove Village, IL; American Academy of Pediatrics; 1994 [p. 232]. Reprinted by permission.

Table 3
Recommendations for *Haemophilus influenzae* type b Conjugate Vaccination in Children Immunized Beginnig at 2 to 6 Months of Age

Vaccine Product at Initiation*	Total Number of Doses to Be Administered	Currently Recommended Vaccine Regimens*
HbOC or PRP-T	4	3 doses at 2-mo intervals When feasible, same vaccine for doses 1-3 Fourth dose at 12 to 15 mo of age Any conjugate vaccine for dose 4†
PRP-OMP	3	2 doses at 2-mo intervals When feasible, same vaccine for doses 1 and 2 Third dose at 12-15 mo of age Any conjugate vaccine for dose 3†

*See text. The HbOC, PRP-T, or PRP-OMP should be given in a separate syringe and at a separate site from other immunizations unless specific combinations are approved by the FDA. HbOC is also available as a combination vaccine with DTP (HbOC-DTP). This combination can be used in infants scheduled to receive separate injections of DTP and HbOC. PRP-T may be reconstituted with DTP, made by Connaught Laboratories; other licensed formulations of DTP may not be used for this purpose.

† The safety and efficacy of PRP-OMP, PRP-D, PRP-T, and HbOC are likely to be equivalent in children 12 mo and older.

NOTE: From American Academy of Pediatrics. [Summaries of Infectious Diseases]. In: Peter G, ed. 1994 Red Book: Report of the Committee on Infectious Diseases. 23rd ed. Elk Grove Village, IL; American Academy of Pediatrics; 1994 [p. 211]. Reprinted by permission.

Table 4
Reportable Events Following Immunization[a]

Vaccine/ Toxoid[b]	Adverse Event	Interval From Vaccination to Onset of Event	
		For Reporting[c]	For Compensation[d]
DTP, P, DTP/ Poliovirus combined	A. Anaphylaxis or anaphylactic shock	24 h	24 h
	B. Encephalopathy (or encephalitis)[e]	7 d	3 d
	C. Shock-collapse or hypotonic-hyporesponsive collapse[f]	7 d	3 d
	D. Residual seizure disorder[g]	(See footnote g)	3 d
	E. Any acute complication or sequela (including death) of above events	No limit	Not applicable
	F. Events described as contraindications to additional doses of vaccine (see manufacturer's package insert[h])	(See package insert[h])	
Measles, Mumps, and Rubella; DT, Td, T	A. Anaphylaxis or anaphylactic shock	24 h	24 h
	B. Encephalopathy (or encephalitis)[e]	15 d for measles, mumps, and rubella vaccine; 7 d for DT, Td, and T	15 d for measles, mumps, and rubella vaccine; 3 d for DT, Td, and T
	C. Residual seizure disorder[g]	(see footnote g)	15 d for measles, mumps, or rubella vaccine; 3 d for DT, Td, and T
	D. Any acute complication or sequela (including death) of above events	No limit	
	E. Events described as contraindications to additional doses of vaccine (see manufacturer's package insert[h])	(See package insert[h])	
OPV	A. Paralytic poliomyelitis		
	• in a nonimmunodeficient recipient	30 d	30 d
	• in an immunodeficient recipient	6 mo	6 mo
	• in a vaccine-associated community case	No limit	Not applicable
	B. Any acute complication or sequela (including death) of above events	No limit	Not applicable
	C. Events described as contraindications to additional doses of vaccine (see manufacturer's package insert[h])	(See package insert[h])	

Table 4 (continued)
Reportable Events Following Immunization[a]

Vaccine/ Toxoid[b]	Adverse Event	Interval From Vaccination to Onset of Event	
		For Reporting[c]	For Compensation[d]
Inactivated Polio Vaccine	A. Anaphylaxis or anaphylactic shock	24 h	24 h
	B. Any acute complication or sequela (including death) of above events	No limit	Not applicable
	C. Events described as contra-indications to additional doses of vaccine (see manufacturer's package insert[h])	(See package insert[h])	

[a] As of December 1993.

[b] The vaccine/toxoid abbreviations, in alphabetical order, are: DT = diphtheria and tetanus toxoids; DTP = diphtheria and tetanus toxoids and pertussis vaccine (pediatric); OPV = oral poliovirus vaccine, live, trivalent; P = pertussis vaccine; T = tetanus toxoid; and Td = tetanus and diphtheria toxoids (for adult use).

[c] Adverse events that are required by *National Childhood Vaccine Injury Act of 1986* (NCVIA) to be reported to Vaccine Adverse Events Reporting System (VAERS) if their onset is within the indicated interval after vaccination.

[d] Adverse events that may be compensable under NCVIA if the onset is within this interval after vaccination.

[e] Encephalopathy means any significant acquired abnormality of, injury to, or impairment of function of, the brain. Among the frequent manifestations of encephalopathy are focal and diffuse neurologic signs, increased intracranial pressure, or changes lasting at least 6 h in level of consciousness, with or without convulsions. The neurologic signs and symptoms of encephalopathy may be temporary with complete recovery or may result in various degrees of permanent impairment. Signs and symptoms such as high-pitched and unusual screaming, persistent inconsolable crying, and bulging fontanel are compatible with an encephalopathy, but in and of themselves are not conclusive evidence of encephalopathy. Encephalopathy can usually be documented by slow-wave activity on an electroencephalogram.

[f] Shock-collapse or hypotonic-hyporesponsive collapse may include signs or symptoms such as decrease or loss of muscle tone, paralysis (partial or complete), hemiplegia, hemiparesis, loss of color or turning pale white or blue, unresponsiveness to environmental stimuli, depression of or loss of consciousness, prolonged sleeping with difficulty being aroused, or cardiovascular or respiratory arrest.

[g] Residual seizure disorder may have occurred if no other seizure or convulsion unaccompanied by fever or accompanied by a fever of < 102°F occurred before the first seizure or convulsion after the administration of the vaccine involved, and if, in the case of measles-mumps, or rubella-containing vaccines, the first seizure or convulsion occurred within 15 d after vaccination, or, in the case of any other vaccine, the first seizure or convulsion occurred within 3 d after vaccination, and, if 2 or more seizures or convulsions unaccompanied by fever or accompanied by a fever of 102°F occurred within 1 y after vaccination. The terms "seizure" and "convulsion" include grand mal, petit mal, absence, myoclonic, tonic-clonic, and focal motor seizures and signs.

[h] Refer to the CONTRAINDICATION section of the manufacturer's package insert for each vaccine/toxoid. Adapted from Update on adult immunization: recommendations of the Immunization Practices Advisory Committee (ACIP). *MMWR.* 1991;40(RR-12):53-54.

NOTE: From American Academy of Pediatrics. [Active and Passive Immunization]. In: Peters, G, ed. *1994 Red Book: Report of the Committee on Infectious Diseases.* 23rd ed. Elk Grove Village, IL; American Academy of Pediatrics; 1994 [p. 33]. Reprinted by permission.

- Key Concepts—Health Promotion 1 Week to 1 Year
  1. Emphasize infant's strengths/abilities
     a. Discuss time away from infant for parents, caregivers; need for responsible babysitters
     b. Anticipatory guidance for next developmental level; include safety measures
     c. Breastfed infants, vitamins with iron, may start at 10 to 14 days; add fluoride if needed in specific locale
     d. Formula fed infants do not require supplemental vitamins; fluoride requirements may vary depending upon whether "ready to feed" formula is used and specific locale
  2. Laboratory Screening
     a. Bilirubin as needed
     b. Hemoglobin, preterm infant, as needed
     c. Routine hemoglobin; lead screening (normal range 0-10 μg/dl); Sickle Cell if family history is positive, or applicable according to agency protocol
  3. Nutrition
     a. Nutritional requirements
        (1) 110/120 calories/kg/day
        (2) Consumption of 32 oz of formula per day usually an indicator of need for solids
        (3) Formula recommended up to 1 year of age; whole milk until two years of age
        (4) Judicious use of juices (some fortified with vitamin C)
     b. Introduction of solids
        (1) Usually between 4 to 6 months of age
        (2) Cereal usually the first food added to diet followed by vegetables, fruits
     c. Introduction of cup
        (1) Usually can be introduced between 8 months to 11 months
        (2) When infant loses interest in bottle

   (3) Spout cup may be used initially

  d. Stopping bottle by 1 year of age

   (1) Gradually decrease number of bottles over several weeks

   (2) Nighttime bottle usually the last one to be taken away

 4. Safety Factors for Each Developmental Level

  a. Injury prevention

   (1) Electrical wires out of reach; outlets covered; cabinet safety locks; medicines, poisons out of reach

   (2) Smoke detectors in household; keep syrup of Ipecac readily available, to be used in case of accidental poisoning; Poison Control telephone number available, other emergency phone numbers

   (3) Car seats appropriate for child's weight, age

   (4) Avoid walkers and stairs; use gates to barricade doorways and unsafe areas, e.g., kitchen and bathroom

  b. Water safety

   (1) Do not leave child unattended in bathtub

   (2) Do not allow child to play in water unattended, e.g., toilet bowls, sinks, buckets of water

   (3) Use of safety devices around swimming pools, lakes and in boats, e.g., life jackets

   (4) Lock fences around swimming pools

   (5) Continuous supervision around water

   (6) Do not leave other children in charge of infants and toddlers around any body of water

  c. Sun safety, sunburn prevention

   (1) Use lotion with sun protective factor (SPF) of 15 or higher

   (2) Avoid area around eyes

   (3) Use caps with sun visors or bonnets to protect eyes

   (4) Infants under 1 year should be kept in shade, even with sunscreen

   (5) Avoid sun between hours of 10 am to 2 pm

5. Issues of Alternative Child Care

   a. Babysitters

   b. Day care

   c. Need for appropriate supervision in all settings

   d. Adequate language, visual and motor stimulation

   e. Need for adequate motor activities

Health Maintenance: Toddler/Preschooler (1 to 4 Years)

- Subjective Data

  1. Appetite, nutrition, elimination, sleep, development

  2. Parental concerns

- Objective Data

  1. Assess parent/child interaction and effects on child's behavior; parenting style

  2. Physical examination

     a. Height, weight; head circumference (up to 3 years of age)

     b. Blood pressure (3 years and above)

     c. Vision, hearing screening, can be subjective by history; objective standardized testing method can be used for 4 year olds

  3. Laboratory—hematocrit, hemoglobin, urinalysis; lead levels at age 3, or at any time if not previously checked

  4. Tuberculin Test—between 12 and 15 months of age

- Anticipatory Guidance/Plan of Care

  1. Update immunizations (See Tables 1 to 3 for routine immunizations and Tables 5 and 6 for those children not immunized during the first year)

  2. Side-effects of immunizations

  3. Medications, include vitamins, fluoride

  4. Nutrition (foods from five major food groups; 1/4 to 1/3 of adult portion or one measuring tablespoon for each year of child's age)

  5. Discuss toilet training

6. Safety and injury prevention

7. Reinforce earlier safety factors

8. Discuss temper tantrums

9. Discuss aspects of parenting

    a. Limit setting; use of time-out

    b. Praise good behavior

    c. Emphasize consistency

    d. Remove temptations from child's environment

    e. Prepare for sibling rivalry

    f. Avoid strangers; teach child methods to avoid encounters with strangers which can be harmful

    g. Prevention of sexual abuse—talk to child about inappropriate touching; advise parents to reinforce prevention

- Child Care Arrangements
  1. Day care
  2. Head start programs
  3. Nursery school; pre-school programs
  4. Babysitters

- Dental Care
  1. Use of tooth brush
  2. Visit to dentist (age 3)

- Speech
  1. Refer to speech therapist if child is unable to communicate clearly by age 3

- Developmental Tasks (See Growth and Development Chapter)
  1. Name pictures in book
  2. Draw circles, lines, squares, person in three parts

- Assign chores appropriate to developmental level (See Growth and Development Chapter)
  1. Set/clear table
  2. Put toys away

Table 5
Recommended Immunization Schedules for Children Not Immunized in the First Year of Life

Recommended Time/Age	Immunization(s)[a,b]	Comments
Younger Than 7 Years		
First visit	DTP, Hib[c], HBV, MMR, OPV	If indicated, tuberculin testing may be done at same visit. If child is 5 y of age or older, Hib is not indicated.
Interval after first visit:		
1 mo	DTP, HBV	OPV may be given if accelerated poliomyelitis vaccination is necessary, such as for travelers to areas where polio is endemic.
2 mo	DTP, Hib,[c] OPV	Second dose of Hib is indicated only in children whose first dose was received when younger than 15 mo
≥ 8 mo	DTP or DTaP,[d] HBV, OPV	OPV is not given if the third dose was given earlier
4-6 y (at or before school entry	DTP or DTaP,[d] OPV	DTP or DTaP is not necessary if the fourth dose was given after the fourth birthday; OPV is not necessary if the third dose was given after the fourth birthday.
11-12 y	MMR	At entry to middle school or junior high school.
10 y later	Td	Repeat every 10 y throughout life.
7 Years and Older[e,f]		
First visit	HBV,[g] OPV, MMR, Td	
Interval after first visit:		
2 mo	HBV,[g] OPV, Td	OPV may also be given 1 mo after the first visit if accelerated poliomyelitis vaccination is necessary
8-14 mo	HBV,[g] OPV, Td	OPV is not given if the third dose was given earlier
11-12 y	MMR	At entry to middle school or junior high.
10 y later	Td	Repeat every 10 y throughout life.

[a] Abbreviations for vaccines are explained in the footnotes to Table 1. If all needed vaccines cannot be administered simultaneously, priority should be given to protecting the child against those diseases that pose the greatest immediate risk. In the U.S., these diseases for children younger than 2 y usually are measles and *Haemophilus influenzae* type b infection; for children older than 7 y, they are measles, mumps, and rubella (MMR).

[b] DTP or DTaP, HBV, Hib, MMR, and OPV can be given simultaneously at separate sites if failure of the patient to return for future immunizations is a concern.

[c] See *Haemophilus influenzae* Infections, p. 210, including Table 3.9 (p 212) in AAP "Red Book" and Table 6 in this chapter.

[d] DTaP is not currently licensed for use in children younger than 15 mo of age and is not recommended for primary immunization (i.e., first 3 doses) at any age.

[e] If person is 18 y or older, routine poliovirus vaccination is not indicated in the U.S.

[f] Minimal interval between doses of MMR is 1 mo.

[g] Priority should be given to hepatitis B immunizatin of adolescents (see Hepatitis B, p. 232 in AAP "Red Book").

NOTE: From American Academy of Pediatrics. [Active and Passsive Immunization]. In: Peter G, ed. 1994 Red Book: Report of the Committee on Infectious Diseases. 23rd ed. Elk Grove Village, IL: American Academy of Pediatrics; 1994: [p. 24]. Reprinted by permission.

Table 6
Recommendations for *Haemophilus influenzae* type b Conjugate Vaccination in Children in Whom Initial Vaccination Is Delayed Until 7 Months of Age or Older

Age at Initiation of Immunization (mo)	Vaccine Product at Initiation	Total Number of Doses to Be Administered	Currently Recommended Vaccine Regimens[a]
7-11	HbOC, PRP-T, or PRP-OMP	3	2 doses at 2-mo intervals[b] When feasible, same vaccine for doses 1 and 2 Third dose at 12-18 mo, given at least 2 mo after dose 2 Any conjugate vaccine for dose 3[c]
12-14	HbOC, PRP-T PRP-OMP, or PRP-D	2	2-mo interval between doses[b] Any conjugate vaccine for dose 2[c]
15-59	HbOC, PRP-T PRP-OMP, or PRP-D	1[d]	Any conjugate vaccine
60 and older[e]	HbOC, PRP-T, PRP-OMP, or PRP-D	1 or 2[d]	Any conjugate vaccine

[a] See text. HbOC, PRP-T, or PRP-OMP should be given in a separate syringe and at a separate site from other immunizations unless specific combinations are approved by the FDA. HbOC is also available as a combination vaccine with DTP (HbOC-DTP). This combination can be used in infants scheduled to receive separate injections of DTP and HbOC. PRP-T may be reconstituted with DTP, made by Connaught Laboratories; other licensed formulations of DTP may not be used for this purpose. In children 15 mo or older eligible to receive DTaP (containing acellular pertussis vaccine), however, separate injections of conjugate vaccine and DTaP are acceptable because of the lower rate of febrile, minor local and systemic reactions associated with DTaP.

[b] For "catch up," a minimum of a 1-mo interval between doses may be used.

[c] The safety and efficacy of PRP-OMP, PRP-D, PRP-T, and HbOC are likely to be equivalent for use as a booster dose in children 12 mo or older.

[d] Two doses separated by 2 mo are recommended by some experts for children with certain underlying diseases associated with increased risk of disease and impaired antibody responses to *H influenzae* type b conjugate vaccingation (see AAP "Red Book").

[e] Only for children with chronic illness known to be associated with an increased risk for *H influenzae* type b disease (see AAP "Red Book").

NOTE: From American Academy of Pediatrics. [Summaries of Infectious Diseases]. In: Peter G, ed. *1994 Red Book: Report of the Committee on Infectious Diseases.* 23rd ed. Elk Grove Village, IL: American Academy of Pediatrics; 1994: [p. 212]. Reprinted by permission.

■ Key Concepts—Health Promotion (1 to 4 Years)

    1. Good parenting practices

        a. Time-out used appropriately

        b. Parents/caregivers as role models

        c. Spend time with child, read to child

        d. Nutrition—parent education regarding "food jags", and "picky eaters"

2. Safety and prevention of injury

   a. Home safety/streets/playgrounds

   b. Water safety

   c. Sunburn prevention

   d. Continued use of car seats according to weight

   e. Use of helmets with any type of bicycle use either as a passenger or alone

3. Dental care

   a. Prevention of dental caries

   b. Record tooth development on examination findings

      (1) Malocclusion

      (2) Baby bottle mouth syndrome (caused by prolonged use of the bottle or allowing infant to use bottle in bed)

      (3) Oral infections

   c. Referrals to dentist—age 3 years

4. Socialization

   a. Promotion of good health habits

   b. Parents/caregivers provide interaction with other children

   c. Limit television viewing to appropriate children's programs; limit time spent watching TV

Health Maintenance: School Age (5 to 12 Years)

- Subjective Data

1. Habits

   a. Appetite; quality of food presented to child; amounts consumed

   b. Sleep—number of hours, accommodations, e.g., single bed, youth bed, sleep alone, etc.

   c. Elimination, especially constipation, enuresis

   d. Development, activity, exercise, school progress, friends

2. Parental/Child's concerns—family relationships; child's feelings of anxiety, anger, sadness

3. Illnesses, review of systems

■ Objective Data

   1. Physical examination

      a. Vital signs, blood pressure

      b. Height,weight percentiles

      c. Vision—objective, by a standard testing method 5, 6, 8 and 12 years of age

      d. Hearing

         (1) Objective, by a standard testing method 5, and 12 years of age

         (2) Subjective, by history 6, 8, and 10 years of age unless problem suggestive of need for standard testing method

      e. Tanner staging

      f. Scoliosis screening

      g. School reports as needed

   2. Review immunization status—update boosters

   3. Laboratory data

      a. Hemoglobin, hematocrit, urinalysis

      b. Tuberculin skin test between 4 and 6 years

      c. Cholesterol, at the discretion of provider, e.g., family history or obesity

   4. Behavioral assessment

      a. Parent/Child interaction

      b. Shows interest in school, recreation, hobbies, friends, peers

      c. Adequate adult supervision

      d. Communication with health care provider, e.g., shyness or disruptive activities

      e. School adjustment, achievements

      f. Level of independence; separation from parents

■ Anticipatory Guidance/Plan of Care

   1. Side-effects of immunizations

   2. Safety

      a. Bicycle; use of helmets

      b. Seat belt use

      c. Prevention of sexual abuse, e.g., inappropriate touching; what to do if occurs

      d. Water safety; swimming

      e. Fire prevention safety; home fire drill

      f. Sunburn prevention

      g. Prevention of violence in the home; lock up guns, ammunition; teach child gun safety

3. Encourage development of self-esteem and responsibility

4. Discuss prevention of drug, alcohol, tobacco use

5. Promote outside activities

      a. Sports

      b. Hobbies

6. Discuss onset of puberty

      a. Prepare child for menarche, night-time ejaculations

      b. Discuss parents preparation for child's questions on puberty

7. Discuss parenting practices

      a. Parental supervision—establish fair rules

      b. Respect for child's privacy

      c. Allow for decision making

8. Referrals as necessary

- Key Concepts—Health Promotion (5 to 12 Years)

1. Update immunizations

2. Establishing good health habits

      a. Balanced nutrition; avoid junk food; maintain appropriate weight

      b. Dental health

      c. Regular exercise

      d. Sufficient sleep

      e. Avoidance of drugs, alcohol, tobacco

f. Limit television; appropriate films

3. School adjustment

    a. Emphasize regular attendance

    b. Peer relationships

    c. Involvement in outside supervised activities

4. Safety

    a. Inside home—fire prevention; fire drills; proper use of appliances

    b. Outside home—automobile safety, bicycle, pedestrian

5. Promote good parenting practices

    a. Importance of spending time with child; communicate with child

    b. Discuss methods of discipline—use of positive reinforcement

    c. Appropriate adult supervision

    d. Parents' expectations of child's abilities and level of achievement

    e. Discussion of parents as role models

    f. Promote responsibility through completion of chores and care of pets

    g. Discuss need to provide child with an allowance

    h. Discuss selection of television/films that are appropriate to child's developmental level

    i. Encourage school attendance

    j. Praise child for achievements

    k. Show affection

Health Maintenance: Adolescent (13 to 18 Years)

- Subjective Data

    1. Interim History

        a. Review past history

        b. Review health history; accidents, hospitalizations, surgery, illnesses, dental history, vision, hearing, weight; review of systems

- Review of Habits

    1. Diet

2. Elimination

3. Activity, exercise

4. Sleep patterns

5. Stress factors

6. School attendance, achievement

7. Use of drugs, alcohol, tobacco

- Developmental History

  1. Onset of menarche, menstrual history, e.g., intervals of periods, duration

  2. Night-time ejaculation—12 to 14 years

  3. Enuresis

- Social History

  1. Peer relationships, friends

  2. Boyfriend, girlfriend

  3. Sports, hobbies

  4. Work

  5. Driver's license

- Parental Interview—separate from adolescent

  1. Family communication; stresses

  2. Parental concerns

  3. Parent's perception of adolescent's strong points, attitudes, moods; expectations of adolescent

  4. Discipline practices

- Adolescent Interview—separate from parent; includes review of systems

  1. Assure confidentiality

  2. Health concerns

  3. Sexual activity

  4. Personal concerns identity; goals for self; future goals; adolescent plans to reach goals

  5. Strong points, weak points

6. Independence
7. Methods of handling feelings of anger, sadness, worry, anxiety
8. Development of secondary sex characteristics; concerns
9. Tobacco, drug, alcohol use

■ Objective Data
1. Vital signs, blood pressure, height, weight percentiles
2. Vision
   a. Objective by a standard testing method at 14, 18 and 20 years of age
   b. Subjective, by history at 16 years of age
3. Hearing
   a. Subjective, by history at 14, 16 and 20 years of age
   b. Objective by a standard testing method at 18 years of age
4. Physical examination
5. Tanner stage
6. Scoliosis screen
7. Dental assessment
   a. Caries
   b. Malocclusion
   c. Infections
   d. Dental referral
8. Breast or testicular self-examination
9. Pelvic examination (at discretion of provider); recommended after age 16 unless sexually active or having irregular menses
10. Laboratory
    a. Urinalysis
    b. Hemoglobin, hematocrit, cholesterol
    c. GC, VDRL, HIV, Chlamydia (if sexually active)
    d. Pap smear
    e. Liver function tests (if on drugs)

- Key Concepts—Health Promotion Adolescence (13 to 18 Years)
  1. Review; update immunization status; recommend Hepatitis B vaccine
  2. Legal/ethical considerations
     a. Reportable information to parents includes
        (1) Self-destructive behavior
        (2) Attempted suicide
        (1) Pregnancy, abortion; birth control information depends on state laws
  3. Risk taking behavior—promote safety in all areas (driving, personal)
  4. Promote responsibility for self-care
     a. Good health habits
     b. Self-breast examination, self-testicular examination
     c. Regular health maintenance
  5. Encourage communication
     a. Family
     b. Peers
     c. School personnel
  6. Discuss plans for the future
     a. Further education
     b. Work; recreation; hobbies
     c. Marriage
     d. Parenthood
  7. Anticipatory guidance/plan
     a. Diet; maintain appropriate weight
     b. Physical activities; appropriate exercise; sufficient sleep
     c. Discuss issues of safety
        (1) Drinking, driving
        (2) Personal safety, sexuality; disease and pregnancy prevention
        (3) Dating; peer pressure
        (4) Drugs, alcohol, tobacco abuse

    d. Academic activities

       (1) Discuss issues of satisfactory school performance; graduation

       (2) College, vocational training; work

    e. Discuss issues of good parenting practices with parents

       (1) Fairness in rules

       (2) Allow decision making

       (3) Respect adolescent's privacy

       (4) Expect periods of estrangement (be available; adolescent needs supportive family)

       (5) Praise achievements at home, school, extracurricular

       (6) Supervision as needed

       (7) Encourage independence, new experiences, after-school activities, including part-time job

       (8) Promote family communication

       (9) Serve as role model (practice good health habits, e.g., parents should not smoke if they do not want child to imitate their behavior)

8. Issues related to family functioning

    a. Non-traditional families

       (1) Common-law marriages, e.g., social contract

       (2) Reconstituted or blended families

       (3) Homosexual couples

       (4) Joint custody arrangements

       (5) Single parent families—the most common, e.g., by divorce, death, separation, personal choice, unplanned pregnancy in single women (often adolescents); mother is most often the single parent

       (6) Number of single parent families is increasing

    b. Risks related to single parenting

Parent	Child
(1) Lack of emotional support	(1) Responses are affected by other relationships, e.g., of the parents to

       each other; relationships between each parent/child; presence of surrogate parent, extended families involved in care giving

(2) Lower incomes, usually mother

(2) Effect on child is dependent upon the cognitive developmental level of the child

(3) Social isolation

(3) In early childhood developmental progress may be arrested or regress; acute separation anxiety may develop, e.g., fear of abandonment

(4) Responsibilities of work/study; lack of appropriate childcare

(4) School-age children (5-12) may become depressed; blame themselves for the separation (see Depression)

(5) Limited access to social support systems, e.g.; language barriers transportation, financial, limited education

(5) Adolescents may present with depression; become involved in substance abuse; become suicidal or run away.
Boys are more vulnerable than girls in experiencing father's absence; boys tend to act out distress by becoming disruptive. Girls may exhibit precocious sexual behavior if there is no father figure

(6) Adolescent mothers who drop out of school have more difficulty extricating themselves and their children from the cycle of poverty

(6) Both mother and child may develop cognitive developmental delays

(7) All ages affected by parental high stress levels and inconsistencies of parenting; changes within the household membership; poverty

    c. Assess the availability of parents to

       (1) Nurture child

       (2) Provide attention, love

       (3) Provide guidance; protection of child (children)

    d. Assess the impact of social risks upon the family

(1) Access to health care, social support systems (location, feasibility, e.g., how to access, time available)

(2) Means of transportation

(3) Ability to seek appropriate care, e.g., language barrier, education level can prevent persons from seeking help

   e. Recognize traits of parental dysfunction

(1) Individual parent illness

(2) Personality disorders

(3) Addiction/alcoholism

(4) Mental retardation

(5) Excessive child-rearing responsibilities

(6) Chronically-ill or disabled child, e.g., excessive emotional, financial and energy demands

(7) Multiple births

(8) Temperament of child that conflicts with parents' temperament

   f. Assume advocacy role; connect family to community resources

(1) Refer to appropriate health care, social agency, e.g., early intervention programs; home visiting

(2) Refer family for financial planning assistance

(3) Refer for educational assistance, e.g., job-corps; schools that assist with acquiring high school diploma

(4) Refer for recreational opportunities

(5) Refer and advocate for quality, affordable child care

(6) Parent support groups

(7) Schedule frequent follow-up for reassessment

Issues of Health Maintenance and Health Promotion

See Zimmerman, M. L. (1994). Behavioral and emotional disorders of childhood and adolescence. In C. Houseman (Ed.), Psychiatric certification review guide for the generalist and clinical specialist in adult, child and adolescent psychiatric and mental health nursing (pp. 409-490). Potomac, MD: Health Leadership Associates, for additional information on the following disorders

School Avoidance/Phobias/Refusal Syndrome

- Definition: Applies to symptoms or anxiety in a school-aged child who resists going to school
- Etiology/Incidence
  1. Existing interdependence between parent-child
  2. Children who have suffered early deprivation
  3. Children who are fearful or depressed
  4. Chronic or acute illness which leads to excessive or unwarranted school absence
  5. Involves all socioeconomic levels, intellectual levels, ethnic origins
  6. More common in girls than boys
- Clinical Findings
  1. Complaints that do not support frequent absences or school refusal
  2. Symptoms subside when child is able to remain at home (weekends and holidays)
  3. Child expresses anxiety or fear of a specific school-related situation
  4. Separation from home, parent, caregiver
     a. Change in home situation
     b. New neighborhood
     c. New sibling, ill sibling
     d. Divorce or death
  5. Miscommunication between parents
  6. Overprotection from one or both parents
- Differential Diagnosis

1. Depression

2. Substance abuse

3. Psychopathological condition

4. Acute/chronic illness

5. Psychosomatic factors

6. Abuse/neglect

- Diagnostic Tests/Findings

    1. History and physical examination

    2. Data from school

    3. Interview with parent, caregiver, child

- Management/Treatment

    1. Return child to school as soon as possible; discuss problem with school nurse, administrator to prevent child being sent home inappropriately

    2. Consultation/Referral to psychological/psychiatric services, if refusal is greater than two weeks

    3. Referral for family counseling

    4. Support family's short/long term goals for consistent attendance

    5. Allow child to express concerns

    6. Counsel parents on interpreting child's behavior; teach parents about signs, symptoms of illness that need intervention

    7. Educate, reassure, prepare child for new experiences

Aggression

- Definition: Behavior that attempts to injure another person or destroy property

- Etiology/Incidence

    1. Correlation between violence on television and children's aggression

    2. Displacement of anger

    3. Modeling of aggressive behavior

        a. Type of discipline at home

        b. Parental role models, violent behavior at home

4. Parental reinforcement of aggressive behavior, e.g., showing approval for inappropriate aggression

   a. Permission given child to be violent

   b. Encouragement of aggressive behavior

5. Males more aggressive than females

- Clinical Findings

  1. Repeated number of occurrences of aggression with documentation

  2. Activity which interferes with social or cognitive functioning

  3. Different manifestations of aggression, e.g., may become progressively violent, or hitting may become biting as the aggressive act of choice

  4. Duration of four weeks or longer

- Differential Diagnosis

  1. Temporary state of anger

  2. Substance abuse

  3. Child abuse/neglect

  4. Depression

- Diagnostic Tests/Findings

  1. Observation of child

  2. Interview with parent, child, caregiver

  3. Physical examination

- Management/Treatment

  1. Refer for counseling, psychologic, psychiatric intervention, as needed

  2. Educate, counsel parents in appropriate guidelines to minimize misbehavior, e.g., is child acting out due to sibling rivalry

  3. Refer to social services agencies as needed to eliminate family stress and/or violence

Depression in Middle Childhood and Adolescence

- Definition: A psychosocial dysfunction manifested by a sad, withdrawn manner; sometimes irritability and/or tearfulness; adolescents often express boredom or emptiness

- Etiology
    1. Traumatic event, e.g., accidents, disasters
    2. Loss or separation from relative, friend, pet, key persons of childhood, adolescence
    3. Chronic illness, disability
    4. Low self-esteem
    5. History of depressive illness in one or both parents
    6. Alcohol, drug abuse; physical abuse; sexual abuse within the household of child/adolescent
    7. Parental dysfunction, e.g., inability to nurture child, adolescent appropriately
- Clinical Findings
    1. Appetite, sleep disturbances or hypersomnia
    2. Poor concentration; academic achievement impaired
    3. Severe or exaggerated adolescent mood swings lasting longer than one week
    4. Increased time spent alone brooding over issues of life, death; guilt; ideation of suicide
    5. Dependent or aggressive, disruptive, angry behavior
    6. Truancy; school refusal
    7. Expressed loneliness, fearfulness
    8. Frequent complaints of headache, stomachache without specific pathology
    9. Associated injuries due to inadequate adult supervision before or after school hours
    10. Possibly drugs or alcohol abuse—not a consistent finding
- Differential Diagnosis
    1. Normal transient moodiness of adolescence
    2. Grieving process, e.g., loss due to separation, death, divorce which resolves spontaneously or with minimal counseling
    3. Physical disorders
        a. Seizure disorder

    b. Metabolic disorder

    c. Viral/bacterial infections

    d. Endocrine disorder

    e. Cerebral lesions

    f. Migraine headaches

    g. Unwanted pregnancy

- Diagnostic Tests/Findings

   1. Sad, withdrawn behavior with 4 to 5 or more additional symptoms, e.g., loss of appetite, insomnia, etc. lasting more than two weeks (see clinical findings)

   2. Interview/observation/history includes social, family; review school records for attendance and achievement; review of current medications (some may cause depression)

   3. Height, weight percentiles; blood pressure, vital signs; possible weight loss; blood pressure and vital signs changes consistent with drug abuse

   4. Physical examination; neurological screening

   5. Laboratory tests as clinically indicated; may include thyroid function tests, UA; toxicity for drugs, alcohol, BUN, CBC; glucose, electrolytes, pregnancy tests

- Management/Treatment

   1. Early identification/referral for psychological, psychiatric evaluation, counseling, intervention

   2. Pharmacotherapy for chronic depression; usually tricyclic anti-depressants

   3. Monitor for side effects of specific drug

   4. Refer/treat for underlying physical disorder

   5. Provide/promote child and family social support through referrals and counseling

   6. Promote opportunities to assist child to develop strong self-esteem

   7. Advocate for children for safe alternative care, e.g., after-school programs, day care, etc.; refer parents/child to existing programs

   8. Teach/counsel parents about children's safety according to the developmental level of the child

Suicide Attempt

- Definition: A deliberate act of self-injury with the intent of killing oneself; all threats of suicide must be taken seriously; all troubled adolescents should be questioned about suicidal ideation

- Etiology/Incidence
  1. Increase in numbers of dysfunctional families contributing to feelings of vulnerability
  2. Increased competition in society which fosters insecurity
  3. Severe adolescent mood swings and limited resources for resolving difficulties
  4. Unrealistic parental expectations of child and adolescent
  5. Parental rejection and/or hostility
  6. History of suicide, psychosis, substance abuse or sexual abuse in the family
  7. Usually there is a loss of communication links between child and parent
  8. More boys than girls commit suicides
  9. Many accidental deaths may actually be suicides and need to be carefully investigated
  10. Increasing numbers of children ages 5 to 9 attempt suicide

- Clinical Findings
  1. Suicidal ideation includes thoughts, or plans for suicide
  2. Hopelessness expressed
  3. Suicidal gesture is serious attempt to cause severe injury or death; sends signal for help
  4. Attempt may be serious enough to cause bodily harm or death
  5. Depression; withdrawal; chronic depression
  6. May have a contagion effect, e.g., when one suicide appears to trigger others
  7. High-risk behavior, such as substance abuse

- Differential Diagnosis
  1. Psychosis manifested by suicidal gestures

    2.   Unintentional "accidental" injuries

- Diagnostic Tests/Findings

    1.   Evidence of pre-existing psychosocial problems or depression

    2.   Clinical evidence of substance abuse may confirm suicidal attempt (overdose, increasing evidence of addiction)

    3.   Previous attempts, threats, gestures, verbalized ideation, expression of hopelessness

    4.   Physical evidence of serious injury

    5.   Observation by peers of suicidal ideation or behavior

- Management/Treatment

    1.   Refer immediately for intervention; use 24-hour crisis intervention resources

    2.   Remove child/adolescent from acute situation; hospitalization may be necessary

    3.   Refer for psychiatric intervention

    4.   Treat underlying depression

    5.   Provide/refer for counseling or program for preventing suicide

    6.   Report incident to family, other professionals; inform child/adolescent of the report

- Resources for Referrals
  American Association of Suicidology
  2459 South Ash
  Denver, CO 80222
  (303) 692-0985

  The Youth Suicide National Center*
  1825 I Street NW
  Washington, DC 20006
  (202) 429-0190

  *Provides information about 24-hour crisis intervention centers

Substance Abuse/Tobacco/Alcohol/Drugs

- Definition: The use of substances to produce an altered state of consciousness or alter the real self-image to that of the ideal self-image

    1.   Drug abuse, misuse, addiction are voluntary behaviors

2. Drug tolerance, physical dependence are involuntary physiologic changes

- Etiology/Incidence
    1. Psychological factors/motivational influences
        a. Socioeconomic status; cost, availability
        b. Parental approval, e.g., smoking, use of alcohol
        c. Media advertising
        d. Child abuse, sexual abuse
    2. Biologic factors, physiologic dependence, addiction
    3. Developmental factors
        a. Stress related to puberty
        b. Peer pressure
        c. Prestige associated with glamorous people/role models
    4. More girls than boys smoke
    5. Two categories of adolescents who use drugs/alcohol
        a. Experimenters
        b. Compulsive users
    6. Substance abuse is widespread among children/adolescents
        a. Alcohol is drug of choice
        b. Drug abuse increase is related to availability/affordability
        c. Methamphetamine is becoming more widespread and popular

- Clinical Findings

Substance	Physical/Behavioral Symptoms
Tobacco use	Decreased breathing capacity; teeth staining; odor of tobacco on breath and clothing
CNS depressants Alcohol use	Marked mood changes/impaired judgement; Gastritis-symptoms or history
Alcohol abuse, e.g., goal is intoxication	Muscle incoordination; memory decrease; vomiting; respiratory depression; hypoglycemia; coma
Barbiturates	Impaired judgement; slurred speech; slowed reflexes, ataxia

Non-Barbiturates (quaalude; placidyl)	Incoordination, tremors; hyporeflexia; diplopia

Narcotics/Opiates
  Heroin
  Morphine
  Meperidine hydrochloride
  (Demerol)
  Methadone
  Codeine
	Constricted pupils, respiratory depression, cyanosis; needle marks may or may not be visible on skin; various infections may be present (skin, septicemia, HIV); related poor nutrition from neglect; lack of cleanliness; dental caries

Stimulants
  Hallucinogens
  Cannabis (marijuana,
  hashish)
	May have tachycardia; may have slow reflexes or incoordination

Lysergic acid diethylamide (LSD)	Dilated pupils, reddened eyes; may have hypertension; may have increased appetite; user may describe or experience flashbacks, hallucinations

CNS Stimulants
  Amphetamines
  Cocaine
  Crack
	Hypertension; weight loss, anorexia, insomnia; violent behavior, aggression, psychotic episode, hyperflexia, tachycardia, nausea and vomiting; nasal irritations, perforated septum associated with cocaine, crack inhalations

Any sudden change in behavior/school performance/ peer group may indicate substance abuse

- Differential Diagnosis
  1. Chronic depression
  2. Experimental versus substance abuse
  3. Neurologic disorders
  4. Gastrointestinal disorders
  5. Learning problems
  6. Head trauma

- Diagnostic Tests/Findings
  1. History—past, present, social; review of systems
  2. Interviews with child/adolescent, school personnel, parents, peers
  3. Description of observations from others, especially from peers are

valuable for identification of substance

4. Height, weight, vital signs, blood pressure, physical examination

5. Presence of Ethanol breath—alcohol abuse

6. Laboratory Tests—Ast (formerly SGOT), ALT (formerly SGPT) (elevated in heroin use); CBC; serum and urine toxicology and HIV testing of intravenous drug users

- Management/Treatment

  1. Referral to appropriate source for detoxification

  2. Monitor long-range management—all substances

  3. Educate and counsel about important legal consequences of substance abuse

  4. Use non-judgmental approach with child/adolescent in counseling

  5. Assess risk-taking behavior, include driving

  6. Discuss prevention; initiate referral to smoking, drug, alcohol prevention programs (or, for assistance in overcoming tobacco addiction)

  7. Refer
     National Institute on Drug Abuse (NIDA)
     Hotline: (800) 662HELP

     Other Resources:
     National Clearinghouse for Alcohol and Drug Abuse Information
     P.O. Box 2345
     Rockville, MD 20852
     (800) 729-6686

     National Institute on Drug Abuse Prevention Branch
     (800) 638-2045 or
     (301) 443-2450 (Maryland)

     National Federation of Parents for Drug-Free Youth
     (800) 544-KIDS or
     (301) 585-5437 (Maryland)

  8. Monitor infants born to substance user mothers, e.g., excessive jitteriness, seizure disorder, abnormal neurological findings, developmental delays; test mothers who are intravenous drug users for HIV; HIV testing of infants born to HIV positive mothers

  9. Educate children, parents, community on prevention

10. Become aware of subliminal advertising that glamorizes or encourages children, adolescents to use alcohol, tobacco or drugs

11. Use role as health care provider to boycott products, change advertising that subtly or overtly encourages substance use, abuse

12. Provide support, counseling for child/parent in locating, utilizing appropriate, affordable treatment modalities for substance abuse

13. Utilize health care team approach; involve all members in the care of the child/family

Anorexia Nervosa

- Definition: A chronic eating disorder characterized by loss of 15% of body weight (or weight proportionately below ideal weight), characteristic psychologic changes and in females (amenorrhea), without evidence of any other physical or psychiatric disorder (Harper & First, 1994).

- Etiology/Incidence

    1. The psychologic components consist of

        a. A disturbed body image

        b. An inaccurate perception of hunger

        c. Cultural emphasis on slimness through advertising/current fashion

        d. An overwhelming sense of ineffectiveness

        e. Individual may be a high achiever

    2. Affects mostly adolescent females

        a. Most frequently occurs in middle/upper middle income families

        b. Few attain complete recovery

        c. Younger children may be anorexic

- Clinical Findings

    1. Profound weight loss from self-imposed starvation

    2. Vigorous exercise is often undertaken to lose weight

    3. Lowered body temperature, blood pressure, bradycardia

    4. Altered metabolism; fatigue

    5. May have anemia, jaundice, secondary amenorrhea

    6. May have dry skin, brittle nails

7. May present with diminished reflexes

- Differential Diagnosis
    1. Endocrine dysfunction
    2. Psychotic disorders, depression
    3. Gastrointestinal diseases

- Diagnostic Tests/Findings
    1. History includes diet history, past medical, social; review of systems
    2. Height, weight percentiles; vital signs, blood pressure
    3. Physical examination; Tanner Staging
    4. CBC, electrolytes, thyroid function tests, cholesterol, glucose, urinalysis; any others deemed necessary by health care provider

- Management/Treatment
    1. Treatment is often not satisfactory
    2. Utilize team approach (patient, family, nurse practitioner, nutritionist, psychiatrist) and refer for immediate counseling
    3. Treatment for underlying disorder revealed on laboratory data
    4. Refer for hospitalization when necessary (severe dehydration)
    5. Refer for psychotherapy
    6. Psychoactive medications; tricyclics, MAO inhibitors
    7. Promote adequate nutrition and fluid intake
    8. Support, reassure child to help increase self-esteem
    9. Utilize team approach in behavior modification techniques
    10. Refer child and family to outside counseling services

       The American Anorexia/Bulimia Association, Inc.
       418 East 76th Street
       New York, NY 10021
       (212) 734-1114

       The National Association of Anorexia Nervosa and Associated Disorders, Inc. (ANAD)
       P.O. Box 7
       Highland Park, IL 60035
       (312) 831-3438

The National Anorectic Aid Society, Inc.
5796 Karl Road
Columbus, OH 43229
(614) 436-1112

Anorexia Nervosa and Related Eating Disorders (ANRED)
6125 Clayton Avenue
Suite 215
St. Louis, MO 63139
(314) 567-4080 or (800) 762-3334 (crisis hotline)

11. Promote public awareness through education

Bulimia Nervosa

- Definition: Chronic eating disorder characterized by episodic dyscontrol, with gorging on food followed by self-induced vomiting, use of laxatives, diuretics, excessive dieting and/or exercise; considerable overlap between anorexia and bulimia

- Etiology/Incidence

  1. Psychological/behavioral components consist of

     a. A prevailing feeling of lack of control over eating

     b. Overconcern with body image

  2. Likely to develop in late adolescence or early twenties

- Clinical Findings

  1. Regularly engages in self-induced vomiting or uses laxatives, diuretics

  2. May engage in vigorous exercise to burn off calories

  3. Diminished reflexes; fatigue; cardiac arrhythmias, potassium depletion in diuretic abuse

  4. Bulimics may have sluggish bowel function; cramping in laxative abuse

  5. Dental caries may be increased from enamel erosion caused by stomach acids in persistent vomiting

  6. Fingers, hands may be excoriated from strategies used to induce vomiting

  7. Chronic sore throats

  8. Anemia

- Differential Diagnosis
    1. Psychotic disorders
    2. Gastrointestinal diseases
- Diagnostic Tests/Findings: Same as for Anorexia Nervosa with the addition of cardiac function tests which may reveal abnormalities related to loss of electrolytes
- Management/Treatment
    1. Hospitalization may be necessary; treatment is directed toward symptoms; intravenous fluids; replacement of potassium; cardiac monitoring
    2. Refer for immediate counseling and psychotherapy
    3. See management/treatment of Anorexia Nervosa
    4. Treatment is often not satisfactory as in Anorexia Nervosa

Obesity
- Definition: Result of an intake of calories which exceeds the energy expenditure for a specific individual
- Etiology/Incidence
    1. Abundance of available food, especially high caloric snack foods
        a. Attitudes of parents regarding food; increased consumption of fast foods within the culture; increased number of snacks allowed
        b. Educational; socioeconomic factors; quality of food presented
        c. Emotional, e.g., using food as a reward or pacification
        d. Lack of physical exercise; excessive television viewing and snacking
        e. Heredity; size and type of build of parents, siblings
        f. Nutritional knowledge deficits
        g. Highest incidence occurs in urban areas of the Northeastern U.S.
        h. More prevalent in winter months
- Clinical Findings
    1. Two standard deviations above appropriate weight for height, sex, age on percentile chart

2. Emotional disturbances, especially adolescents

3. Pickwickian syndrome

4. Orthopaedic disorders contributing to inactivity

5. Underlying genetic disorders

6. Depression

7. May be taller than peers due to earlier maturity

- Differential Diagnosis

    1. Endocrine dysfunction

    2. Genetic disorders

- Diagnostic Tests/Findings

    1. History includes dietary, past, present, social; review of systems; developmental milestones; weight, height of parents, siblings

    2. Onset of obesity

    3. Height, weight percentiles, blood pressure, vital signs, physical examination

    4. CBC, UA; consider electrolytes, blood glucose, cholesterol, thyroid function

    5. Skin fold thickness measurements of triceps above the 85th percentile (subscapular measurements may be in combination with triceps)

- Management/Treatment

    1. Prevention in infancy through parental education of dietary requirements, limits of intake

    2. Discuss diet modification; exercise plan with child/family

    3. Goal in growing children is to maintain weight while linear growth continues; weight reduction is appropriate for adolescents who have completed linear growth

    4. Use team approach (school personnel/nutritionist)

    5. Refer to appropriate, affordable community support groups

    6. Provide monitoring of weight, dietary intake through log keeping; supportive environment

    7. Enlist child, family cooperation; encourage child, family in long term life style changes in nutritional, exercise habits

Child Abuse and Neglect

- Definition
    1. Physical or mental injury, sexual abuse, negligent treatment or maltreatment of a child younger than 18 years by a person responsible for the child's welfare under circumstances indicating that the child's health or welfare is harmed or threatened (Martin, 1992)
    2. Munchausen Syndrome by Proxy (MBP)—a form of child abuse in which parent or caregiver creates the impression the child is ill by either giving false information or inflicting harm on the child

- Etiology/Incidence
    1. Characteristics of the mistreating adult—adult has difficulty controlling anger, aggression, violence; often is socially isolated; few family supports; dysfunctional parenting; failure of adult to attach emotionally to child; inadequate knowledge of realistic expectations of child's development
    2. Characteristics of child that unintentionally place child at risk— physically, mentally disabled; unwanted child; hyperactive child; child's personality perceived as difficult by adult
    3. Social context that increases risk
        a. Stress which becomes chronic—divorce, separation, economic problems, inadequate housing, substance abuse/addiction
        b. Birth of an additional child may place other siblings at risk
        c. Working parents with multiple commitments; substitute caregivers may be abusers
    4. Incidence
        a. Approximately 10% of all children are assaulted yearly in the U.S.
        b. Homicide accounts for about 5% of all deaths in children
        c. About 33% of abused children are neglected

- Clinical Findings
    1. History and type of injuries do not match
        a. Conflicting stories of how injuries occurred
        b. Accident described and injury inconsistent with child's developmental ability

2. Pathognomonic physical signs, e.g., marks of object can be seen on child's skin, (burn marks resemble an electric iron)

3. Presence of physical injuries in various stages of healing (multiple bruises or fractures)

4. Undernutrition, poor hygiene

5. Indications of untreated illness (secondarily infected injuries; unhealed old injuries)

6. Developmental delays in children less than five years of age (may be the result of neglect or abuse)

- Differential Diagnosis

   1. Accidents

   2. Organic failure to thrive (OFTT)

   3. Disease processes, e.g., hemophilia, osteogenesis imperfecta

   4. Cultural practices, e.g., Asian practice of coining

   5. Sudden Infant Death Syndrome (SIDS)

   6. Normal skin pigment variants, e.g., mongolian spots

- Diagnostic Tests/Findings

   1. History to determine onset, types of injuries, neglect; precise documentation required

   2. X-rays, photographs may be necessary for documentation; laboratory tests to determine bleeding disorders; CBC, electrolytes

   3. Complete physical examination and neurodevelopmental screening

   4. Observation of child's behavior (extremes of behavior)

- Management/Treatment

   1. Refer for hospitalization, if necessary (severe, life threatening injuries, dehydration)

   2. Refer, report to Child Protective Services (moderate to severe injuries, neglect or if child is further threatened by situation); reporting is mandatory in most states

   3. Describe in detail all injuries, marks and document precisely

   4. Utilize team approach—nurse practitioner, physician, social services personnel; parent support groups

5. Utilize prevention by identifying potentially abusive situations

    a. Identify negative attitudes toward pregnancy/child

    b. Identify the vulnerable child

    c. Identify predisposing social, environmental factors

    d. Identify dysfunctional parenting

    e. Identify violent behavior, substance abuse

    f. Recognize knowledge deficits in nutrition, child behavior, development

6. Educate parents, e.g., realistic expectations of child; need for parents to take time for themselves periodically; point out strengths of child; teach parenting strategies

7. Initiate intervention

    a. Appropriate referrals to child care agencies, programs

    b. Refer to Child Protective Agency in potentially explosive situations, e.g., substance abuse of one or more adults; battering of a parent, violence, before abuse of child is noted, when possible

    c. Refer to appropriate agency for an evaluation of the home situation before, after child is born and periodically if situation warrants, e.g., adolescent mothers, or if abuse is suspected

    d. Refer to agencies concerned with violent families

    e. Discuss with school personnel; refer to counselor, psychologist

    f. Refer parents to support groups, self-help groups, e.g., parents anonymous deals with prevention

    g. Develop a high level of awareness of the signs, symptoms of abuse and initiate follow-up

Failure To Thrive

- Definition

1. Infants and children who without obvious cause fail to gain weight and often lose weight OR

2. Progressive decrease in weight to below the 5th percentile OR

3. A decrease in expected rate of growth along the child's previous growth curve irrespective of a relationship to the 5th percentile

- Etiology/Incidence
  1. Organic Failure to Thrive (OFTT)— affects 10-15%, is usually due to
     a. Congenital cardiac defects
     b. Neurologic defects, microcephaly
     c. Endocrine dysfunction
     d. Malabsorption syndrome, gastroesophageal reflux
     e. Renal insufficiency, chronic urinary tract infections
     f. Cystic fibrosis
     g. Congenital malformations
     h. Intrauterine growth retardation (IUGR)
     i. Fetal alcohol syndrome (FAS)
     j. Pica in toddler or older child
  2. Non-Organic Failure to Thrive (NOFTT), affects 50-90%, usually attributed to
     a. Disturbances in maternal/child attachment in early infancy
     b. Parents' inadequate nutritional information
     c. Deficiency in infant care, e.g., lack of commitment to parenting
- Clinical Findings
  1. Height may fall below the 5th percentile on growth chart
  2. Persistent deviation from an established growth curve
     a. Weight loss occurs first
     b. Linear growth slows
     c. Head circumference decreases
  3. Usually noted in children under 2 years of age
  4. Applicable to older children
  5. Applies to any age with developmental delays
- Differential Diagnosis
  1. Preterm low-birth weight infant
  2. Term infant small-for-gestational-age (SGA)—child usually catches up in growth by 9 months of age

3. Infants of drug-addicted mothers

4. Genetic factors (parents are of small stature)

5. Social factors

6. Mouth trauma or malformation, e.g., cleft palate or short frenulum which inhibits sucking reflex

■ Diagnostic Methods/Findings

1. History—prenatal, perinatal, neonatal; past, present; review of systems; social

2. Height, weight, head circumference; vital signs including blood pressure for children 3 years of age and over

3. Physical examination; neurological data; developmental assessment

4. CBC, UA, if applicable; tuberculosis test; blood lead levels; sweat test; electrolytes profile; other tests at the discretion of the provider include stool specimen for parasites; skull, chest, long bones radiographs in an older child; liver function tests; buccal smear analysis in delayed adolescence

5. Determination of caloric intake calculated over 24 hours

6. Psychosocial evaluation related to issues of NFTT

7. Home visit to assess situation and provide daily weights; assessment of child's health

■ Management/Treatment

1. Provide adequate nutrition

2. May be necessary to hospitalize child to prevent further deterioration

3. Multidisciplinary approach is often required

   a. Information/intervention

   b. Other referrals to community agencies, e.g., women, infants, children (WIC), supplemental nutritional programs; community agencies involved in nutritional and/or parenting programs

   c. Consultation with pediatrician

   d. Child Protection Services, if other interventions fail

   e. Social services to assist in reversal of family stresses; welfare services

   f. Mental health professional

4. Teach parents the nutritional/caloric requirements; feeding strategies to promote optimal growth

5. Monitor child's growth and development; social environment; care (schedule biweekly/weekly follow-up, if necessary)

6. Consult on weekly basis with personnel from other agencies involved with interventions

7. Involve all family members in the solution of the problem

Attention Deficit Hyperactivity Disorder (ADHD)

- Definition: A complex syndrome which includes high motor activity, problems with concentration, attention and impulsivity; often resistant to behavior modification; may experience extremes of emotions with little provocation

- Etiology/Incidence

  1. May be related to illness or trauma in prenatal, perinatal or postnatal periods

  2. Usually multiple causes exist, including genetic factors

  3. Recent theories suggest the underlying genetic cause is centered on dysfunctions in monoamine neurotransmitters; thyroid disorders recently implicated (Hauser et al. 1993)

  4. More boys than girls are affected

- Clinical Findings: According to the *Diagnostic Criteria from DSM-IV*™ (1994) published by the American Psychiatric Association, a diagnosis of ADHD may be made based upon *either* set of symptoms of inattention or hyperactivity and other considerations noted below.

  1. Inattention—at least 6 (or more) of the following have persisted for at least 6 months; inconsistent and/or maladaptive with developmental level

     a. Often fails to give close attention to details or makes careless mistakes

     b. Has difficulty sustaining attention

     c. Does not seem to listen

     d. Does not follow through with directions

     e. Has difficulty organizing tasks and activities

  f. Reluctant to engage in activities that require sustained attention

  g. Loses things frequently

  h. Easily distracted by external stimuli

  i. Often forgetful

 2. Six or more of the following have persisted for at least 6 months; maladaptive and/or inconsistent with developmental level

  a. Hyperactivity

   (1) Fidgets with hands or feet, squirms

   (2) Will not sit still in classroom setting

   (3) Often runs about or climbs excessively

   (4) Has difficulty engaging in quiet play

   (5) "On the go"; can't seem to stop moving

   (6) Often talks continuously

  b. Impulsivity

   (1) Often blurts out answers before questions have been completed

   (2) Has difficulty waiting turn

   (3) Often interrupts others' conversations or games

 3. Other considerations include

  a. Some of the signs and symptoms existed prior to 7 years of age

  b. Some of the impairment from the signs and symptoms have existed in two or more settings

  c. Clear evidence exists that there is a significant impairment that interferes with social and academic activities

  d. The impairment is not a result of other psychological or pathological disorders

■ Differential Diagnosis

 1. Genetic disorders

 2. Behavior in response to stressful situations which is misinterpreted by adults

 3. Abuse, neglect affecting child's behavior

4. Neurologic disorder

5. Mismatch between environmental factors and the child's temperament

6. Childhood/adolescent depression

7. Dysfunctional parenting

8. Endocrine disorders

- Diagnostic Tests/Findings

  1. History—past, present, social; review of systems; developmental, parenting styles

  2. Supplemental information from parents, relatives, babysitters

  3. Questionnaires from school personnel (Connor's abbreviated parent-teacher questionnaire)

  4. Psychological evaluation

  5. Height, weight, percentiles, blood pressure, vital signs

  6. Physical examination; neurological screening; laboratory data

  7. Vision, hearing screening (impairments may affect behavior and school performance)

- Management/Treatment

  1. CNS stimulant medication

     a. Methylphenidate (Ritalin)

     b. Dextroamphetamine (Dexedrine)

     c. Pemoline (Cylert)

  2. Starting doses are small and adjusted as needed until beneficial effects are noted

  3. Provide explanations of syndrome and medications to parents, child, school personnel; side effects of medication

  4. Short-acting stimulants usually produce immediate effects; at least 4 days should elapse before the dose is adjusted; continue for 1 month to several years

  5. Medication often is combined with behavior modification strategies and remedial tutoring

  6. Side effects of stimulant medication include appetite reduction, weight loss; other side effects include sleepiness

7. Contraindications to prescribed CNS-stimulant medication include

    a. History or indication of possible drug abuse in family

    b. Children younger than 5 years; side effects are more severe

    c. Adolescents who indicate their intention of noncompliance

    d. Treatment of underlying thyroid disorder

8. Medication may be discontinued when a 2 to 3 month trial off the stimulant results in no behavioral deterioration

9. Monitor children treated with stimulant medication every 3 to 4 months for continued need for medication

10. Assess, monitor child's growth every 3 to 4 months

11. Coordinate, review child's behavior and medication compliance with parent, school personnel, health care provider, psychologist

12. Review child's/family's understanding of the effects of medication and compliance with therapeutic regimes

Teenage Pregnancy

Adolescent pregnancy and epidemic sexually transmitted diseases are currently major health problems in the U.S. The number of sexually active teenagers has increased dramatically during the past 20 years, thus the inclusion of the topic in this chapter. Sexually transmitted diseases can be found in the Genitourinary/Gynecological Disorders chapter

Pregnancy/Subjective Changes

■ Amenorrhea (any adolescent whose menstrual cycle is overdue or who is concerned about the diagnosis of pregnancy should have a pregnancy test)

    1. Differential Diagnosis

        a. Endocrine dysfunction

        b. Metabolic disorders

        c. Psychologic factors

        d. Systemic diseases, (e.g., tuberculosis, or malignancy)

        e. Nonestablished regularity of cycles

■ Nausea/Vomiting

    1. Differential Diagnosis

       a. Gastrointestinal disorders

       b. Acute infections

       c. Emotional disorders

       d. Anorexia nervosa/Bulimia

■ Urinary Frequency

    1. Differential Diagnosis

       a. Infection

       b. Pathology of urinary tract

       c. Emotional causes

■ Breast Tenderness

    1. Differential Diagnosis

       a. Premenstrual tension

       b. Chronic cystic mastitis

       c. Unusual growth of any type

       d. Trauma

■ Quickening, or the mother's perception of fetal movements

    1. Differential Diagnosis

       a. Increased peristalsis

       b. Flatulence

       c. Abdominal muscle contractions

■ Obtain data through complete history

    1. Name, age, address, phone; height, usual weight

    2. Age of menarche, menstrual history; include date of last menstrual period, use of contraceptives

    3. Number of pregnancies, number of living children; problems during labor or delivery with other children

    4. Review prescription/nonprescription medications; use of drugs, alcohol, tobacco

    5. History of illnesses; sexually transmitted diseases, includes HIV; immunization status

    6. Mother's education (level of schooling); occupation

7. Mother's acceptance of pregnancy; plans for outcome

8. Family history; number of siblings, health status of each member

9. Father's name, age, education, occupation

10. Health status of father; use of prescription/ nonprescription medications, use of alcohol, drugs, tobacco

11. Housing—type, number of persons occupying the dwelling, number of smokers in household

12. Available supportive persons

■ Diagnostic Methods

1. Document vital signs, blood pressure, height, weight

2. Laboratory tests—urine, blood, over-the-counter pregnancy tests (if used, confirm with laboratory tests); ultrasound of abdomen, CBC, UA

3. Perform physical examination, pelvic examination for detectable changes

   a. Goodell's sign—softening of the cervix

   b. Chadwick's sign—purple to blue discoloration of mucous membranes of the cervix, vagina, vulva; due to increased vaso-constriction

   c. Uterine enlargement

■ Differential Diagnosis

1. Use of contraceptives may cause softening of cervix, hyperpigmentation of skin

2. Hyperemia of vulva, vagina, mucous membranes may be caused by infections

3. Obesity, ascites, pelvic or uterine tumors

Risk Factors and Effect on Neonate

Maternal Factors	Neonatal Implication
Poor nutrition	Low birth weight (LBW)
Inadequate nutrition (2300-2400 calories per day throughout pregnancy is considered adequate)	Intrauterine growth retardation (IUGR), fetal malnutrition, prematurity

Maternal age younger than 16 (difficult labor, delivery, e.g., cephalopelvic disproportion)	LBW, Birth injuries
Maternal age over 35	Congenital anomalies Chromosomal aberrations
Maternal smoking (one pack or more per day)	LBW IUGR Preterm birth
Maternal use of addicting drugs	Congenital anomalies; LBW; neonatal withdrawal syndrome; HIV
Alcohol consumption	Fetal Alcohol Syndrome (FAS)

- Management/Treatment
    1. Refer to appropriate obstetrical/gynecological facility as soon as diagnosis is confirmed for prenatal care
    2. Assist pregnant adolescent with decisions; support her decisions
    3. Encourage early prenatal care, education
    4. Discuss risks, plans for care of infant, mother
    5. Encourage participation, if possible, of grandparents, father, in processes of prenatal care, labor and delivery
    6. Refer pregnant adolescent and family to social services if necessary

Questions

Select the best answer

1. What components of a health maintenance visit are essential to each visit?

   a. Laboratory tests
   b. Initial health history
   c. Immunization review
   d. Vision and hearing screening

2. Which of the following immunizations is not recommended for all children?

   a. Pneumovax
   b. MMR, OPV, or IPV
   c. HIB
   d. DPT, Td

3. In a newborn physical examination, the PNP would expect to elicit all of the following neurological responses except?

   a. Rooting/sucking
   b. Parachute reflex
   c. Gag Reflex
   d. Moro

4. Susie Bryan is a healthy 12 month old infant whose mother brought her to the pediatric facility for immunizations. What immunizations would you expect to find documented on susie's record?

   a. MMR, DPT (4 doses)
   b. OPV (4 doses)
   c. HIB (3 doses)
   d. Hepatitis B (4 doses)

5. What immunizations would you select to administer to Susie when she returns at 18 months of age, if her record states that she has received DPT (3 doses) Hepatitis B (2 doses), MMR (1 dose), OPV (2 doses) and HIB (4 doses)?

   a. MMR, Td
   b. DPT, or DTaP, OPV and Hepatitis B
   c. HIB booster
   d. OPV, Hepatitis B, Tine

6. At what age should the health maintenance visit for a normal, healthy infant include laboratory screening with a hemoglobin and hematocrit?

   a. At 4 months of age when iron stores decrease
   b. Not necessary until age 3
   c. Nine months of age is recommended
   d. Between 6 and 9 months of age

7. Andrew Henderson is a healthy 4 month old infant weighing 14 lb 6 oz (birth weight 7 lb 4 oz). According to his mother, he is taking 38 oz of formula in 24 hours and seems hungry. She says he has begun waking at night after previously sleeping 10 hours. What advice would you give Andrew's mother?

   a. Decrease his formula intake to 32 oz. in 24 hours, start small amounts of cereal and juice
   b. Introduce vegetables, fruits and cereal. Decrease his formula to 20 oz in 24 hours
   c. Begin whole milk
   d. Increase Andrew's formula intake

8. Which of the following best describes the most important aspect of anticipatory guidance during the health maintenance visits of infants and toddlers?

   a. Discussion of limiting TV viewing time
   b. Preparation for sibling rivalry
   c. Day care and head start programs
   d. Prevention of injury

9. Anticipatory guidance for all school age (5-12 years) children should include

   a. Prevention of sexual abuse
   b. Discussion of future dating practices
   c. How much allowance a child should receive for household chores
   d. Encouraging competitive sports

10. Jane Lucas is 13 years old. She has recently reached menarche and is a normal, healthy adolescent. She has many friends but denies sexual activity. During your examination of her you promote self-care. What is most important to teach Jane at this age?

   a. Self-breast examination
   b. Birth control, pregnancy prevention
   c. Proper dental care
   d. Avoidance of HIV transmission

11. What immunization(s) would you recommend for Jane?

   a. DPT, HIB
   b. MMR booster
   c. Td

d. b and c

12. Which of the following should alert the nurse practitioner to the potential for childhood, adolescent suicide?

    a. Mood swings
    b. Experimentation with alcohol
    c. Impulsivity
    d. Expressed hopelessness

13. Which of the following is not a typical characteristic of ADHD?
    a. Inattentiveness, disruptiveness
    b. Impulsivity
    c. Variation of symptoms from day to day
    d. Frequent mood swings

14. Symptoms of depression in childhood, adolescence requiring immediate intervention are

    a. Transient mood swings of one week duration
    b. Weight loss
    c. Sad, withdrawn behavior with 4 to 5 significant clinical findings
    d. Headache, nausea, refusal to attend school

15. The following clinical findings are associated with substance abuse
    a. Sudden change in behavior, school performance
    b. Hyperglycemia, tachycardia, tremors, moodiness
    c. Hyperactivity, increased alertness, hyporeflexia
    d. Weight loss, increased endurance, hypersomnia

16. Sylvia, 16, weighs 100 lbs and is 5 feet 4¾ inches tall. The last time you examined her was 1 year ago. At that visit Sylvia weighed 120 lbs and was at the 50th percentile for height and weight. Menarche occurred at age 13 with regularity of menses until 6 months ago when menses ceased. The history is negative for recent infections. She denies sexual activity. Sylvia does not smoke or use alcohol or drugs. She is an excellent student, a cheerleader and plays basketball on a girls team at her school. She lives with her 12 year old brother and both parents who are professionals. On examination, Sylvia's blood pressure is normal, her temperature is 97 degrees fahrenheit and her heart rate is 60/minute. Lab studies are incomplete. You suspect that Sylvia is anorexic. What is the first question that is most appropriate to ask at this time?

    a. Is there anything that is causing her to be depressed?
    b. What does Sylvia think about her size, is she too fat or too thin?
    c. What is the ideal weight Sylvia wants to achieve?
    d. What do her friends say about Sylvia's size?

17. What is one of the major clinical findings in child physical abuse?

    a. Findings of physical neglect are outstanding features of abuse
    b. Child's developmental ability correlates with the injuries
    c. The abuser tells conflicting stories of how the injuries occurred
    d. More than one child in the family is usually abused

18. In order to diagnose NFTT it is most important to:

    a. Discuss the home situation with the caregiver
    b. Calculate the caloric intake over 24 hours
    c. Graph the child's weight over a period of 3 months
    d. Assess the caregiver's nutritional knowledge

19. Colin, age 8, has been diagnosed as ADHD. Although his parents and Colin are compliant with the prescribed pharmacotherapeutic regime and behavior modification, they have concerns about the medication. What information can you give them which will help them understand it better?

    a. It modifies the impulses transmitted to the musculoskeletal system and slows hyperactivity
    b. It has a reversed action on the mood swings that affect ADHD
    c. The action is poorly understood but increased amounts are required to reach the maximum benefit
    d. It is possible the medication can be discontinued if there is no deterioration in behavior after a 2 to 3 month trial off the medication

20. The risks of pregnancy that negatively impact the neonate are

    a. Sociocultural beliefs
    b. Geographic areas
    c. Nutrition deficits
    d. Educational level

21. Jeff, age 18, tells you during his routine health maintenance visit that he has been experimenting with marijuana. He asks you not to tell his parents as he will be living away from them soon. You remind him that

    a. There are legal consequences to the use of illegal drugs no matter what age you are
    b. Marijuana use may lead to health problems
    c. You are obligated by law to tell his parents
    d. He should be straightforward with his parents and tell them himself

22. Jeff's younger brother, Jay, age 15, has become disruptive and aggressive over the past 2 weeks. His grades at school have dropped and he takes little interest in his friends or former activities. During his visit you note that his appearance is

disheveled. He has lost weight, he says he has no appetite and he is not sleeping very much. On examination, you note that he is tachycardic, his reflexes are exaggerated and he has persistent clear nasal drainage without evidence of upper respiratory infection. You suspect substance abuse. Which drug is Jeff most likely using?

a. LSD
b. Marijuana
c. Heroin
d. Cocaine or crack cocaine

23. By what method would you suspect Jeff is using the drug?

a. Swallowing the drug
b. Injections into the muscle
c. Nasal inhalation
d. Intravenous injections

24. What laboratory tests would be most helpful in making a diagnosis of drug abuse?

a. HIV testing
b. Serum/urine toxicology
c. CBC, UA
d. AST, ALT

25. Seventeen-year-old Mary T. is on the track team at high school. She has been running 5 miles a day for the past 2 months. Since she started to run regularly, her periods have stopped. What would you consider first as a probable cause?

a. That Mary T. is a victim of Anorexia Nervosa
b. That the amenorrhea is a result of the increased exercise
c. That Mary T. may be pregnant
d. That Mary T. should be further examined for a thyroid dysfunction

Answers

1. c
2. a
3. b
4. c
5. b
6. d
7. a
8. d
9. a
10. a
11. d
12. d
13. d
14. c
15. a
16. b
17. c
18. b
19. d
20. c
21. a
22. d
23. c
24. b
25. c

Bibliography

American Academy of Pediatrics. (1994). Committee on Infectious Diseases. *1994 Red Book: Report of the Committee on Infectious Diseases* (23rd ed.). Elk Grove Village, IL: The American Academy of Pediatrics.

American Psychiatric Association. (1994). *Diagnostic criteria from DSM-IV™*. Washington, DC: American Psychiatric Association.

Behrman, R. E., Kliegman, R. M., Nelson, W. E. & Vaughn, V. C. (Eds). (1992). *Nelson textbook of pediatrics* (14th ed.). Philadelphia: W. B. Saunders.

Carruth, B. R., Skinner, J. D., & Nevling, M. S. (1993). Eating readiness: Reading the cues. *Pediatric Basics*. 63, 2-8.

Committee on Psychosocial Aspects of Child and Family Health (1988). *Guidelines for health supervision* (2nd ed.). Elk Grove Village, IL: The American Academy of Pediatrics.

Eichenwald, H. F, Stroder, J., & Ginsburg, C. (Eds.). (1993). *Pediatric therapy* (3rd ed.). St. Louis: Mosby Year Book.

Friedman, S. B., Fisher, B., & Schonberg, S. K. (Eds.). (1992). *Comprehensive adolescent health care*. St. Louis: Quality Medical Publishing.

Greene, M. G. (Ed.). (1991). *The Harriet Lane handbook*. (12th ed.). St. Louis: Mosby Year Book.

Harper, G., & First, L. R. (1994). Eating disorders (anorexia nervosa and bulimia nervosa). In M. E. Avery & L. R. First (Eds.). *Pediatric medicine* (pp. 79-80). Baltimore, MD: Williams & Wilkins.

Hauser, P., Zametkin, A. J., Martinez, P., Vitiello, B., Matochik, J. A., Mixson, A. J., & Weintraub, B. D. (1993). Attention-deficit-hyperactivity disorder in people with generalized resistance to thyroid hormone. *New England Journal of Medicine, 328*, 997-1001.

Hoekelman, R. A., Friedman, S. B., Nelson, N. M., & Seidel, H. M. (Eds.). (1992). *Primary pediatric care*. (2nd ed.). St. Louis: Mosby Year Book.

Martin, H. P. (1992). Child abuse and neglect. In R. A. Hoekelman, S. B. Friedman, N. M. Nelson & H. M. Seidel (Eds.). *Primary pediatric care* (2nd ed.) (pp. 560-565). St. Louis: Mosby Year Book.

Schmitt, B. (1992). *Instructions for pediatric patients*. Philadelphia: W. B. Saunders.

Stockman, J. A., Corden, T. F., & Kim, J. J. (1991). *The Pediatric book of lists*. St. Louis: Mosby Year Book.

Sweds, S. E., Retlew, D. C., Kuppenheimer, M., Lum, D., Dolan, S., & Goldberger E. (1991). Can adolescent suicide attempters be distinguished from at-risk adolescents? *Pediatrics*, 88, 620-629.

Whaley, L. & Wong, D. (1991). *Nursing care of infants and children* (4th ed.). St. Louis: Mosby Year Book.

Wong, D., & Whaley, L. (1990). *Clinical manual of pediatric nursing* (3rd ed.). St. Louis: Mosby Year Book.

Endocrine Disorders

Jacalyn P. Dougherty

Gynecomastia

- Definition: Visible or palpable glandular enlargement of the male breast occurring commonly in healthy adolescent males (pubertal gynecomastia). Occasionally indicative of underlying disease (pathologic gynecomastia). Seen frequently in newborns (neonatal gynecomastia).

- Etiology/Incidence

  1. Neonatal gynecomastia—secondary to cross-placental transfer of maternal hormones

  2. Pubertal gynecomastia—influence of too little androgen and/or too much estrogen on mammary tissue

      a. Affects 40% of boys 10 to 16 years

      b. Peak incidence in 14 year old boys

  3. Pathologic gynecomastia—secondary to drug side effects, underlying disease, injury to the nervous system, chest wall or testes; or, may be idiopathic

- Clinical findings

  1. Neonatal—usually bilateral, often asymmetric breast tissue enlargement, resolves within days

  2. Pubertal (physiologic) gynecomastia

      a. Breast tissue enlargement glandular, movable, disk-shaped, below areola, non-adherent to skin or underlying tissue

      b. Typically breasts unequal in size and < 3 cm diameter

      c. Breasts may be tender, nipples irritated secondary to rubbing clothing

      d. Tanner stages II to IV of pubertal development with testes ≥ 3 cm length

      e. If tissue ≥ 4 to 5 cm/diameter and breasts dome-shaped, macrogynecomastia present

  3. Pathologic gynecomastia

      a. Malnourishment

      b. Lymphadenopathy

      c. Delayed sexual maturity with undermasculinization

d. Signs of chronic disease, (e.g., goiter, liver or renal disease, endocrinopathies, cancer, colitis, CF, AIDS)

e. Absent, underdeveloped or asymmetric testes

f. Breast tissue $\geq$ 3 cm/diameter, asymmetric, hard, fixed, indurated, not directly beneath areola

- Differential Diagnosis

  1. Obesity (lipomastia)

  2. Tumors (lipoma, neurofibroma, cancer)

  3. Breast infection

  4. Fat necrosis secondary to injury

- Diagnostic Tests/Findings

  1. Endocrinologic investigation if appropriate

  2. Imaging techniques if appropriate

     a. Ultrasonography of testes- identification of impalpable testicular tumor

     b. CT, MRI of abdomen-identification of adrenal tumors

- Management/Treatment

  1. Neonatal gynecomastia—parental education and reassurance about etiology, transience and normalcy of condition

  2. Pubertal (physiologic) gynecomastia < 4 cm—explanation, reassurance and observation. Regression usually spontaneous and within a few months, rarely beyond 2 years

  3. Physiologic macrogynecomastia ($\geq$ 4 cm mass)—medical or surgical treatment usually required as regression rare, especially if gynecomastia present for > 4 years

  4. Pathologic gynecomastia—treatment of underlying cause, (e.g., surgical removal of tumors, discontinuance of causative drugs, euthyroidism treatment, testosterone for hypogonadism [Mahoney, 1990]); refer to appropriate specialist

  5. Gynecomastia usually very upsetting to adolescent but often not discussed because of embarrassment; reassure about transience and spontaneous regression

Hypothyroidism

- Definition: Genetic or acquired metabolic disorder resulting in absent or insufficient production of thyroxin by thyroid gland

- Etiology/Incidence

  1. Endemic cretinism—common, endemic congenital thyroid disorder caused by iodine deficiency; leading world-wide cause of mental retardation and permanent central nervous system damage in children

  2. Sporadic congenital hypothyroidism—congenital thyroid disorder occurring in 1:4000 births; permanent or transient

     a. Causes of permanent congenital hypothyroidism

        (1) Absence, underdevelopment or atrophy (dysgenesis) of thyroid gland most common

        (2) Inherent problems with iodine transport or assimilation or thryroid hormone synthesis (dyshormonogenesis)

        (3) Inherent deficiencies in production of thyrotropin or thyroid releasing hormone; rare inherited disorder (Gruters, 1992)

     b. Causes of transient congenital hypothyroidism

        (1) Pre- or post-natal exposure to iodine-containing drugs and agents including potassium iodine

        (2) Use of maternal antithyroid drugs

        (3) Placental crossing of maternal antibodies to thyroid

  3. Acquired hypothyroidism—due to insufficient production of thyroid hormone

- Clinical Findings: Signs and symptoms may be nonspecific and insidious

  1. Neonate

     a. History of lethargy, poor feeding, prolonged jaundice, vomiting, constipation

     b. May have increased birth weight (> 4000 g)

     c. Hypothermia, mottling

     d. Large fontanels, especially posterior; wide sutures; hirsute forehead; coarse facial features

     e. Normal, slightly enlarged, or goitrous thyroid gland

     f. Hoarse cry

     g. Distended abdomen, umbilical hernia or hypotonia

2. Older infant, child

    a. May have growth retardation or growth deceleration; delayed bone maturation and dentition

    b. Increased weight for height

    c. Developmental delay; delayed puberty, occasionally precocious puberty or pseudoprecocity

    d. Increased pigmentation of skin; pale, cool, gray, mottled, coarse, thickened

    e. Hair dry, brittle

    f. Myopathy

    g. Mental and physical sluggishness, poor motor coordination

    h. Galactorrhea, menstrual problems

    i. Infants with sporadic congenital hypothyroidism are at increased risk for congenital heart disease

- Differential Diagnosis: Differentiate primary hypothyroidism due to intrinsic thyroid gland defects from secondary thyroid deficiency caused by pituitary and hypothalamic disorders

- Diagnostic Tests/Findings

    1. Newborn (NB) screening—low T_4 (serum thyroxine) and/or elevated TSH levels; positive screen may be first indication of disease; if NB screening tests positive, confirmatory tests needed

    2. Most accurate screening results with T_4 and TSH levels occur with samples obtained 3 to 5 days after birth. Validate NB screen done at 2-week visit

    3. Low T_4 or high TSH levels obtained birth to 5 days of life should be followed up with confirmatory tests

    4. Confirmatory tests include serum TSH, T_4, free T_4, T_3, thyroxine-binding globulin (TBG). Other tests indicated after consultation with physician or upon referral may be antithyroid antibodies and urinary iodine excretion; thyroid releasing hormone (TRH), other pituitary tests to check thyrotropin levels; thyroid ultrasound, bone age determinations and radionuclide imaging (Gruters, 1992)

- Management/Treatment

    1. Physician consultation or referral to pediatric endocrinologist for

neonates and children with suspected or confirmed hypothyroidism

2. Rapid, adequate thyroid hormone replacement critical to avoid permanent mental retardation

3. Thyroid hormone (oral L-thyroxine) treatment for infants with permanent congenital hypothyroidism needed for life

4. Thyroid therapy in older children and adolescents gradually increased to avoid undesirable side effects and clinical symptoms of thyrotoxicosis

5. Give L-thyroxine before meals to prevent reduced absorption

6. Diagnosis and treatment within first month of life gives best prognosis for normal intellectual development

7. Parental and child education about disease, treatment regimen and routine monitoring

8. Genetic counseling indicated if genetic etiology

Hyperthyroidism

- Definition: Excessive production and secretion of thyroid hormone by the thyroid gland resulting in increased basal metabolism, goiter, autonomic nervous system disorders and problems with creatinine metabolism

- Etiology/Incidence

  1. Autoimmune response most common cause in children → body produces antibodies which stimulate TSH receptors, causing overproduction of thyroid hormone and thyromegaly (acquired Graves' disease)

  2. Antibody formation in Graves' may be triggered by body's reaction to bacterial or viral infections, although exact etiology of immune response unknown

  3. Girls have higher incidence of Graves'

- Clinical Findings: May have some or all of following signs and symptoms of thyrotoxicosis

  1. Nervousness, irritability, decreased attention span, school difficulty, behavior problems

  2. Sleep restlessness, insomnia, nightmares

  3. Weight loss although adequate or increased dietary intake

  4. Heat intolerance, diaphoresis

5. Visual disturbances, (e.g., increased lacrimation, diplopia, photophobia, blurring)

6. Palpitations

7. Increased frequency in urination and stooling, occasional enuresis

8. Muscle weakness, fatigue

9. Restlessness

10. Warm, moist, diaphoretic skin

11. Eye findings (proptosis, lid lag, lid retraction, stare, chemosis, periorbital and conjunctival edema)

12. Enlarged, tender or non-tender, spongy or firm thyroid with bruit or thrill

13. Tachycardia, systolic hypertension, increased pulse pressure

14. Muscle weakness, diminished fine motor control, tremor, brisk DTRs

15. With subacute thyroiditis, may have positive history of preceding URI

16. In neonate, goiter may be present; symptoms usually present shortly after birth or may present days or weeks later

17. Severely affected neonates may have craniosynostosis, ophthalmopathy, jaundice, thrombocytopenia, hepatosplenomegaly, cardiac problems, other signs of severe illness (Zimmerman & Gan-Gaisano, 1990) and may be preterm, small for dates, tachycardic

- Differential Diagnosis

    1. Neonates—systemic illness, sepsis and narcotic withdrawal

    2. Children and adolescents—nodular thyroid disease, thyroid cancer, other chronic diseases, (e.g., pituitary disease), thyroiditis, accidental or deliberate excessive thyroid hormone or iodine ingestion

- Diagnostic Tests/Findings

    1. T_3 or T_4 levels— elevated

    2. TSH—normal or abnormal depending upon underlying etiology

    3. If signs or symptoms of thyrotoxicosis or enlarged thyroid— confirmatory laboratory studies include thyroid function tests (total and free T_4, T_3 and TSH), thyroidantibody tests including thyrotropin receptor antibody (TRAb), and complete blood and differential counts (Foley, 1992b). Also, sedimentation rates and tests for circulating

antibodies

- Management/Treatment

    1. Physician consultation or referral to pediatric endocrinologist for suspected or confirmed hyperthyroidism

    2. Treatment dictated by identified etiology for hyperthyroidism and thyrotoxic state

    3. Goal of treatment prompt return to euthyroidism with short term use of beta-adrenergic receptor blockers, use of anti-thyroid drugs (ablative therapy), radioiodine treatment of the thyroid gland, or thyroid surgery

    4. Prompt diagnosis and treatment especially important in neonates as condition may be life-threatening

    5. Parental and child education about disease and adherence to treatment regimen

    6. Genetic counseling indicated if etiology genetic

Amenorrhea

- Definition

    1. Primary amenorrhea—failure of onset of menarche in females who are 16 years and have normal pubertal growth and development; 14 years with absence of normal pubertal growth and development; or in girls who have not begun menstruation 2 years after completed sexual maturation (Polaneczky & Slap, 1992)

    2. Secondary amenorrhea—absence of menstruation for > 3 cycles or at least 6 months after menstruation established (Polaneczky & Slap, 1992)

- Etiology/Incidence

    1. Primary amenorrhea

        a. Constitutional/familial (common)

        b. Frequently associated with delayed puberty

        c. Organic hypothalamic or pituitary disorders, e.g., tumors, CNS irradiation)

        d. Functional hypothalamic or pituitary disorders, e.g., decreased gonadotrophin secretion; effects of chronic diseases such as DM, CF, anorexia; endocrinopathy

        e. Decreased, absent or abnormal ovarian function, e.g., gonadal dysgenesis, pelvic irradiation, oopherectomy

   f. Anatomic anomalies, e.g., cervical atresia, imperforate hymen

   g. Pharmacologic agents, e.g., cytotoxins, opiates

   h. Pregnancy (rare)

2. Secondary amenorrhea

   a. Pregnancy (most common)

   b. Many causes of primary amenorrhea may also cause secondary amenorrhea (see above)

   c. Hypothalamic, pituitary and adrenal disorders or tumors; chromosomal abnormalities, endocrinopathies and chronic illness, especially those causing severe weight loss or malnutrition; conditions affecting gonadal function

   d. Pharmacologic agents (discontinuance of birth control pills, use of tranquilizers)

   e. Significant emotional stress

   f. Strenuous exercise programs, especially with runners, ballet dancers and gymnasts

   g. Uterine dysfunction after abortion, infection, C-section

   h. Hysterectomy

■ Clinical Findings

1. Primary amenorrhea

   a. May have normal examination or multiple system involvement

   b. May have findings associated with

      (1) Marked psychosocial stress

      (2) Pituitary or hypothalamic disease

      (3) Chronic illness

      (4) Adrenal disease

      (5) Gonadal disease or injury

      (6) Chromosomal abnormalities

      (7) Anorexia nervosa or bulimia

      (8) Pregnancy

2. Secondary amenorrhea: May have sudden or gradual cessation of

menses. Findings vary depending on underlying etiology. See findings as listed under Primary amenorrhea

- Differential Diagnosis
    1. Primary amenorrhea—constitutional/familial etiology and pregnancy
    2. Secondary amenorrhea—pregnancy
- Diagnostic Tests/Findings: Pregnancy test and careful family history to rule-out constitutional/familial delay, then consultation with physician and/or referral to specialists
- Management/Treatment
    1. Constitutional/familial primary amenorrhea—education, reassurance, monitoring
    2. Amenorrhea associated with other etiologies requires further evaluation, physician consultation or referral to appropriate specialist, e.g., reproductive endocrinologist, surgeon, pediatric neurologist, obstetrician, psychologist
    3. Treatment directed at management or correction of underlying cause of abnormal menstrual processes
    4. Sensitivity to significant concern of delayed development by child and family very important
    5. Parental and child education regarding amenorrhea and adherence to treatment regimen, if any
    6. Genetic counseling may be indicated if genetic etiology

Dysmenorrhea

- Definition: Crampy abdominal or back pain related to menstrual blood flow
    1. Primary dysmenorrhea is not associated with pelvic pathology
    2. Secondary dysmenorrhea is associated with underlying pelvic pathology
- Etiology/Incidence
    1. Most common gynecologic problem in adolescent female and leading cause of school absenteeism
    2. Primary dysmenorrhea
        a. Caused by excessive endometrial synthesis or prostaglandins F_{2x} and E_2 which causes myometrium to contract producing pain

    b. Usually associated with ovulatory cycles which begin 6 to 18 months after menarche, thus incidence increases through adolescence

    c. Most dysmenorrhea during adolescence is primary

  3. Secondary dysmenorrhea

    a. Associated with underlying pelvic pathology including endometritis, endometriosis, presence of intrauterine device (IUD), congenital anomalies, pelvic infection or abdominal adhesions

    b. Uncommon in adolescents

    c. Usually occurs a few years after menarche onset

- Clinical Findings

  1. Primary dysmenorrhea

    a. Pain characteristically begins with or after beginning of menstrual flow; may begin several hours prior to onset of flow

    b. Pain usually crampy, spasmodic and localized over lower abdomen and suprapubic region

    c. Rectal examination should be an integral part of examination to identify abnormalities of Müllerian system

    d. Normal physical examination findings with possible tenderness on abdominal palpation

  2. Secondary dysmenorrhea

    a. Characteristically severe pain occurs at time of menses; may start 1 to 2 days prior to onset of menses

    b. Physical examination may show

      (1) Regional adenopathy

      (2) Abdominal pain or tenderness

      (3) Vaginal or cervical discharge, erythema

      (4) Vaginal or uterine anomalies with outflow obstruction or other pelvic abnormalities (masses, cysts)

- Differential Diagnosis

  1. Acute abdomen

  2. Complications of pregnancy

- Diagnostic Tests/Findings
  1. If congenital anomalies or endometriosis suspected, gynecologic examination with ultrasound, hysteroscopy or laparoscopy
  2. Cervical cultures to rule out infection
- Management/Treatment
  1. Primary dysmenorrhea
     a. Education about normal menstrual processes
     b. Exercise throughout cycle, relaxation, warm baths, heat
     c. Mild pain—use non-prescriptive analgesics
     d. Moderate pain—use OTC or prescriptive prostaglandin synthetase inhibitors or low dose oral contraceptives
  2. Secondary dysmenorrhea
     a. Treatment contingent upon etiology and may require referral to a gynecologist or surgeon, e.g., for congenital anomalies
     b. Antibiotics for infection, pelvic inflammatory disease, salpingitis
     c. Hormonal therapy or surgery for endometriosis
     d. Analgesics/prostaglandin inhibitors
  3. Immediate consultation and/or referral for adolescents with suspected acute abdomen or complications of pregnancy
  4. Careful teaching regarding use of oral contraceptives and prostaglandin inhibitors
  5. Periodic monitoring important, especially for girls placed on oral contraceptives

Premenstrual Syndrome (PMS)

- Definition: A condition characterized by irritability, mood swings, depression, edema, cramps approximately 7 to 14 days prior to onset of menstruation with resolution after menstrual flow has begun
- Etiology/Incidence
  1. Cause is unknown
  2. Syndrome seems to be related to fluctuations in estrogen and

progesterone but no consistent hormonal abnormalities have been found

3. Prevalence is variable; does not seem to be related to dysmenorrhea which is more common in the adolescent female

- Clinical Findings
    1. May include
        a. Breast fullness, tenderness; bloating
        b. Fatigue, irritability, mood swings, depression
        c. Inability to concentrate; tearfulness
        d. Headache
        e. Increased appetite, especially for sweets and salty foods
    2. Physical findings usually negative
    3. Bimanual pelvic examination to determine pelvic pathology
- Differential Diagnosis
    1. Anemia
    2. Diabetes
    3. Thyroid disorder
    4. Pregnancy
    5. Endometriosis
    6. Pelvic inflammatory disease
    7. Depression; anxiety disorders
    8. Prolactin-producing tumors
- Diagnostic Tests/Findings
    1. CBC—identify bleeding disorders, diabetes, anemia, etc.
    2. Thyroid function tests—identify thyroid dysfunction
    3. Glucose tolerance test—if diabetes suspected
- Management/Treatment
    1. No single treatment is effective for all patients
    2. For the adolescent first-line therapy includes
        a. Education and reassurance

b. Well-balanced diet with restriction of salt, sugar, and caffeine

c. Regular aerobic exercise

d. Caution should be used in prescribing diuretics

e. Progesterone suppositories should be reserved for severe cases

f. Prostaglandin inhibitors, e.g., ibuprofen

g. Oral contraceptives may be used in the sexually active patient

Hypoglycemia

- Definition: A syndrome characterized by symptoms provoked by an abnormally low plasma glucose level

- Etiology/Incidence

  1. Transient neonatal hypoglycemia

     a. Decreased production of blood sugar from physiologic immaturity; most common in premies, small-for-gestational age (SGA) infants; highest in SGA preemies

     b. Increased glucose use from physiologic stressors (asphyxia, anoxia, respiratory illness, heart disease, infection, cold injury, starvation)

     c. Hyperplasia of beta cells of pancreas (hyperinsulinism) due to chronic intrauterine exposure to elevated maternal blood sugars (infant of diabetic mother [IDDM])

     d. Common during first week of life

  2. Persistent neonatal hypoglycemia

     a. Inherited defects (inborn errors) in carbohydrate metabolism

     b. Hormone deficiencies

     c. Pancreatic defects

  3. Childhood hypoglycemia

     a. Causes as identified under persistent neonatal hypoglycemia

     b. Other acquired causes include diminished glucose production from hepatic disease, injury; hormonal or substrate deficiency

     c. Ketotic hypoglycemia most common cause > 1 year with onset 9 months to 5½ years, peaks at age 2 years (Kogut, 1992); associated with prolonged fast during concurrent URI

d. Hyperinsulinism from pancreatic and abdominal tumors; growth hormone (GH) or glucocorticoid deficiency

■ Clinical Findings

1. Transient neonatal hypoglycemia

   a. Findings variable and may include

      (1) Cachexic or macrosomic infant

      (2) Irritability, lethargy

      (3) Hypothermia, cyanosis, diaphoresis

      (4) Weak cry

      (5) Uncoordinated eye movements, eye-rolling

      (6) Apnea, irregular breathing

      (7) Twitching, jitteriness, convulsions and coma

2. Persistent neonatal or childhood hypoglycemia

   a. Findings as with transient neonatal hypoglycemia

   b. May also include diminished growth, difficulty talking, signs of other systematic illness, abdominal or pelvic masses

3. Ketotic hypoglycemia

   a. Symptoms vary—occur in early morning following prolonged fast or illness and may include CNS symptoms, pallor, vomiting, unresponsiveness

■ Differential Diagnosis: Hyperviscoscity; for ketotic hypoglycemia rule out other endocrinopathies such as GH deficiency

■ Diagnostic Tests/Findings

1. Transient neonatal hypoglycemia—whole blood glucose levels < 35 mg/dL in first 24 hours or < 40 mg/dL thereafter or when plasma glucose level < 40 mg/dL in first 24 hours or < 45 mg/dL thereafter (Marks & Maisels, 1992)

2. Persistent neonatal or childhood hypoglycemia—blood or serum glucose level < 45 mg/dL or whole blood glucose level of < 40 mg/dL after first month of life (Kogut, 1992)

3. Ketotic hypoglycemia—abnormal blood glucose levels at time of symptoms

■ Management/Treatment

1. Management defined by blood glucose levels requires consultation and referral to physician for delineation of etiology and treatment

2. Immediate return of blood glucose levels to within normal range, especially in neonates and infants, to avoid permanent damage to the brain

3. Educate children, adolescents and parents to regularly monitor blood glucose levels, to correlate levels with concomitant physical feelings, and to know guidelines for when to contact health care providers

4. Hypoglycemic reactions in children with diabetes

   a. Mild reactions (hunger at unusual time)—treat with extra sugar, juice or food

   b. Moderate reactions (shakiness or irritability)—treat with simple sugar, then retest child. If level > 80 mg/dL, give food; if < 80 mg/dL, give more juice before solid food

   c. Severe reactions (confusion, pallor, marked shakiness)—use Instant Glucose® or Reactose® or simple sugar

   d. Very severe reactions (loss of consciousness, convulsion)—use Instant Glucose® Reactose®, then Glucagon (Chase, 1992)

5. Children with ketotic hypoglycemia—treat with liberal carbohydrate diet and bedtime snack, avoid prolonged overnight fasting, especially if child ill. Parents may need to check urinary ketones

6. On-going support and education needed for children with diabetes and their families to reduce likelihood of hypoglycemic reactions associated with too little food, too much exercise or too much insulin

Diabetes Mellitus

- Definition: Hereditary metabolic disorder characterized by insulin deficiency resulting in abnormal metabolism of carbohydrate, protein, and fat (Insulin dependent diabetes mellitus [IDDM] or Type I diabetes)

- Etiology/Incidence

  1. Basic cause is decreased secretion of insulin

  2. Mechanisms that cause failure of pancreatic beta-cell function thought to include

     a. Genetic predisposition

     b. Autoimmune response

    c. Environmental factors including viruses and chemicals

  3. Develops gradually over months or years secondary to repeated insults from viral infections, stress and exposure to chemical agents although clinical symptoms usually present for short time

  4. Prevalence in school-age children is approximately 1.9/1000 (Sperling, 1992); frequency increases with age

  5. Peak incidence between 5 and 7 years and at puberty

■ Clinical Findings

  1. May initially present with no symptoms or with signs of severe illness from ketoacidosis

  2. Symptoms may include

    a. Behavioral changes, emotional lability, fatigue

    b. Weight loss or failure to gain weight

    c. Polyphagia, polydipsia

    d. Polyuria, nocturia, enuresis

    e. Abdominal or lower extremity cramping

    f. A child in ketoacidosis may also have abdominal pain, nausea and vomiting

  3. Physical examination shows

    a. Signs of weight loss

    b. Lethargy

    c. Dehydration, flushed and dry skin

    d. Fruity odor to breath

    e. Weak, rapid pulse

    f. Confusion

    g. Kussmaul respirations

    h. Coma

■ Differential Diagnosis

  1. Diabetes insipidus

  2. Non-diabetes causes of polyuria, e.g., psychogenic polydipsia, CNS injury, tumors

3. Other causes of fatigue, weight loss, behavioral change, e.g., hypothyroidism, systemic illness

- Diagnostic Tests/Findings

    1. Fasting blood glucose levels— > 120 mg/dL

    2. Oral glucose tolerance test—2 hour value $\geq$ 180 mg/dL (venous whole blood) or $\geq$ 200 mg/dL (capillary whole blood); (glucose dose is 1.75 g/kg [maximum of 75g])

    3. Children with diabetes may initially present with diabetic ketoacidosis with elevated blood glucose; urinary and blood ketones; possible elevated Blood Urea Nitrogen BUN); and depressed sodium, potassium, CO_2, pH and bicarbonate levels

    5. Glycosylated hemoglobin blood test—reliable measurement of long-term glycemic control during preceding 2 to 3 months; HbA_{1c} value of 6 to 9% indicates good metabolic control

- Management/Treatment

    1. Supportive care of patient and family through stages of grieving following diagnosis

    2. Primary goal to maintain blood glucose levels at near normal to prevent complications

    3. Diabetes specialists using multidisciplinary team approach should provide initial care and management, especially for in-patient care

    4. Many children have "honeymoon" period of variable duration after initial diagnosis

    5. Management of blood sugar levels—provided by insulin adjustments in conjunction with careful, frequent blood glucose monitoring

    6. Most children treated with combination of Regular and long-acting insulin usually given twice daily before breakfast and before evening meal

    7. Insulin types, onset, peak action, and duration vary

8. Features of insulin

Type	Onset (Hours)	Peak (Hours)	Duration of action
Short-acting			
Regular	½ hour	1 to 4 hours	4 to 6 hours
Semilente®	1 hour	2 to 5 hours	8 to 12 hours
Long-acting			
NPH®	2 to 4 hours	6 to 12 hours	18 to 24 hours
Ultralente®	4 to 6 hours	8 to 15 hours	18 to 24 hours
Combined (pre-mixed) Lente® (3 parts Semilente® and 7 parts Ultralente®)			
	1 to 2 hours	6 to 12 hours	18 to 24 hours

Note: Human insulin (changed or engineered from pork insulin) is increasingly preferred because it causes fewer localized reactions, has lower antibody response, may prolong "honeymoon period" and requires slightly lower doses (Source: Chase,1992)

9. Blood sugars should be maintained between 100 to 200 mg/dL for children < 5 years; between 80 to 180 mg/dL for children 5 to 12 years; and between 70 to 150 mg/dL for children 13 years and older (Chase, 1992)

10. Normal ranges for blood sugars range from 80 to 120 mg/dL; low blood sugar ranges from 20 to 60 mg/dL

11. Insulin doses are based on body weight and self blood glucose monitoring (SBGM) results; insulin doses after initial diagnosis average 0.5 unit/kg to 1.0 unit/kg (¼ unit/lb to ½ unit/lb) of body weight per day. Amount of insulin may be need to be increased during adolescent growth spurt (Chase, 1992)

12. Glycosylated hemoglobin blood test every 3 months to assess overall blood sugar states (Chase, 1992)

13. Frequent follow-up initially to monitor response to treatment regimen

14. Insulin doses need seasonal adaptations to reflect activity level changes

15. Better blood sugar control at time of puberty decreases likelihood of adverse vessel changes although normal adolescent rebelliousness an issue in adherence

16. Education regarding insulin injections, self-monitoring of blood glucose, signs and symptoms of hypoglycemia and ketoacidosis, care

during illness and stress, complications, regular exercise and need to have sugar, Glucagon® and Regular insulin available

17. Nutritional management—well-balanced, consistent diet and elimination of dietary refined sugar, sucrose, glucose/dextrose, fructose, maltose and syrups (Chase, 1992)

18. Emphasize normalcy; view of child as "child with diabetes" vs. "diabetic child"

19. Transfer of care from provider to parent and child should be based on on-going assessment of capabilities, development and readiness

20. Flu vaccine recommended by American Academy of Pediatrics

21. Referral to pediatric ophthalmologists and other specialists as needed

22. Recently developed insulin infusion systems are used in some children; surgically implanted insulin pumps now available; careful selection of candidates for these therapies is required

23. Concurrent hypothyroidism more common in children with diabetes than in children without diabetes

24. Sexually-active adolescents need instruction regarding pregnancy prevention

Growth disturbances: Short stature or decelerated growth

- Definition: Deviation of growth from previously established channels for weight, height or both, or weight or height falling ≥ 2 standard deviations (SDs) below the mean (Tunnessen, 1988)

- Etiology/Incidence: Multiple etiologies including physiologic, nutritional, environmental, psychosocial and constitutional factors

- Clinical Findings

  1. Normal variants

     a. Familial short stature—small at birth ($\leq 3\%$) but consistent with family pattern

     b. Constitutional growth delay—usually normal size at birth with declining height and weight throughout 1 to 1½ years to $< 5\%$

  2. Pathologic causes

     a. Proportionate growth disturbances

        (1) Pre-natal

(a) Intrauterine growth retardation (IUGR)—Birth weight (BW) > 2 SDs below mean for gestational age, sex, race (Mahoney, 1987)

(b) Dysmorphism including abnormal facies

(c) Chromosomal abnormalities (abnormal examination with stigmata of Down syndrome)

(2) Post-natal

(a) Hypopituitarism—may have immature facies, ophthalmologic defects, CNS malformations; anomalies; signs of CNS tumors; truncal obesity; micropenis, small testes, underdeveloped scrotum; delayed bone maturation and puberty

(b) Signs and symptoms of hypothyroidism or diabetes mellitus

(c) Glucocorticoid excess—fatigue, weakness, easy bruising, back pain, hypertension, plethora, moon facies, purple striae, interscapular fat pad, truncal obesity, muscle wasting, latent diabetes

(d) Hypogonadism—growth retardation after age 10 years in girls, age 12 years in boys (Mahoney, 1987); delayed sexual development, sexual infantilism, small testes

(e) Psychosocial dwarfism—abnormalities in psychosocial development

(f) Systemic illness

b. Disproportionate growth disturbances

(1) Skeletal dysplasia—abnormal upper to lower body ratios, disproportionate features

(2) Rickets—short stature, frontal bossing, leg bowing, etc.

- Differential diagnosis: Normal variants of familial and constitutional delay short stature need to be distinguished from pathologic causes

- Diagnostic Tests/Findings

1. Previous occipital-frontal circumference (OFC), height and weight recordings plotted on age-standardized tests to determine growth percentile and velocity and patterning

2. Careful family history with emphasis on familial growth patterns

3. Growth measurements, radiographic bone age assessment, body segment measurements, upper to lower body ratio measurements

4. Other laboratory tests as indicated to rule out systemic disease or hormonal deficiency, e.g., TSH, Somatomedin-C (SM-C)

5. Home evaluation to rule out psychosocial etiology

- Management/Treatment

1. Physician consultation or referral to appropriate pediatric specialists for children with other than familial or constitutional growth delay

2. If familial or constitutional growth delay, periodic monitoring of growth pattern needed

3. Growth hormone (GH) may be indicated for those children with known deficiency

4. Deviation from established growth channel is unusual after age 2 years and requires further evaluation by appropriate specialist

Questions

Select the best answer

1. The peak incidence for adolescent gynecomastia occurs at age

   a. 12 years
   b. 14 years
   c. 16 years
   d. 17 years

2. Differential diagnoses for adolescent pubertal gynecomastia include all but the following

   a. Obesity with lipomastia
   b. Neurofibromas
   c. Breast cancer
   d. Lymphadenitis

3. The breast enlargement of transient newborn gynecomastia

   a. Usually resolves in several days
   b. Indicates which adolescents are more likely to develop adolescent physiologic gynecomastia
   c. Usually is indicative of underlying disease
   d. Usually resolves in the fourth month of life

4. The most common world-wide cause of congenital hypothyroidism is

   a. Dyshormonogenesis
   b. Endemic cretinism
   c. Deficiencies in TSH production
   d. Thyroid atrophy

5. Newborn screening for hypothyroidism

   a. Has virtually no false positives or false negatives
   b. Should be repeated at the 2 month visit
   c. Is a reliable means to assess hypothyroidism in the newborn
   d. Can differentiate transient from permanent hypothyroidism

6. Infants with congenital hypothyroidism may have all of the following except

   a. Hoarse cry
   b. Coarse features
   c. Frequent stooling
   d. Lethargy

7. School children and adolescents with hypothyroidism often have

   a. Decreased linear growth
   b. Third fontanels
   c. Soft, silky hair
   d. Advanced bone age

8. Adolescents with Graves' disease may present with all of the following except

   a. Behavioral problems
   b. Sleep disturbances
   c. Weak pulses
   d. Tachycardia

9. Secondary amenorrhea may be caused by all of the following except

   a. Pregnancy
   b. Imperforate hymen
   c. Pituitary tumor
   d. Uterine lining scarring after curettage or therapeutic abortion

10. In a teen with secondary amenorrhea, your first suspicion should be

    a. Uterine agenesis
    b. Pituitary tumor
    c. Turner syndrome
    d. Pregnancy

11. Which age adolescent is least likely to experience primary dysmenorrhea?

    a. 11 year old
    b. 12 year old
    c. 15 year old
    d. 18 year old

12. Drugs of choice for primary dysmenorrhea are

    a. Aspirin products
    b. Acetaminophen
    c. Prostaglandin inhibitors
    d. Tranquilizers

13. All of the following are true statements about hypoglycemia except

    a. Idiopathic beta-cell hyperplasia may be a cause of neonatal hypoglycemia
    b. It can be caused by severe infection or injury to the liver
    c. Diabetes with mild hypoglycemia requires no treatment
    d. It occurs when the child has too much exercise, too little food, or too much insulin

14. Transient neonatal hypoglycemia is

    a. Most common in AGA infants
    b. Highest in premature SGA infants
    c. Most common in LGA infants
    d. Least common in LGA infants

15. Another name for Diabetes Mellitus is

    a. Type II diabetes
    b. Type I diabetes
    c. Type II, Insulin-Dependent Diabetes Mellitus
    d. Non-insulin Dependent Diabetes Mellitus

16. Regular insulin

    a. Has a quicker onset of effect and longer duration than NPH®
    b. Has a slower onset of effect and shorter duration than NPH®
    c. Has a quicker onset of effect and shorter duration than NPH®
    d. Has the longest duration of the insulins available

17. Blood levels of children 5 to 12 years with diabetes should be maintained between

    a. 80 to 180 mg/dL
    b. 100 to 200 mg/dL
    c. 60 to 80 mg/dL
    d. Slightly over 200 mg/dL

18. Glucagon® should be used to treat

    a. Children with mild hypoglycemia
    b. Children with moderate hypoglycemia
    c. Children with severe hypoglycemia
    d. Children with very severe hypoglycemia

19. Symptoms of diabetes onset in children include all but the following

    a. Alopecia
    b. Gylcosuria
    c. Polydipsia
    d. Polyuria

20. Abdominal pain and vomiting are particularly critical to monitor in children with diabetes because these findings may represent the onset of

    a. Gastrointestinal infection
    b. Hyperglycemia
    c. Autoimmune response to the pancreas
    d. Ketoacidosis

21. All of the following are true statements about IDDM except
    a. The "honeymoon" period post-diagnosis is of variable duration
    b. Diabetes is a relatively common disease in childhood
    c. Children with IDDM can switch to oral insulin agents once they reach adulthood
    d. Three factors influencing a child's development of diabetes are genetic predisposition, an autoimmune response and exposure to viral or chemical agents

22. Normal variant growth disturbances in children manifest
    a. Only pre-natally
    b. Only at the time of puberty
    c. At any time during the life span
    d. Usually at birth, during the first two years of life or at puberty

23. Growth retardation appearing after age 10 in girls likely may be caused by
    a. Hypogonadism
    b. Periodic dieting
    c. Diabetes, even though the diabetes is well controlled
    d. Occasional use of street drugs

Answer key:

1.   b
2.   d
3.   a
4.   b
5.   c
6.   c
7.   a
8.   c
9.   b
10.   d
11.   a
12.   c
13.   c
14.   b
15.   b
16.   c
17.   a
18.   d
19.   a
20.   d
21.   c
22.   d
23.   a

Bibliography

Cara, J. F., & Johanson, A. J. (1990). Growth hormone for short stature not due to classic growth hormone deficiency. *Pediatric Clinics of North America, 37*(6), 1229-1250.

Chase, H. P. (1992). *Understanding insulin dependent diabetes* (7th ed.). Denver, CO: A. B. Hirschfield Press.

Clark, L. M., & Plotnick, L. P. (1990). Insulin pumps in children with diabetes. *Journal of Pediatric Health Care, 4*(1), 3-10.

Coupey, S. M., & Ahlstrom, P. (1989). Common menstrual disorders. *Pediatric Clinics of North America, 36*(3), 551-558.

DiGeorge, A. M. (1992). The endocrine system. In R. E. Behrman & R. M. Kliegman (Eds.). *Nelson textbook of pediatrics* (14th ed.) (pp. 1397-1472). Philadelphia: W. B. Saunders Co.

Foley, T. P., Jr. (1992a). Hypothyroidism. In R. A. Hoekelman (Ed.), *Pediatric primary care* (2nd ed.) (pp. 1292-1294). St. Louis, MO: Mosby Year Book.

Foley, T. P., Jr. (1992b). Thyrotoxicosis in childhood. *Pediatric Annals, 21(1),* 43-49.

Giordano, B. P., Petrila, A., Banion, C. R., & Neuenkirchen, G. (1992). The challenge of transferring responsibility for diabetes management from parent to child. Journal of Pediatric Health Care, 6(5, Pt. 1), 235-239.

Gotlin, R. W., & Klinginsmith, G. J. (1991). Endocrine disorders. In W. E. Hathaway, J. R. Groothuis, W. W. Hay, Jr. & J. W. Paisley (Eds.), *Current diagnosis and treatment* (10th ed.) (pp. 770-814). Norwalk, CT: Appleton & Lange.

Gruters, A. (1992). Congenital hypothyroidism. *Pediatric Annals, 21*(1), 15-28.

Henry, J. J. (1992). Routine growth monitoring and assessment of growth disorders. *Journal of Pediatric Health Care, 6*(5, Pt. 2), 291-301.

Hoekelman, R. A. (1992). Screening for congenital hypothyroidism. *Pediatric Annals, 21*(1), 9-10.

Joffee, A. (1992). Amenorrhea. In R. A. Hoekelman (Ed.), *Pediatric primary care* (2nd ed.) (pp. 821-824). St. Louis: Mosby Year Book.

Kaplan, D. W., & Mammel, K. A. (1991). Adolescence. In W. E. Hathaway, J. R. Groothuis, W. W. Hay, Jr. & J. W. Paisley (Eds.), *Current diagnosis and treatment* (10th ed.) (pp. 215-253). Norwalk, CT: Appleton & Lange.

Kogut, M. D. (1992). Hypoglycemia. In R. A. Hoekelman (Ed.), *Pediatric primary care* (2nd ed.) (pp. 1626-1632). St. Louis: Mosby Year Book.

LaFranchi, S. (1992). Thyroiditis and acquired hypothyroidism. *Pediatric Annals, 21*(1), 29-39.

Mahoney, C. P. (1987). Evaluating the child with short stature. *Pediatric Clinics of North America, 34*(4), 825-849.

Mahoney, C. P. (1990). Adolescent gynecomastia-Differential diagnosis and management. *Pediatric Clinics of North America, 37*(6), 1389-1404.

Marks, K. H., & Maisels, M. J. (1992). Critical neonatal illnesses. In R. A. Hoekelman (Ed.), *Pediatric primary care* (2nd ed.) (pp. 499-517). St. Louis: Mosby Year Book.

Pinyerd, B. J. (1992). Assessment of infant growth. *Journal of Pediatric Health Care, 6*(5, Pt. 2), 302-308.

Polzaneczky, M. M., & Slap, G. B. (1992a). Menstrual disorders in the adolescent: Amenorrhea. *Pediatrics in Review, 13*(2), 43-48.

Polzaneczky, M. M., & Slap, G. B. (1992b). Menstrual disorders in the adolescent: Dysmenorrhea and dysfunctional uterine bleeding. *Pediatrics in Review, 13*(3), 83-87.

Rosenberg, A. A., & Battaglia, F. C. (1991). The newborn infant. In W. E. Hathaway, J. R. Groothuis, W. W. Hay, Jr. & J. W. Paisley (Eds.), *Current diagnosis and treatment* (10th ed.) (pp. 50-103). Norwalk, CT: Appleton & Lange.

Rudy, C. (1991). 8-year old girl with short stature. *Journal of Pediatric Health Care, 5*(4), 223.

Sperling, M. A. (1992). Metabolic diseases. In R. E. Behrman & R. M. Kliegman (Eds.), *Nelson textbook of pediatrics* (14th ed.) (pp. 390-408). Philadelphia: W. B. Saunders Co.

Tunnessen, W. W., Jr. (1988). *Signs and symptoms in pediatrics* (2nd ed.). (pp. 10-20). Philadelphia: J. B. Lippincott.

Tuttle, J. I. (1991). Menstrual disorders during adolescence. *Journal of Pediatric Health Care, 5*(4), 197-203.

Vessey, J. A. (1992). Diabetes mellitus (Type I). In P. L. Jackson & J. A. Vessey , *Primary care of the child with a chronic condition* (pp. 229-241). St. Louis: Mosby Year Book.

Zimmerman, D., & Gan-Gaisano, M. (1992). Hyperthyroidism in children and adolescents. *Pediatric Clinics of North America, 37*(6), 1273-1288.

Hematological/Oncological/ Immunological Disorders

Jo-Anne Tierney

ABO/Rh/Incompatibility

- Definition: Hemolytic disease in newborns due to incompatibility between mother and baby's blood; maternal antibodies cross placenta and bind to fetal red blood cells causing hemolysis
- Etiology/Incidence
    1. Rh incompatibility—hemolytic anemia occurring in newborn period due to incompatibility between mother and child in the major antigen of rhesus
        a. Rarely occurs in first pregnancy
    2. ABO incompatibility—hemolytic disease occurring when the major blood group antigens of the fetus are different from the mother
        a. Occurs in 20 to 25% of pregnancies
- Clinical Findings
    1. Rh incompatibility
        a. Usually no symptoms in newborns from first pregnancy
        b. Mild to severe anemia
        c. Hepatosplenomegaly
        d. Jaundice usually absent at birth
        e. Severe cases result in cardiomegaly, respiratory distress, circulatory collapse (hydrops fetalis)
    2. ABO incompatibility
        a. Usually milder than Rh incompatibility
        b. Jaundice first 24 hours of life
        c. Mild anemia
- Differential Diagnosis
    1. Infection
    2. Physiologic jaundice
    3. Hemolytic anemias
- Diagnostic Tests/Findings
    1. Maternal/infant blood types—ABO or Rh incompatibility

2. Coomb's test—positive

3. CBC—anemia

4. Reticulocyte count—increased

- Management/Treatment

    1. ABO incompatibility

        a. Rarely requires treatment; phototherapy may be effective

        b. Treatment—single exchange transfusion

    2. Rh incompatibility

        a. Intrauterine direct intravascular transfusion of packed red blood cells

        b. Exchange transfusions for liveborn infants

        c. Prevention of Rh sensitization (1mL of RhoGAM within 72 hours of delivery or abortion

        d. Impossible to reverse sensitization

    3. Support of family

Hyperbilirubinemia

- Definition: An excess of circulating bilirubin in the blood

- Etiology/Incidence

    1. Transition of bilirubin metabolism from fetal stage to adult stage

    2. Unconjugated hyperbilirubinemia occurs in 50% of all newborns

    3. Physiologic jaundice (increased bilirubin concentration [unconjugated])

        a. Immature liver

        b. Decreased RBC survival

        c. Increased bilirubin burden from birth

    4. Nonphysiologic jaundice (due to problem in production and excretion of bilirubin)

        a. Causes

            (1) Hemolytic disease (blood group incompatibility)

            (2) Bacterial sepsis

(3)　Crigler-Najjar syndrome

5. Breast-feeding and jaundice

   a. Associated with unconjugated hyperbilirubinemia

   b. May be due to an increased enterohepatic circulation of bilirubin or inhibition of hepatic glucuronyl transferase

   c. Estimated that 1 in 200 breast-fed term infants develop significant elevation of unconjugated bilirubin

- Clinical Manifestations

  1. Physiologic—jaundice by 2nd day of life; usually peaking between 2nd and 4th day and decreasing between 5th and 7th days of life

  2. Nonphysiologic—significant variation in time of appearance and duration of jaundice from that of physiologic jaundice; kernicterus

  3. Breast-feeding and jaundice—jaundice usually appears after 3rd day of life and may continue for approximately 2 weeks and then gradually clear

- Differential Diagnosis

  1. Unconjugated (indirect) hyperbilirubinemia

     a. Physiologic

     b. Nonphysiologic

  2. Conjugated hyperbilirubinemia

     a. TORCHS infection

     b. Obstructive jaundice

     c. Sepsis

- Diagnostic Tests/Findings

  1. Physiologic

     a. Rule out pathologic causes of jaundice

        (1)　CBC with a peripheral blood smear

        (2)　Maternal and infant blood types—no ABO/Rh incompatibility

        (3)　Coomb test (indirect and direct)—negative

        (4)　Bilirubin level (direct and indirect)—indirect elevated

     b. Serum bilirubin—typically peaks at 3rd day of life (less than 13

(handwritten: table)

mg/dL) and returns to normal in approximately 10 days

    c. Umbilical cord bilirubin less than 2 mg/dL

  2. Nonphysiologic jaundice

    a. Jaundice within first 24 hours of life

    b. Umbilical cord serum bilirubin elevated (greater than 2 mg/dL)

    c. Total serum bilirubin concentration increases by more than 5 mg/dL/24 hours

    d. Total serum bilirubin concentrations exceeding 13 mg/dL in full-term infants; usually lasts longer and reaches higher levels

    e. Direct (conjugated) serum bilirubin concentration exceeding 1.5 to 2 mg/dL

  3. Breast-feeding and jaundice

    a. Bilirubin levels rise progressively from 4th day of life reaching a maximum of 10 to 30 mg/dL by 10 to 15 days; peak at 2 weeks and gradually decline

    b. Serum bilirubin levels of 20 mg/dL have not been associated with kernicterus as a result of breast-feeding alone (Avery & First, 1994; A-kadar & Balistreri, 1993)

- Management/Treatment

  1. Phototherapy

  2. Exchange transfusion

    a. Used in hemolytic disease

    b. High bilirubin concentrations

  3. Support

  4. Education for

    a. Disease process

    b. Treatment modality

  5. Many opinions and limited data regarding management of breast feeding and jaundice; some advocate temporary cessation for 48 hours and others urge continuation since no incidence of kernicterus in otherwise healthy infants

Iron Deficiency Anemia

- Definition: A microcytic anemia characterized by small, pale RBCs and depletion of iron stores with subsequent decrease in bone marrow erythropoiesis
- Etiology/Incidence
    1. Causative factors
        a. Low-birth-weight infants
        b. Rapid growth
        c. Blood loss—GI tract common location
        d. Inadequate dietary intake from 9 to 24 months of age
    2. Most common cause of anemia in children
    3. Most common 9 to 24 months of age
    4. Common in diet composed mostly of milk
- Clinical Manifestations
    1. Mild anemia
        a. Physical examination normal
        b. Pale conjunctiva
    2. Severe
        a. Irritability
        b. Anorexia
        c. Tachycardia; systolic murmur
        d. Brittle concave nails
- Differential Diagnosis
    1. Beta-thalassemia trait
    2. Alpha-thalassemia trait
    3. Anemia of chronic disease
    4. Lead poisoning
- Diagnostic Test/Findings
    1. Serum ferritin— < 10 mg/mL significant
    2. CBC with RBC indices—decreased MCV < 83, decreased Hgb, 6 to

10 g/dL

3. Serum iron— < 30 μg/dl

4. Reticulocyte count—low, normal, slightly elevated

5. Blood smear—RBC microcytic, hypochromic

6. Lead level—low

- Management/Treatment

    1. Elemental iron 6 mg/kg/day in 3 divided doses; absorbed best on an empty stomach and in the presence of ascorbic acid; taking medication through straw minimizes staining of teeth

    2. Measurement of treatment response

        a. Reticulocyte count—increase in 2 to 3 days, peaking 7 to 10 days verifies adequate treatment

        b. Hemoglobin—rechecked in 2 to 4 weeks when indices should have returned to normal

    3. Parenteral iron—in noncompliant situations and in cases of iron malabsorption

    4. Continuation of iron therapy for about 2 to 3 months once normal hemoglobin levels have been confirmed

    5. Severe anemia (Hgb < 3.0 g/dL)—refer for transfusion therapy

    6. Education—side effects of iron therapy; diet high in iron

Sickle Cell Anemia

- Definition: Chronic hemolytic anemia characterized by sickle-shaped RBCs

- Etiology/Incidence

    1. Causative factor—abnormal autosomal gene

        a. Substitution by valine in place of glutamic acid causing erythrocytes to sickle

    2. Most common form of hemolytic anemia in Afro-Americans

    3. 10% of Afro-Americans have sickle cell trait

- Clinical Findings

    1. Clinical course characterized by episodic "crisis"

    2. Asymptomatic in infancy prior to 5 to 6 months of age

3. Acute sickle dactylitis (hand-foot syndrome)—frequently first sign in infant; painful swelling of hands and feet

4. Pain is most predominant and frequent symptom and may require hospitalization in severe cases; usually involves the extremities

5. Jaundice

6. Splenomegaly

7. Cardiomegaly in older children

8. Life threatening problems

    a. Splenic sequestration crisis

    b. Overwhelming infection

9. Poor growth

■ Differential Diagnosis

1. Acute rheumatic fever

2. Pneumonia

3. Osteomyelitis

4. Rheumatoid arthritis

5. Leukemia

■ Diagnostic Tests/Findings

1. Trait

    a. Hgb electrophoresis

    b. Solubility test

2. Anemia

    a. Fetus can be diagnosed in utero

    b. Hgb electrophoresis—Hgb 5%

    c. Peripheral smear—contains target cells, poikilocytes, and sickled cells

3. Liver function tests—abnormal

4. Sedimentation rates—slow

5. Platelet count—usually increased

■ Management/Treatment

1. Prevent Infection

    a. Standard immunizations

    b. Pneumococcal vaccine

    c. Penicillin prophylaxis—125 mg orally twice a day; started at 2 months and continued to 4 years of age (erythromycin for penicillin sensitivity)

    d. Febrile episodes—treat for sepsis

2. Mild to moderate pain

    a. Prevention stressed

        (1) Recognition and avoidance of precipitating factors, e.g., exposure to cold, inadequate fluid intake, exercise at high altitudes, overexertion

        (2) Pain treated with increased fluid intake to correct dehydration, and acetaminophen or ibuprofen

3. Chronic pain

    a. Multidisciplinary approach with support services, e.g., psychologists, social workers, rehabilitative specialists

    b. Nonsteroidal anti-inflammatory drugs

4. Vaso-occlusive crisis

    a. Analgesics

    b. Transfusions

5. Aplastic crisis—transfusions

6. Education about disease process

7. Stress importance of routine health care

8. Psychosocial support

Glucose-6-phosphate dehydrogenase (G-6-PD)

■ Definition: Glucose-6-phosphate dehydrogenase deficiency either in structure or amount which results in decreased life span of red blood cells which in turn can lead to hemolysis following exposure to inciting agents

■ Etiology/Incidence

1. Deficiency of glucose-6-phosphate dehydrogenase; may not be

significant unless exposure to drugs, infection occurs, or in the presence of diabetic ketoacidosis

2. Most common RBC metabolic disorder

3. Incidence

   a. Blacks 10%

   b. Orientals 5%

   c. Mediterranean cultures 2 to 25%

4. Over 150 Variants—most commonly found in areas with an increase in malaria

- Clinical Manifestations

  1. Episodes of hemolytic anemia with varying degrees of severity; may result in shock/death

  2. Jaundice

  3. Back pain

- Differential Diagnosis

  1. Sickle cell anemia

  2. Hemoglobinopathies

  3. Other causes of hemolytic anemia

- Diagnostic Tests/Findings

  1. N.B.T. test—quantitation of N.B.T. (Nitroblue tetrazolium dye reduction)

  2. Electrophoresis—to identify variant

- Management/Treatment

  1. Avoid food and drugs that cause hemolysis

     a. Fava beans

     b. Acetylsalicylic acid

     c. Sulfonamides

     d. Ascorbic acid

     e. Methylene blue

     f. Antimalarials

     g. Chloramphenicol

h. Nalidixic acid

i. Naphthalene mothballs

j. Primaquine

2. If hemolysis present support with transfusions

3. Education regarding food and drugs that cause hemolysis

Acute Idiopathic Thrombocytopenic Purpura (ITP)

- Definition: Usually a self-limited disorder characterized by a reduced platelet count; recurrent episodes may appear in 1 to 4% of children for many months or years

- Etiology/Incidence

  1. Results from production of autoantibodies against platelets

  2. Usually follows viral infection

  3. Peak onset between 2 and 5 years

- Clinical Findings

  1. Onset is usually acute

  2. Bruising and petechial rash occur 1 to 4 weeks following a viral infection; not always however preceded by illness

  3. Rash is asymmetric and usually most prominent over legs

  4. Epistaxis may be severe

- Differential Diagnosis

  1. Systemic lupus erythematosus

  2. Aplastic anemia

  3. AIDS

  4. Lymphoma

  5. Sepsis

- Diagnostic Tests/Findings

  1. CBC—platelet count less than 150,000

  2. Antiplatelet antibodies (found in 60% of children with ITP)

- Management/Treatment

  1. Excellent prognosis without treatment

2. Corticosteroids seem to reduce severity and duration, e.g., prednisone 1 to 2 mg/kg/24 hours in divided doses

3. Intravenous gamma globulin (IVIG)—used for active bleeding and noncompliance regarding activity restrictions (effectiveness controversial); may also be used in place of prolonged corticosteroid therapy

4. Prevention of trauma

5. Education of patient/family

   a. Bleeding precautions

   b. Avoid aspirin, aspirin-containing products

   c. Educate patient and family to report immediately severe, prolonged headaches

Hemophilia

- Definition: Blood coagulation disorders secondary to deficiencies of either factor VIII or factor IX

- Etiology/Incidence

  1. Hemophilia A/ Factor VIII:C deficiency

     a. Most common form of hemophilia (75% of cases)

     b. X linked inheritance

     c. Affects 1 in 10,000 males

  2. Hemophilia B/ Factor IX deficiency

     a. Accounts for 15% of all cases of hemophilia

     a. X linked inheritance

- Clinical Findings

  1. Hemophilia A and B (signs and symptoms depend on severity of factor deficiency)

     a. Prolonged bleeding anywhere in the body

     b. Subcutaneous and intramuscular bleeding is common

     c. Hemarthrosis—spontaneous bleeding into joints

     d. Bleeding from trauma or surgical procedure

        (1) Loss of tooth

        (2)   After circumcision

- Differential Diagnosis

   1.   Thromobocytopenia

   2.   Disorders of other clotting factors

       a. von Willebrand disease

       b. Vitamin K deficiency

   3.   Disseminated intravascular coagulation

- Diagnostic Tests/Findings

   1.   Hemophilia A

       a. PTT—prolonged

       b. Bleeding time—normal

       c. Factor VIII assay—decreased Factor VIII:C with normal Factor VIII:R

   2.   Hemophilia B

       a. PTT—prolonged

       b. Bleeding time—normal

       c. Factor IX—decreased

- Management/Treatment

   1.   Supportive care for bleeding diathesis

   2.   Replacement therapy

       a. Hemophilia A

          (1)   Cryoprecipitate or Factor VIII concentrate

          (2)   1-desamino-8-D-arginine-vasopressin acetate trihydrate (DDAVP)

       b. Hemophilia B—prothrombin complex replacement

   1.   Hepatitis B vaccine in infancy

   2.   Replacement therapy before surgery or tooth extractions

   3.   Regular exercise program to strengthen muscles around joints and to control bleeding

   4.   Genetic counseling after diagnosis is made

Thalassemias

- Definition: A group of hereditary microcytic anemias characterized by defective Hgb synthesis and ineffective erythropoiesis
- Etiology/Incidence
  1. Beta Thalassemia (Thalassemia Major; Cooley Anemia)
     a. Results from decreased synthesis of beta polypeptide chains
     b. Found in Mediterranean backgrounds
     c. Autosomal recessive trait
  2. Alpha Thalassemia (Thalassemia Minor)
     a. Etiology
        (1) Decreased synthesis of alpha chains due to gene deletion
        (2) Inherited in more complex fashion
        (3) Severe form in Asian populations
- Clinical Findings
  1. Beta thalassemia major (Cooley anemia)
     a. Severe hemolytic anemia
        (1) Develops approximately 2nd 6 months of life
        (2) Hepatosplenomegaly
     b. Bone marrow hyperplasia if untreated
        (1) Frontal bossing
        (2) Prominent cheeks
        (3) Maxillary hypertrophy
     c. Hemosiderosis from transfusions/iron therapy
  2. Alpha thalassemia minor (trait)
     a. Usually normal findings
     b. Mild anemia
- Differential Diagnosis
  1. Iron deficiency anemia
  2. Sideroblastic anemia
  3. Lead poisoning

■ Diagnostic Tests/Findings

TEST	MINOR (trait)	MAJOR
1. Hemoglobin electrophoresis	Increased Hgb A	Decreased Hgb A or absent
2. CBC with RBC indices	Microcytosis	Hypochromic microcytic anemia
3. Peripheral smear	Coarse basophilic stippling	Target cells prominent Basophilic stippling

■ Management/Treatment
   1. Major (Cooley's anemia)
      a. Transfusions
      b. Careful type and cross matching (prevent transfusion reactions)
      c. Chelating agents for hemosiderosis
      d. Splenectomy may be considered
   2. Trait (minor)
      a. No therapy
      b. Genetic counseling
   3. Psychosocial support

Cancers

■ Definition: A cellular malignancy which results in unregulated growth with a lack of differentiation

■ Etiology/Incidence
   1. Most occur with unknown etiology, in healthy children
   2. Predisposing factors
      a. Environmental
         (1) Radiation therapy
         (2) Solar radiation
         (3) Drugs e.g., diethylstilbestrol, immunosuppressive agents, anabolic androgenic steroids, chemotherapy
      b. Genetic

              (1)   Immunodeficiencies

                    (a) Wiskott Aldrich

                    (b) Blooms syndrome

                    (c) Fanconi's anemia

              (2)   Chromosome abnormalities—trisomy 21

              (3)   Neurocutaneous disorders—neurofibromatosis

              (4)   Hereditary

                    (a) Retinoblastoma

                    (b) Wilms tumor

         c. Viruses

              (1)   RNA viruses

              (2)   DNA viruses, e.g., Epstein-Barr (EB)

              (3)   Papova viruses

    3.   Incidence 1 out of 600 (1 to 14 year olds)

    4.   Second most common cause of death 1 to 15 year olds in U.S.

    5.   Leukemia is the most common type of childhood cancer

    6.   Brain tumors are the most common solid tumor

■ Clinical Findings (depends upon location)

    1.   Fever

    2.   Lymphadenopathy

    3.   Bone pain

    4.   Abdominal mass

    5.   Pancytopenia

    6.   Bleeding

    7.   Headache

■ Differential Diagnosis

    1.   Infection

    2.   Coagulation disorders

    3.   Trauma

    4.   Migraine/Sinusitis

    5.   Constipation, full bladder

- Diagnostic Tests/Findings
  1. Leukemia—bone marrow aspiration with greater than 25% blasts
  2. Solid tumor—biopsy to confirm a malignancy
- Management/Treatment
  1. Surgery
  2. Radiotherapy
  3. Chemotherapy
  4. Bone marrow transplant
  5. Psychosocial support
  6. Education regarding
     a. Disease process
     b. Side effects of treatment
     c. Compliance with treatment

Leukemia

- Definition: A disease characterized by the uncontrolled proliferation of immature white blood cells
- Etiology/Incidence
  1. Etiology unknown—theories involve environmental and genetic factors
  2. Most common childhood cancer
  3. Approximately 2500 new cases per year in children less than 15 years of age in the U.S.
     a. Majority of cases acute lymphoblastic leukemia (80%)
     b. Acute nonlymphoblastic leukemia (10 to 20%)
     c. Chronic leukemias (< 5%)
  4. Peak incidence 3 to 5 year olds
- Clinical Findings
  1. Early manifestations are anorexia, irritability, lethargy
  2. Later signs are fever, bleeding, pallor
  3. Bone pain

    4.   Lymphadenopathy

- Differential Diagnosis

    1.   Idiopathic thrombocytopenic purpura

    2.   Solid tumor with marrow involvement

    3.   Aplastic anemia

    4.   Acute infectious mononucleosis

    5.   Neutropenic conditions

- Diagnostic Tests/Findings

    1.   Complete blood count with differential

       a. May be normal

       b. Abnormal

          (1)   Anemia (most patients)

          (2)   Thrombocytopenia

          (3)   Neutropenia

          (4)   Leukocytosis

          (5)   Blast cells—present

    2.   Bone marrow aspiration—greater than 25% leukemic blasts

- Management/Treatment

    1.   Chemotherapy

    2.   Radiation therapy; cranial radiation usually for high risk patients only

    3.   Education regarding

       a. Side effects of chemotherapy

       b. Understanding leukemia

       c. Neutropenic/thrombocytopenic precautions

       d. Infection

    4.   Psychosocial support

Hodgkin's Disease

- Definition: A unique malignant disorder usually arising in lymph nodes
- Etiology/Incidence

1. Etiology unknown
2. Bimodal incidence—rare under 5 years; peaks between 15 and 34 years and again after 50
3. Twice as common in boys as in girls

- Clinical Findings

    1. Most common presenting sign is a painless, firm supraclavicular or cervical lymph node; usually no associated inflammation to explain lymphadenopathy
    2. Mediastinal mass—2/3 of patients; usually found "by accident" on chest radiograph; may produce cough
    3. Systemic symptoms—30% of children
        a. Unexplained fever
        b. Night sweats
        c. Weight loss
        d. Lethargy
        e. Easy fatigability

- Differential Diagnosis

    1. Lymphadenopathy—infectious cause
    2. Other malignancies
        a. Leukemia
        b. Soft tissue sarcomas
    3. Normal thymus in children with mediastinal mass

- Diagnostic Tests/Findings

    1. Needle biopsy of enlarged lymph node— presence of Reed Sternberg cells
    2. CBC—depressed level of one or more blood cell lines
    3. ESR—elevated
    4. Serum copper—elevated
    5. Serum ferritin—elevated
    6. Chest radiograph—explore possibility of mediastinal mass

- Management/Treatment

1. Staging (I to IV) made by clinical and laboratory tests
2. Radiation therapy alone or with chemotherapy
3. Chemotherapy
4. Education regarding
   a. Disease process
   b. Side effects of treatment
   c. Sperm banking
5. Psychosocial support

Wilms Tumor (Nephroblastoma)

- Definition: An embryonal adenomyosarcoma of the kidneys
- Etiology/Incidence
  1. Etiology unknown
  2. Most common malignant tumor of kidney in childhood
  3. Occurs primarily in children under 5 years old, median age about 3 years; males and females equally affected
- Clinical Findings
  1. Abdominal mass
     a. Most common presentation
     b. Usually found by a parent
     c. Child asymptomatic
  2. Less common presenting features
     a. Abdominal pain
     b. Hematuria
     c. Anemia
     d. Fever
     e. Malaise
     f. Hyptertension
  3. Can occur in association with congenital anomalies, e.g., hemihypertrophy, aniridia, genitourinary anomalies
- Differential Diagnosis

1. Hydronephrosis
2. Polycystic kidney disease
3. Rhabdomyosarcoma
4. Neuroblastoma
5. Lymphoma

- Diagnostic Tests/Findings
    1. Determine site of origin
    2. Chest radiography for pulmonary metastasis
        a. Ultrasonography—identification of mass
        b. CT abdomen—establish intrarenal origin of tumor and extent of tumor
    3. Bone scan skeletal survey for bone involvement

- Management/Treatment
    1. Therapy depends upon stage and histology of tumor (National Wilms Tumor Study [NWTS] staging criteria)
    2. Surgery
        a. Nephrectomy
        b. Removal of lymph nodes
    3. Radiotherapy to residual disease
    4. Chemotherapy—Actinomycin and Vincristine most common agents
    5. Psychosocial support
    6. Education regarding
        a. Disease process
        b. Side effects of treatment

Infectious Mononucleosis

- Definition: An acute disease characterized by fever, pharyngitis, lymphadenopathy; usually associated with heterophil antibodies and atypical lymphocytosis

- Etiology/Incidence
    1. Caused by Epstein-Barr virus (EBV)

2. Transmitted by oropharyngeal contact

   a. Kissing

   b. Contaminated objects

3. Incubation period 30 to 50 days

4. Commonly diagnosed in adolescents and young adults

- Clinical Manifestations

  1. Fever

  2. Malaise, fatigue

  3. Sore throat with moderate to severe tonsillopharyngitis with marked hypertrophy of tonsils often with exudate

  4. Cervical lymphadenopathy

  5. Hepatosplenomegaly

- Differential Diagnosis

  1. Measles

  2. Leukemia

  3. Viral illness

  4. Streptococcal pharyngitis

  5. Hepatitis

- Diagnostic Tests/Findings

  1. Monospot—positive

  2. Heterophil antibody test—titers greater than 1:28 or 1:40 considered positive (may be negative early in disease)

  3. CBC—leukocytosis with 10,000 to 20,000 cells/mm^3

     a. 60% lymphocytes

     b. 20 to 40% atypical lymphocytes

  4. Throat culture—to identify presence of beta hemolytic streptococcal infection

- Management/Treatment

  1. Reassurance that illness usually follows a self-limited course of about 2 to 3 weeks

  2. Symptomatic measures include

      a. Acetaminophen

      b. Saline gargles

      c. Sufficient fluid intake

3. No isolation

4. Education regarding mode of transmission

5. Positive throat cultures for group A beta hemolytic streptococci treated with penicillin or erythromycin; ampillin or amoxicillin may elicit a generalized rash in some patients

Infection

- Definition: "Invasion and multiplication of microorganisms in body tissues, which may be clinically inapparent or result in local cellular injury due to competitive metabolism, toxins, intracellular replication, or antigen-antibody response" (Dorland, 1988, p. 334)

- Etiology/Incidence

  1. Caused by an infecting pathogen (viruses, bacteria, mycoplasmas, rickettsiae, chlamydiae, fungi, protozoas, and larger parasites such as roundworms and flatworms)

  2. Factors determining susceptibility and manifestation of infection

     a. Virulence, invasiveness and organ preference of infecting organism

     b. Site of the infection

     c. Patient's underlying condition

         (1)   Immunodeficiency

         (2)   Nutritional status

         (3)   Race, sex, temperature, fatigue

     d. Age of the child

         (1)   Neonatal period

             (a) *E. coli* most common pathogen

         (2)   Infants and children, common pathogens

             (a) *H. influenza*

             (b) Pneumococci

             (c) Meningococci

      e. Environmental risks

         (1)   Day care/school

         (2)   Exposure to sick person/animal

         (3)   Trauma

■ Clinical Findings

    1. Local infection

       a. Erythema

       b. Pain

       c. Edema

       d. Warm to touch

       e. Fever

    2. Systemic

       a. Fever

       b. Malaise

       c. Anorexia

       d. Rash

       e. Poor feeding

       f. Lymphadenopathy

■ Differential Diagnosis

    1. Allergy

    2. Immunodeficiency disease

    3. AIDS

    4. Cancer

    5. Autoimmune disease

■ Diagnostic Tests/Findings

    1. Culture/gram stain of infected site— positive

    2. CBC—increased or decreased WBC count

       a. Bacteria—shift to the left

       b. Viral—lymphocytosis

       c. Fungal—associated with immune deficiencies with prolonged antibiotic therapy

3. ESR—elevated

4. Physical examination—abnormal findings suggestive of infection

5. Radiographic studies

- Management/Treatment

  1. Antimicrobial therapy

  2. Symptomatic support

     a. Fluids

     b. Acetaminophen

     c. Rest

  3. Follow-up

  4. Reassurance/support

  5. Education for

     a. Isolation

     b. Drug, dose, side effects

Septicemia

- Definition: Systemic disease associated with the presence and persistence of pathogenic microorganisms or their toxins in the blood

- Etiology/Incidence

  1. Uncommon in children over 3 months of age with normal immune systems

     a. Most common organisms

        (1) *H. influenzae* type b

        (2) *N. meningitides*

     b. Decreased incidence with *H. influenzae* vaccine

  2. Common in immunosuppressed child

     a. Causative organisms

        (1) *Pseudomonas aeruginosa*

        (2) Staph aureus

- Clinical Findings

1. Normal immune system
   a. Fever
   b. Irritability
   c. Child will appear ill
2. Immunosuppressed—fever may be only sign

■ Differential Diagnosis
   1. Infectious disease
      a. Rocky mountain spotted fever
      b. Toxic shock syndrome
      c. Viral sepsis
      d. Fungal infections
   2. Non-infectious
      a. Hemorrhagic shock
      b. Anaphylactic shock

■ Diagnostic Tests/Findings
   1. CBC—WBC count greater than 15,000/mm³ (shift to the left)
   2. Blood cultures—positive; cerebrospinal fluid culture—positive
   3. Chest radiograph—identify pneumonia
   4. Prothrombin time-prolonged
   5. Fibrinogen levels—reduced

■ Management/Treatment
   1. Broad spectrum antibiotics for gm(+), gm(−) bacteria
   2. Septic shock—refer
   3. Education regarding
      a. Disease process
      b. Treatment
      c. Follow-up
   4. Prevention against *H. influenzae* type b (see Health Maintenance and Promotion chapter)

Acquired Immunodeficiency Syndrome (AIDS)

- Definition: A secondary immunodeficiency syndrome characterized by opportunistic infections, malignancies, neurologic dysfunction and a variety of other syndromes

- Etiology/Incidence

  1. Caused by RNA cytopathic human retroviruses, specifically, human immunodeficiency virus type 1 (HIV-1) and less commonly HIV-2

  2. Seventh leading cause of death in children 1 to 4 years old

  3. Sixth leading cause of death in 15 to 24 years old

  4. Transmission

     a. Most infected children in U.S. have been born to families in which one or both parents have HIV infection (AAP, 1994)

     b. 80% of pediatric AIDS cases acquire infection perinatally

     c. 15 to 20% infected with contaminated blood

  5. Infants usually develop symptoms before age 2

- Clinical Manifestations

  1. Recurrent infections

  2. Failure to thrive

  3. Low birth weight (small for gestational age)

  4. Interstitial pneumonia

  5. Lymphadenopathy

  6. Hepatosplenomegaly

  7. Oral candidiasis

  8. Developmental delay

  9. Skin rashes

  10. Parotitis

  11. Diarrhea

  12. Gastrointestinal bleeding

  13. Facial dysmorphism

  14. Encephalopathic manifestations, e.g., visual impairment, motor

abnormalities, seizures, microcephaly, speech and language, disabilities, ataxia, spasticity, peripheral neuropathies

- Differential Diagnosis

    1. Congenital infections—TORCHS

    2. Primary cellular immunodeficiencies

        a. SCID—severe combined immunodeficiency disease

        b. D. Jorge syndrome

    3. Hematologic disorders

    4. Secondary immunodeficiency

- Diagnostic Tests/Findings

    1. Enzyme-linked immunosorbent (ELISA) HIV screening test—positive assays

    2. Western blot assay—confirmatory test

    3. Rising HIV antibody titer—maternal vs infant

    4. HIV antigen detection

        a. HIV culture

        b. Detection of p24 antigen

        c. Polymerase chain reaction (PCR)

    5. Serum IgG—over 1800 mg/dL at 1 year of age or 2300 mg/dL at 2 years of age typical of AIDS

- Management/Treatment

    1. Current therapy limited to date

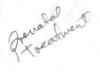

    2. Antiretroviral therapy—a standard of care for all children with symptomatic HIV infection

        a. Zidovudine (formerly AZT)

            (1) Children < 12 years, 720 mg/m²/day (maximum 800 mg/day)

            (2) Children ≥ 12 years, 500 to 600 mg/day in 3 to 6 divided doses (AAP, 1994)

        b. Didanosine (DDI)

            (1) Alternative therapy for children who cannot tolerate zidovudine or with disease progression on zidovudine

therapy

    (2)   Oral—200 to 300 mg/m^2/day in 2 to 3 divided doses

    (3)   Adequate buffering of stomach acid and no food or drink 30 minutes before and after drug administration (AAP, 1994)

3.   Prophylaxis with immune globulin for recurrent bacterial infections or demonstration of B cell dysfunction

4.   Education regarding transmission, prevention of viral infection

5.   Psychosocial/emotional support

6.   Nutritional support

7.   Immunizations

Questions

Select the best answer

1. A 1-day old infant is noted to be jaundiced while his mother is breast feeding him. The most likely cause of this would be

   a. Breast feeding
   b. ABO incompatibility
   c. Physiologic jaundice
   d. Sepsis

2. Most children with ABO incompatibility are managed by

   a. Phototherapy
   b. Exchange transfusion
   c. No therapy
   d. Discontinuing breast feeding

3. Rh negative mothers should be immunized with RhoGam for all the following except

   a. After delivery of first baby only
   b. After an abortion
   c. After delivery of a stillborn
   d. After delivery of first baby and subsequent babies

4. A 2-year old infant is pale, fat, tachycardic with a systolic murmur. His CBC reveals a Hgb < 3 g/dL. Immediate treatment for this child includes

   a. Diet counseling
   b. Immediate iron therapy
   c. Refer for transfusion therapy
   d. Decrease milk consumption

5. Differential diagnosis for iron deficiency anemia includes all the following except

   a. Lead poisoning
   b. Beta-thalassemia trait
   c. Alpha-thalassemia trait
   d. Idiopathic thrombocytopenia purpura

6. Diagnostic tests for sickle cell anemia include

   a. Hgb electrophoresis
   b. Complete blood count
   c. N.B.T. test

   d. Coomb's test

7. Clinical findings in children with sickle cell disease begin

   a. 1½ to 2 months of age
   b. At birth
   c. After 4 to 6 months of age, usually
   d. After a year

8. Which food or drugs should be avoided in G-6-PD disease

   a. Acetylsalicylic acid
   b. Kidney beans
   c. Penicillin
   d. Foods high in calcium

9. Clinical manifestations of G-6-PD may include all the following except

   a. Jaundice
   b. Lymphadenopathy
   c. Anemia
   d. Back pain

10. The most common course of thrombocytopenia in children is

   a. Follows trauma
   b. Follows autoimmune diseases
   c. Follows a viral illness
   d. Follows drug ingestion

11. Which drug should be avoided in children with thrombocytopenia

   a. Tylenol
   b. Ceclor
   c. Aspirin
   d. Amoxacillin

12. Clinical findings in a child with beta-thalassemia may include all but

   a. Hepatosplenomegaly
   b. Mild anemia
   c. Severe anemia
   d. Frontal bossing

13. Diagnostic findings for beta-thalassemia major include all the following except

   a. Decreased or absent Hgb A on electrophoresis
   b. Target cells on the peripheral smear
   c. Hypochromic, microcytic anemia
   d. Heinz bodies

14. Which of the following is consistent with physiologic jaundice

    a. Onset of jaundice within first day of life
    b. Onset of jaundice after third day of life
    c. Onset of jaundice after first week of life
    d. Onset of jaundice 2nd to 3rd day of life

15. Important laboratory tests to exclude pathologic causes of jaundice include all the following except

    a. Blood typing of infant only
    b. Coomb's test
    c. Bilirubin level
    d. CBC with peripheral blood smear

16. The majority of children diagnosed with leukemia have

    a. Acute non-lymphoblastic leukemia
    b. Chronic lymphoblastic leukemia
    c. Lymphoma
    d. Acute lymphoblastic leukemia

17. The diagnosis of leukemia is made by

    a. A complete blood count with peripheral blasts
    b. A bone marrow aspirate
    c. Biopsy of an enlarged lymph node
    d. The presence of hepatosplenomegaly, lymphadenopathy and petechiae on physical examination

18. The most common infectious pathogen in the neonatal period is

    a. *S. aureus*
    b. *C. difficile*
    c. Group B strep
    d. *E. coli*

19. Which of the following would be consistent with a systemic infection

    a. Pain
    b. Increased WBC
    c. Poor feeding
    d. Edema

20. John is a 20-year old college student with a severe sore throat. On physical exam you note enlarged tonsils with large patches of exudate, pharynx inflamed and non-tender posterior cervical adenopathy. John states he feels tired all the time. What is the most likely diagnosis?

a. Infectious mononucleosis
b. Leukemia
c. Streptococcal pharyngitis
d. Tonsillitis

21. Three of John's roommates are concerned that they will catch what John has. What can you tell them about the transmission of this disease.

a. Not very contagious
b. Highly contagious
c. Only contagious if you are immunosuppressed
d. Contagious by direct contact with skin

22. Important diagnostic laboratory studies to obtain in a patient most likely to have infectious mononucleosis includes

a. Blood culture
b. Heterophil antibody test
c. A chest radiograph
d. Complete blood count with a differential

23. Common clinical findings in patients with Hodgkin's disease at diagnosis include

a. Painful lymphadenopathy
b. Soft, non-tender lymphadenopathy
c. Firm, painful lymphadenopathy
d. Painless, firm lymphadenopathy

24. Important information to obtain in the initial history of a patient with probable Hodgkin's disease would be

a. History of fatigue
b. History of bruising
c. History of weight gain
d. History of recent infection

25. The most common clinical presentation in a child with Wilms tumor is

a. Hematuria
b. Abdominal pain
c. Abdominal mass
d. Anemia

26. Which malignancy in childhood is associated with aniridia?

a. Wilms tumor
b. Neuroblastoma
c. Leukemia

  d. Hodgkin's disease

27. Most children with AIDS acquire the infection through

  a. Contaminated blood
  b. Breast feeding
  c. Prenatal transmission
  d. Perinatal transmission

28. All of the following are clinical manifestations of AIDS except

  a. Interstitial pneumonia, diarrhea, lymphadenopathy
  b. Night sweats, interstitial pneumonia, conjunctivitis
  c. Interstitial pneumonia, failure to thrive, skin rashes
  d. Lymphadenopathy, oral candidiasis, developmental delay

29. A predominant clinical finding in hemophilia is

  a. Hemarthrosis
  b. Fatigue and weight loss
  c. Developmental delay
  c. G.I. bleeding

30. The diagnostic evaluation of a child suspected of septicemia would include all of the following except

  a. CBC with differential
  b. EKG
  c. Blood culture
  d. Urine culture

31. Treatment of Hemophilia A consists of

  a. Prothrombin complex replacement
  b. Platelet replacement
  c. Factor VIII concentrate
  d. Plasma concentrate

Answer Key

1.	b	17.	b
2.	c	18.	d
3.	a	19.	c
4.	c	20.	a
5.	d	21.	a
6.	a	22.	b
7.	c	23.	d
8.	a	24.	a
9.	b	25.	c
10.	c	26.	a
11.	c	27.	d
12.	b	28.	b
13.	d	29.	a
14.	d	30.	b
15.	a	31.	c
16.	d		

Bibliography

A-Kader, H. H., & Balistreri, W. F. (1993). Unconjugated hyperbilirubinemia. In F. D. Burg, J. R. Ingelfinger & E. R. Wald (Eds), *Gellis & Kagan's current pediatric therapy* (14th ed.). (pp. 218-219). Philadelphia: W. B. Saunders.

American Academy of Pediatrics, (1994). *Report of the committee on infectious diseases* (23rd ed.). Elk Grove Village, IL: American Academy of Pediatrics

Avery, M. E., & First, L. R. (1994). *Pediatric medicine* (2nd ed.). Baltimore: Williams & Wilkins.

Corrigan, J. J. (1992). Hemorrhagic disorders. In R. Behrman, V. C. Vaugan (Eds.), *Nelson textbook of pediatrics* (pp. 1275-1287). Philadelphia: W. B. Saunders

Dorland, W. A. (1988). *Dorland's illustrated medical dictionary* (27th ed.). Philadelphia: W. B. Saunders

Edelson, P. J. (1991. Childhood AIDS. *Pediatric Clinics of North America, 38*(1).

Esposito, N. W. (1992). Thalassemias: Simple screening for hereditary anemias. *Nurse Practitioner, 17*, 50-61.

Feigin, R. D. (1990). Bacterial infections. In F. Oski (Ed.), *Principles and practice of pediatrics* (pp. 1053-1150). Philadelphia: J. B. Lippincott.

Gotoff, S. P. (1992). The Fetus and the neonatal infant. In R. Behrman, V. C. Vaugan (Eds.), *Nelson textbook of pediatrics* (pp. 476-486). Philadelphia: W. B. Saunders.

Hockenberry, M., Coody, D., & Bennett, B. (1990). Childhood cancers: Incidence, etiology, diagnosis and treatment. *Pediatric Nursing, 16*, 239-245.

Leventhal, B. G., & Kato, G. J. (1990). Childhood Hodgkin and non-Hodgkin lymphomas. *Pediatrics in Review, 12*, 171-179.

Palis, J. (1992). Iron deficiency anemia. In R. A. Hoekelman (Ed.), *Primary pediatric care* (pp. 1308-1313). St. Louis: Mosby Year Book.

Ruccione, K. S. (1992). Wilms' tumor: A paradigm, a parallel, and a puzzle. *Seminars in Oncology Nursing, 8*, 241-251.

Segal, G. B. (1988). Anemia. *Pediatrics In Review, 10*, 77-88.

Dermatological Disorders and Contagious Diseases

Ellen Rudy Clore

Atopic Dermatitis (Eczema)

- Definition: Chronic inflammatory skin disorder
- Etiology/Incidence
    1. Exact cause unknown
    2. Contributing factors consist of
        a. Family history of atopy, allergic rhinitis or asthma
        b. Emotional factors
        c. Environmental factors (allergens, food, fungi, viruses)
        d. Pharmacologic factors
    3. Acute form (infantile) develops between 2 months and 5 years of age
    4. 5 to 7% of all children affected (Cohen, 1992)
    5. 50% of children will have resolution by adolescence
- Clinical Findings
    1. Infantile
        a. Erythematous, weeping vesicles with crusting
            (1) Common sites—face, scalp, extensor aspects of the arms and legs
        b. Intense pruritis
    2. Childhood/adolescence
        a. Increased dryness
        b. Fissures and lichenification
        c. Intense pruritis
        d. Common sites of involvement are wrists, ankles and antecubital and popliteal fossae
- Differential Diagnosis
    1. Allergic contact dermatitis
    2. Scabies
    3. Psoriasis

4. Seborrheic dermatitis

5. Papular acrodermatitis

6. Immune disorders

7. Metabolic diseases

■ Diagnostic Tests/Findings

1. Usually by clinical manifestations

2. IgE antibodies—elevated

3. Culture if secondary infection present

■ Management/Treatment

1. Burow solution or plain tap water compresses or baths

2. Decrease bathing to a few times a week only

3. Benadryl or atarax for pruritis

4. 0.5 to 1% hydrocortisone creme every 4 hours

5. Antibiotics for secondary infections

6. Lubricate skin after bathing or swimming

7. Medical referral for poor response to therapy

8. Dietary management

9. Decrease stress

10. Emotional support—refer to counselor if decreased self-esteem or coping problems

11. Avoid offending agents

12. Emphasize that management involves compliance with total regime

Contact Dermatitis

■ Definition: An acute or chronic inflammation, produced by substances in contact with the skin

■ Etiology/Incidence

1. Contributing factors consist of

    a. Exposure to sensitizing agents such as:

    (1) Plants (poison ivy)

    (2) Pollen/dust

        (3)   Soaps, detergents, fabrics

        (4)   Perfume, cosmetics

        (5)   Mildew, fungus

        (6)   Foods

    b. May develop within 7 to 10 days up to years following initial exposure; once area has become sensitized, re-exposure to offending allergen may result in acute dermatitis in 8 to 12 hours

    c. Direct contact by an irritant (nonallergic reaction)

        (1)   Most common in infancy when skin integrity is easily compromised with irritants such as urine, feces, soaps, detergents

- Clinical Findings: Range from transient redness to severe swelling with bulla formation; pruritis and vesiculation

- Differential Diagnosis

    1. Drug reactions

    2. Atopic dermatitis

- Diagnostic Tests/Findings:

    1. Patch testing—to detect chemical allergen and distinguish allergic contact dermatitis from other forms

- Management/Treatment

    1. Antipruritics

        a. Calamine lotion

        b. Benadryl

        c. Atarax

    2. Medical referral for intense cases—steroids may be indicated

    3. Cool baths or compresses to relieve pruritis

    4. Avoidance of causative agent

Diaper Dermatitis

- Definition: Erythema, scaling, and/or ulceration of the skin in the diaper area

- Etiology/Incidence

1. Contributing factors include

    a. Prolonged contact with urine and feces

    b. Friction

    c. Synthetic components of paper diapers, or rubber or plastic pants, diaper wipes or laundry products

    d. Caregiver neglect

    e. *C. albicans*

2. Common before age of 2 years; usually begins between 1st and 2nd month; peak age 9 to 12 months

- Clinical Findings

    1. *Candida albicans* (monilia)

        a. Perianal inflammation

        b. Beefy-red, shiny, confluent erythema involving inguinal creases, genitalia, with satellite oval lesions

    2. Contact diaper dermatitis

        a. Erythema in convex surfaces of thighs, buttocks, perineum, waist area, lower abdomen; sparing of inguinal folds unless oils or lotions are offending agents

        b. In severe irritation, maceration; oozing and crusting

    3. Seborrheic diaper dermatitis

        a. Sharply demarcated rash with satellite lesions and yellowish-oily scales—skin folds involved

- Differential Diagnosis

    1. Eruptions associated with HIV or immune deficiencies

    2. Atopic dermatitis

- Diagnostic Tests/Findings: KOH preparation—budding yeast present if monilia

- Management/Treatment

    1. Primary treatment drying involved area and prevent contact with irritant

    2. Candida infections

        a. Nystatin cream with each diaper change

      b. Oral Nystatin if thrush present in mouth

  3. Neosporin-G cream q.i.d.

  4. Low-potency anti-inflammatory steroid cream t.i.d.

  5. Alternate use of hydrocortisone 1% cream and Nystatin cream usually results in considerable improvement

  6. Education

      a. Prevention and management

         (1) Frequent diaper changes (incidence decreased with 8 or more changes)

         (2) Keep skin dry-expose to air frequently

         (3) Wash diaper area with warm water at each change; limit use of soap

         (4) Proper laundering of diapers

         (5) Plastic and rubber pants avoided when possible

  6. Encourage fluids

  7. Assess for allergies

  8. Medical referral if diaper rash does not improve within 2 days

Seborrheic Dermatitis

- Definition: An inflammatory scaling disorder of the scalp, face
- Etiology/Incidence

  1. Cause unknown; thought to be related to dysfunction of sebaceous glands

  2. Occurs in neonate, infant and resolves spontaneously by 8 to 12 months of age

- Clinical Findings

  1. Most common site is scalp with erythematous, greasy salmon-colored oval scaly lesions (cradle cap)

  2. Rash may extend to face, neck, intertriginous and flexural areas; trunk and diaper area

- Differential Diagnosis: Atopic dermatitis; contact dermatitis; tinea corporis; scabies, tinea capitis, psoriasis

- Diagnostic Tests/Findings: None
- Management/Treatment
  1. Antiseborrheic shampoo—requires contact with scalp for 5 to 10 minutes to soften and loosen scales; avoid contact of shampoo with eyes
  2. Instruct parents that gentle scrubbing is safe and necessary. Use of toothbrush will facilitate scale removal
  3. Topical steroids for treatment of facial involvement

Sunburn

- Definition: Erythema and skin tenderness secondary to sun exposure
- Etiology/Incidence
  1. Results from overexposure of the skin to ultraviolet rays of 290-320 nm wavelength
  2. Contributing factors include
     a. Certain medications, foods, and diseases
     b. Fair-skinned children with less melanin protection
     c. Intense sun exposure can also produce sunburn in children with dark skin
- Clinical Findings
  1. Erythema and skin tenderness begin 30 minutes to 4 hours after sun exposure
  2. Intense exposure—edema and blistering occur
  3. Severe burns
     a. Nausea
     b. Chills/fever
     c. Abdominal cramping
     d. Headache
     e. Dehydration
- Differential Diagnosis
  1. Chemical burns
  2. Allergic reaction

- Diagnostic Tests/Findings: None
- Management/Treatment
  1. Inhibitors of prostaglandin synthesis such as aspirin and indomethacin may decrease symptoms if given soon after exposure
  2. Cool compresses or tepid baths for 20 minutes
  3. Encourage fluids
  4. Avoid use of topical anesthetic agents; sensitizing and transient in their relief
  5. Medical referral for severe burns
  6. Education
     a. Premature aging of skin
     b. Cancer—melanoma; blistering sunburns in childhood and adolescence increase risk of melanoma in later years
     c. Avoid sun exposure between 10:00 a.m. and 2:00 p.m.
     d. Use of sunscreen agents with sun protection factor (SPF) of 15 or greater
     e. Use of protective clothing, hats and umbrellas

Burns

- Definition: Injury to skin from thermal energy
- Etiology/Incidence
  1. Approximately 1 million children affected each year; 10% require hospitalization
  2. 3rd leading cause of accidental deaths
  3. 80-90% of injuries are potentially preventable
  4. Boys are burned twice as often as girls
  5. Scald burns most common during 1st two years
  6. Flame burns most common in children over 3 year
- Clinical Findings
  1. First-degree
     a. Erythematous epidermis
     b. Pain

2. Second-degree

   a. Mottled red skin appearance

   b. Blistering

   c. Moist to touch

   d. Extremely painful to touch and exposure

3. Third-degree

   a. Dry or waxlike, black or white appearance of skin

- Differential Diagnosis: Accidental vs purposeful child abuse

- Diagnostic Tests/Findings: None

- Management/Treatment

   1. Remove clothing to stop burning process

   2. Wound cleansing with water or saline and mild antibacterial solution

   3. Blisters should be left intact; open blistered areas should be debrided

   4. Silver sulfadiazine cream topically b.i.d.

   5. Dry, sterile occlusive dressing

   6. Acetaminophen or codeine for pain relief

   7. Encourage oral fluids

   8. Tetanus immunization if necessary

   9. Follow-up wound assessment

   10. Refer more extensive burns

Pityriasis Rosea

- Definition: An acute, self limiting disease characterized by superficial scaly lesions on the trunk and extremities

- Etiology/Incidence

   1. Unknown, although thought to be viral in origin

   2. Frequently seen in children, adolescents, and young adults, but rarely in infants

   3. Common in spring and autumn

- Clinical Manifestations

   1. Herald patch—scaly with central clearing, salmon colored,

erythmatous border; usually precedes generalized eruption (resembles ring worm infection, initially)

2. Rash—lesions smaller than herald patch, scaly and papulovesicular

    a. Localized to back, neck, extremities, rarely on face, hands, or feet

    b. Axes of lesions follow cleavage lines, creating a "Christmas tree" configuration on the back

3. Systemic symptoms are usually absent

4. Pruritis

5. Hypopigmentation may occur following clearing of rash; more pronounced in black population but eventually disappears

- Differential Diagnosis

1. Secondary syphilis (most important)

2. Tinea corpris

3. Viral exanthems

4. Drug reactions

- Diagnostic Tests/Findings: None

1. VDRL only to rule out secondary syphilis not a confirmation test for Pityriasis rosea

- Management/Treatment

1. Relief of pruritis

    a. Cool compresses, calamine lotion, antihistamines

    b. Sunlight exposure (artificial or natural)

2. Educate parents

    a. No need to isolate child

    b. Keep child's fingernails short

    c. Rash disappears in reverse order that it appears in 6-8 weeks

Cellulitis

- Definition: Deep locally diffuse infection of the skin with systemic manifestations; usually involves the face or an extremity

- Etiology/Incidence

1. Caused by streptococci, or *H. influenza* type b

2. May be hematogenous or lymphatic source

■ Clinical Findings

1. Lymphangitis "streaking" common

2. Regional lymphadenopathy

3. Fever, swelling; heat, tenderness of involved skin

4. Malaise

5. Violaceous (bluish) hue in *H. influenzae* type b facial cellulitis

6. Localized skin trauma may be present

■ Differential Diagnosis

1. Trauma

2. Thrombophlebitis

3. Pressure erythema

4. Giant urticeria

5. Contact dermatitis

6. Erythema infectiosum

■ Diagnostic Tests/Findings

1. CBC—leukocytosis

2. Cultures from skin, blood—identify pathogen

3. Cerebrospinal fluid culture—identify pathogen in facial cellulitis

■ Management/Treatment

1. Cellulitis of extremity—home management

   a. Oral antibiotics e.g., erythromycin, dicloxacillin, cephalexin

   b. Warm soaks

2. Rest

3. Immobilization of affected area

4. Hot moist compresses to area

5. Extensive cellulitis, especially around a joint or on the face—hospitalization

   a. Oral antibiotics for mild involvement, e.g., amoxicillin-clavulanate or trimethoprim-sulfamethoxazole (for facial cellutis)

      b. Parenteral therapy specific to offending organism, e.g., cephalosporin (2nd or 3rd generation) for more advanced disease

  6. Educate concerning complications

      a. Meningitis

      b. Septic arthritis

Impetigo

- Definition: A superficial vesiculopustular skin infection; begins with discrete or grouped vesicles, on an erythematous base resulting in golden crusted erosions

- Etiology/Incidence
  1. Group A ß hemolytic streptococcus, staphylococci; *S. aureus* more recently implicated
  2. Transmitted by person to person contact
  3. Most prevalent in hot, humid summer months

- Clinical Findings
  1. Multiple lesions of varying sizes and shapes, with vesicles, blebs, and yellow crusts on an erythematous base
  2. Regional lymphadenopathy not uncommon with extensive involvement
  3. Face, neck and limbs are usual site, but lesions may appear on other parts of body

- Differential Diagnosis
  1. Insect bites
  2. Herpes simplex (most common)
  3. Contact dermatitis, eczema, seborrhea, fungal infections

- Diagnostic Testing/Findings
  1. None routinely done
  2. Positive culture for staphylococci and/or streptococci

- Management/Treatment
  1. Regular local cleansing with antibacterial soaps
  2. Mupirocin topical therapy (pseudomonic acid cream) applied sparingly t.i.d.

3. Oral antibiotic therapy with erythromycin is often used in the absence of constitutional symptoms

4. Semisynthetic penicillins or cephalosporin are useful, especially with *S. aureus* infection

5. Assessment of siblings and friends because of communicability

6. Educate parents concerning proper hand washing and separate linens

7. Shorten fingernails to discourage scratching and minimize secondary infections

8. Review most common complication of acute glomerulonephritis

9. Refer to physician if no improvement seen after 24 hours

Tinea

- Definition: Superficial infections caused by dermatophytes-fungi that invade dead tissues of the skin

  1. Tinea Corporis—ringworm infection of the body

  2. Tinea Pedis—ringworm of the feet (athlete's foot)

  3. Tinea Capitis—ringworm of the scalp

  4. Tinea Cruris—"jock itch"

- Etiology/Incidence

  1. Tinea Corporis—*Microsporum canis, Trichophyton mentagrophytes*; acquired by direct contact with infected persons or contact with infected scales or hairs

  2. Tinea Pedis—*Trichophyton mentagrophytes* and *Tricophyton rubrum;* uncommon in young children

  3. Tinea Capitis—*Microsporum canis* or *Trichophyton tonsurans*; usually limited to prepubertal children

  4. Tinea Cruris—*Trichophyton mentagrophytes* and *Epidermophyton flocossum*; unusual before adolescence

- Clinical Findings

  1. Tinea Corporis—usually consists of one or several circular erythematous patches with papular, scaly, annular borders with clear centers on the body

  2. Tinea Pedis

   a. Affects interdigital spaces and plantar surface of the arch

   b. Pruritis

   c. Toe web lesions are often macerated with erythema and scaling borders

   3. Tinea Capitis

   a. Inflamed, circumscribed pustules or inflamed scaly dry patches with broken hairs

   b. Hair loss is common manifestation

   c. Secondary bacterial infection and scarring may occur

   4. Tinea Cruris: Scaly, erythematous pruritic lesions on inner thighs and inguinal creases

- Differential Diagnosis

   1. Tinea Corporis

   a. Pityriasis rosea (herald patch), dermatitis

   b. Psoriasis, secondary syphilis, lupus erythematosus

   2. Tinea Pedis: Atopic and contact dermatitis; scabies

   3. Tinea Capitis

   a. Traction alopecia

   b. Alopecia areata

   c. Trichotillomania

   d. Seborrheic dermatitis

   4. Tinea Cruris

   a. Intertrigo

   b. Contact allergic dermatitis

   c. Candidiasis

- Diagnostic Tests/Findings

   1. Tinea Corporis—KOH wet mount preparations positive

   2. Tinea Pedis—KOH wet mount preparations positive

   3. Tinea Capitis

   a. Wood's light examination—*M. canis* fluoresces, but *T. Tonsurans* does not

 b. KOH examination—if positive hyphae may be seen

 c. Fungal culture—positive if culture turns color

 4. Tinea Cruris—KOH examination for hyphae will confirm the diagnosis

- Management/Treatment

 1. Tinea Corporis, Pedis, Cruris—

  a. Topical therapy in the form of clortrimazole, econazole, miconazole, tolnaftate; 2 to 4 weeks of therapy

 2. Tinea Capitis—griseofulvin for 8 to 12 weeks recommended for all forms

 3. Education

  a. Proper hygiene

  b. Transmission

  c. Clean clothes and socks; well ventilated foot wear; loose cotton underwear (Jock itch)

  d. Medication compliance and side effects

 4. Assess close contacts

 5. Follow-up every 2 weeks depending upon response to therapy

Warts

- Definition: Epidermal, virus-induced tumors of the skin with a variety of clinical presentations

- Etiology/Incidence

 1. Human papillomavirus (HPV)

 2. Incidence of all types of warts is highest in children and adolescents

 3. Transmitted by direct contact and by autoinoculation

- Clinical Findings

 1. Common warts (almost universal in the population)

  a. Solitary flesh-colored papule with an irregular, scaly surface; may be found anywhere on the skin but mostly on hands, knees, elbows

  b. Firm, may have black pinpoint spots (thrombosed capillaries)

 2. Plantar warts

      a. Common on the plantar surface of foot

      b. Papule is pushed in to the skin and results in the verrucous surface appearing level with the skin surface; can be exquisitely tender, especially with weight-bearing such as normal walking

   3. Genital warts (condyloma acuminata)

      a. Can be, but are not always acquired by sexual contact

      b. Multiple confluent papules with an irregular surface; appear on genitals, genital mucosa and adjacent skin or both

- Differential Diagnosis

   1. Callus, corn from Plantar warts

   2. Syphilitic lesions from Genital warts

   3. Foreign body reaction from Common and Plantar warts

- Management/Treatment

   1. A wide variety of treatment modalities exist

   2. Curettage; electrocautery; cryotherapy (liquid nitrogen)—effective at any cutaneous site

   3. Common warts—cryotherapy, salicylic acid paints, cantharidin

   4. Plantar warts—salicylic acid paints, salicylic acid plasters, cantharidin

   5. Genital warts—podophyllin, cryotherapy, trichloracetic acid

   6. Education

      a. Repeated irritation may cause enlargement of warts

      b. Most warts will disappear without treatment

      c. Wear shoes that fit to avoid pressure

Insect Bites or Stings

- Definition: A wound inflicted by the bite or sting of an insect

- Etiology/Incidence

   1. Bites

      a. Caused by the bite of insects, such as mosquito (most common), flies, fleas, gnats, bedbugs, spiders

      b. Usually found on exposed, unclothed body

      c. Common in warmer months

2. Stings—caused by the sting of venomous insects belonging to the order of Hymenoptera (wasps, bees, fire ants)

- Clinical Findings
  1. Bites
     a. Discrete number of scattered erythematous papules and plaques all in same stage of development. May have puncta or vesicles
     b. Papular uticaria possible
     c. Pruritis
  2. Stings—four common categories
     a. Small local reaction, short lived, painful, pruritic uticarial reaction
     b. Large local reaction—diameter of swelling exceeds 5 cm; may last up to a week
     c. Mild systemic reaction—cutaneous and GI symptoms
     d. Severe systemic reaction—cardiovascular symptoms
- Differential Diagnosis
  1. Bullous impetigo
  2. Chickenpox
- Diagnostic Tests/Findings: None
- Management/Treatment
  1. Remove stinger if present by scraping, not squeezing
  2. Treat local reaction with ice, calamine lotion, topical corticosteroid creams, antihistimines, oral analgesics
  3. Education
     a. Avoidance of wearing bright colored and flowered patterned clothes, scented cosmetics and perfumes
     b. Keep food and garbage covered
     c. Use adequate foot protection
     d. Use screening for windows and doors

Animal Bites

- Definition: A wound inflicted by the bite of an animal
- Etiology/Incidence

1. 2 million persons bitten by animals annually
2. 90% of bites by dogs
3. 50% of bites require no medical treatment; 10% require suturing, 2% require hospitalization
4. Peak age is children aged 5 to 14 years; boys bitten twice as much as girls
5. Most instances of bites are provoked by humans

- Clinical Findings
    1. Skin lacerations or avulsions or punctures
    2. Risk of infection depends upon
        a. Location of bite
        b. Type of wound
        c. Time of bite before seeking medical attention
        d. Type of animal

- Differential Diagnosis: None

- Diagnostic Tests/Findings: None, unless wound becomes infected

- Management/Treatment
    1. Meticulous wound care: Clean with soap and water, irrigate with saline
    2. Debride devitalized tissue
    3. Elevation and immobilization for extremity injuries
    4. Tetanus prophylaxis if indicated
    5. Education
        a. Responsible pet care
        b. Avoidance of strange animals

Cat Scratch Disease

- Definition: An infection characterized by subacute regional adenitis following the bite or scratch of a cat

- Etiology/Incidence: Caused by a small gram negative pleomorphic baccili

- Clinical Findings
    1. History of contact with cat or kitten
    2. Painless, nonpruritic erythematous papule at inoculation site—may

pustulate

3. Regional lymphadenitis usually follows within weeks, usually associated with fever, malaise, and other systemic symptoms

- Differential Diagnosis

    1. Bacterial lymphadenitis caused by *S. aureus, S. pyogenes, Francisella tularensis; Brucella* infection

    2. Plague

    3. Tularemia

    4. Lymphogranuloma venereum

    5. Rat bite fever

    6. Sarcoidosis

    7. Lymphomas

- Diagnostic Tests/Findings

    1. CSD skin test—positive

- Management/Treatment

    1. Analgesics for discomfort and fever

    2. Bedrest and limited activity

    3. Animals that transmit disease are not ill and therefore, do not need to be destroyed

    4. Skin tests remain positive for years

Scabies

- Definition: A highly contagious ectoparasite infestation

- Etiology/Incidence

    1. Female mite, *Sarcoptes scabiei*; burrows into stratum corneum to lay eggs which hatch within 2 to 4 days and move to the skin surface

    2. Skin sensitivity to eggs and mites' feces occurs in one month

    3. Transmitted directly by close personal contact and indirectly by infested clothing and linens

- Clinical Findings

    1. Pruritis—more intense at night; restlessness

    2. Rash

      a. Linear, threadlike, grayish burrows 1 to 10mm long with minute papule at open end

      b. Common sites

          (1) Infants < 2 years—eruption usually vesicular; usually appears on head, neck, palms and soles

          (2) Older children and adults—eruptions are usually in finger webs, genitalia, buttocks, thighs, abdomen, extensor surfaces of joints

      c. Persistent pruritis is not always indicative of treatment failure

- Differential Diagnosis

    1. Insect bites; chicken pox; viral exanthems

    2. Drug reaction; atopic dermatitis

- Diagnostic Tests/Findings: Skin scraping and microscopic examination for mites and eggs

- Management/Treatment

    1. Permethrin—a synthetic pyrethroid (Elimite®); alternatives are lindane (use with caution), crotamiton, 6% sulfur in petroleum

    2. Secondary infections—neosporin ointment

    3. Antipruritics—topical corticosteroids for persistent pruritis

    4. Educate parents concerning

      a. Mode of transmission

      b. Bedding and clothing washed in hot water with hot drying cycle on dryer

      c. All nonwashable items stored for several days (mites cannot survive more than 3 to 4 days without skin contact)

    5. Return to school or day care after treatment has been completed

    6. Prophylactic therapy for household members

    7. Medical referral for infants and pregnant females

    8. Retreat for persistent pruritis only if continued evidence of mite manifestations

Pediculosis (Lice)

- Definition: Infestation by lice

  1. Pediculosis capitis—infestation of the hair and scalp

  2. Pediculosis corporis—presence of lice on the body and clothes; usually infests clothes until feeding time

  3. Pediculosis pubis—infestation of genital hair, axillary hair, beard, mustache, eyebrows, eyelashes

- Etiology/Incidence

  1. *Pediculus humanus capitis* (head lice)

     a. Transmission occurs by direct contact or indirectly by contact with personal belongings, e.g., combs, brushes, hats, headphones, carpeting, bedding

     b. Infestation highest in child care and school-aged children

     c. All socioeconomic groups affected; less common in blacks; *not* associated with poor hygiene

  2. *Pediculus humanus corporis* (body lice)

     a. Fomites source of transmission; generally found on individuals with poor hygiene

     b. Vectors of disease, e.g., trench fever, typus

     c. Rare in children

  3. *Pthirus pubis* (pubic lice)

     a. Transmitted through sexual contact and by contaminated items, e.g., towels

     b. Common in adolescents and young adults

     c. May be found on eyelashes of younger children and may be evidence of sexual abuse

  4. Incubation period of louse eggs is 6 to 10 days

- Clinical Findings

  1. Pediculosis capitis

     a. Itching is most common symptom except in those with slight infestations

        b. Lice or eggs (nits) found on hair and behind ears, nape of neck

        c. Skin excoriation caused by itching

        d. Lymphadenopathy due to secondary bacterial infection

    2. Pediculosis corporis

        a. Intense itching, especially at night

        b. Body lice and eggs can be found in seams of clothing

    3. Pediculosis pubis

        a. Pruritis of anogenital area is common

        b. Many hairy areas can be infested

        c. Characteristic sign of heavy pubic lice infestation is bluish or slate-colored macules on chest, abdomen, thighs (AAP, 1994)

■ Differential Diagnosis

    1. Pediculosis capitis—dandruff, hair spray, hair casts, dirt/sand

    2. Pediculosis corporis and Pediculosis pubis—scabies, insect bites, cutaneous larva migrans (creeping eruption), eczema

■ Diagnostic Tests/Findings

    1. Identification of eggs, nymphs and lice is possible with the naked eye; further confirmation can be made with magnifying glass or microscope

■ Management/Treatment

    1. Pediculosis capitis

        a. Permethrin 1% creme rinse for 10 minutes

        b. Pyrethrin shampoo to dry hair for 10 minutes

        c. Education

            (1) Apply only to infested area

            (2) Avoid contact with eyes

            (3) Do not treat in bathtub or shower

            (4) Wash clothes and bedding in a hot water wash and dry for 20 minutes in a hot air dryer

            (5) Soak brushes, combs, etc. in pediculicidal agent for 1 hour

            (6) Store unwashables in plastic bag for 2 weeks

            (7) Notify contacts

(8) Vacuum carpets, rugs, car seats, furniture

   d. Check family members; only treat if infested

   e. Remove nits by hand or with fine tooth nit comb

   f. Medical referral for infants, pregnant or nursing females

   g. Discourage children from sharing personal items

   h. Discourage use of pesticidal sprays

   i. Re-evaluate after 7 days; if nits or lice are present, re-treat

2. Pediculosis corporis

   a. Improvement of hygiene and cleaning clothes is primary

   b. Wash clothes in hot water and dry at hot temperature to kill lice

3. Pediculosis pubis

   a. Pediculosis capitis treatment effective

   b. Retreatment recommended 7 to 10 days later

   c. Petrolatum ointment t.i.d. or q.i.d. for 8 to 10 days for eyelash infestation; remove nits (AAP, 1994)

   d. Education—all sexual contacts treated

Lyme Disease

- Definition: A tick-transmitted, spirochetal, inflammatory disorder

- Etiology/Incidence

  1. Caused by the *Borrelia burgdorferi* spirochete transmitted primarily by the *Ixodes dammini* deer tick

  2. Usually occurs during the summer and early fall

  3. Occurs at any age and in either sex, although most frequent in children and young adults living in heavily wooded areas

- Clinical Findings

  1. Early disease usually begins with a typical rash called erythema migrans at site of recent tick bite

  2. Lesion begins as a red macule or papule and expands, with often central clearing; multiple secondary lesions, red blotches or diffuse erythema can develop

  3. Fever, malaise, headache and mild neck stiffness and arthralgia can

occur

    a. These symptoms are typically intermittent and variable for a period of several weeks

    b. Occasionally early Lyme disease presents as a flulike illness without erythema migrans since the rash is either absent or unrecognized

  4. Weeks to months later

    a. Migratory pain in joints, bursae, tendons, muscles and bones

    b. Transient but severe headache and stiff neck

    c. Poor memory, mood changes, somnolence

    d. Muscle weakness and uncoordinated movements

    e. Chest pain/numbness

    f. Slow, fast, or irregular heartbeat

    g. Dizziness/fainting

    i. Facial palsies

    j. Chronic arthritis uncommon in children

- Differential Diagnosis

  1. Rocky Mountain Spotted Fever

  2. Pauciarticular juvenile arthritis

  3. Multiple sclerosis

  4. Acute rheumatic fever

  5. Influenza

  6. Aseptic meningitis

- Diagnostic Tests/Findings

  1. Culture of erythema migrans positive for *B. burgdorferi*

  2. Enzyme-linked immunosorbent assay (ELISA)—detects presence of antibodies

  3. Immunofluorescence assay (IFA)—detects presence of antibodies

  4. Western blot—confirmation of weak positive titers

  5. ESR—may be elevated

- Management/Treatment

1. Early-stage disease

   a. Amoxicillin or doxycycline at time of appearance of erythema migrans or shortly therafter is drug of choice for children 9 years and older

   b. Amoxicillin or penicillin V is recommended for children younger than 9 years

   c. Cefuroxime axetil and erythromycin for the penicillin-allergic individual, although erythromycin may be less effective (AAP, 1994)

2. Early treatment of erythema migrans should prevent development of later disease stages

3. Late-stage disease for persistent arthritis, carditis and CNS disease treated with parenteral antibiotics

   a. Ceftriaxone

   b. Penicillin G

4. Education—prevention

   a. Ticks that carry Lyme disease are sesame-seed size, not like larger ticks sometimes found on dogs

   b. Avoid tick-infested areas if possible

   c. Wear protective clothing

   d. Tuck clothing—shirts in pants, pants in shoes, socks, or boots; ticks cannot bite through clothes

   e. Use insect repellant

   f. Examination for ticks following outdoor activities in tick-infested areas is required

   g. Check pets regularly for ticks

5. Prompt removal of tick

   a. Use blunt-end tweezers to grasp tick as close to skin surface as possible

   b. Wear rubber gloves—do not touch tick with bare hands

   c. Put tick in bottle of alcohol and bring to health care provider for identification

   d. Disinfect skin area where tick bite occurred

6. Medical referral

Acne Vulgaris

- Definition: Common chronic disorder of the pilosebaceous unit usually initiated by the hormonal stimuli of puberty
- Etiology/Incidence
  1. Stimulation of androgens during puberty results in increased sebaceous gland size and sebum production. Accumulation of epidermal debris (keratin) and presence of bacteria irritate and obstruct the hair follicle
  2. *Propionibacterium acnes* an inhabitant of sebaceous follicle causes inflammation
  3. Commonly occurs on the face, back, and chest of adolescents and young adults
  4. Contributing factors consist of
     a. Cosmetics, environmental irritants, poor hygiene
     b. Mechanical trauma (picking/squeezing)
     c. Menstrual cycle; progesterone-dominant anovulatory agents
     d. Stress; hereditary factors
- Clinical Findings: Combination of open and closed comedones, inflammatory papules, pustules, nodules, cysts with inflammation and pain
- Differential Diagnosis
  1. Impetigo
  2. Eczema
  3. Insect bites
  4. Folliculitis
  5. Steroid acne
  6. Flat warts
- Diagnostic Tests/Findings: None
- Management/Treatment
  1. Avoid manipulating, squeezing, harsh scrubbing
  2. Mild soap for cleaning 2 to 3 times/day
  3. Stress management techniques

4. Controlled ultraviolet light exposure

5. Comedolytics—typical retinoic acid and benzoyl peroxide and antibiotics most effective combined treatment regime

   a. Mild to severe acne

     (1) Topical benzyl peroxide

     (2) Topical tetracycline, erythromycin, clindamycin

     (3) Topical retinoic acid

   b. Severe acne

     (1) Systemic oral retinoids (Accutane isotretinoin)

     (2) Systemic antibiotics, e.g., tetracycline (over 9 years of age), erythromycin

6. Psychological support

7. Reinforce compliance with medical regime—skin may worsen initially; increased dryness

8. Education concerning skin care management

9. Referral to dermatologist if severe

Neonatal Acne

- Definition: Skin condition of neonate, characterized by follicular pustular lesions usually involving face, shoulders and sometimes back

- Etiology/Incidence

1. Thought to be caused by hormonal stimulation of sebaceous glands

2. Occurs in the late neonatal period about 1 month of age

3. Usually disappears over a few weeks

- Clinical Findings: Coalescing erythematous tiny papules mostly over cheeks and chin, forehead, upper chest

- Differential Diagnosis: Milia

- Diagnostic Tests/Findings: None

- Management/Treatment: None, usually resolves in 4 to 8 weeks

Malignant Melanoma

- Definition: Pigmented nodules of variegated colors

- Etiology/Incidence: Rare in childhood, usually first appearing in late adolescence or young adulthood
- Clinical Findings
  1. Red, white and blue colors as well as brown and tan (Weston & Lane, 1991)
  2. Most important feature is rapid progressive growth of a pigmented lesion
  3. Notching of the border of a pigmented nodule and nonuniform irregular surface should cause suspicion
  4. Ulceration and bleeding are far-advanced signs
- Differential Diagnosis
  1. Dermal melanocytic nevus
  2. Compound melanocytic nevus
  3. Blue nevus
  4. Spindle and epithelioid cell nevus
  5. Dermatofibroma
  6. Hemangioma
  7. Pyogenic granuloma
  8. Mastocytoma
  9. Juvenile xanthogranuloma
- Diagnostic Tests/Findings—biopsy
- Management/Treatment
  1. Refer to surgeon for excision
  2. Follow-up any lesion or birthmark for change in color or size
  3. Education
     a. Protection and screening from natural and artificial tanning
     b. Watch for signs suggesting malignancy in pigmented lesions
        (1) Change in color
        (2) Change in characteristics of border of lesion
        (3) Change in suraface characteristics
        (4) Development of pruritis, tenderness, pain

Roseola (Exanthem subitum)

- Definition: An acute disease characterized by high fever and appearance of rash simultaneously with, or immediately following, decrease in temperature
- Etiology/Incidence
  1. Human herpesvirus-6
  2. Most common in spring and fall
  3. Most cases seen between 6 and 24 months
- Clinical Findings
  1. Abrupt onset of high fever (102-105 °F) for 3 to 4 days with possible convulsions
  2. Irritability
  3. Slight edema of eyelids
  4. Mild pharyngitis
  5. Lymphadenopathy in cervical, postauricular and suboccipital areas
  6. Rash appears after temperature returns to normal—macular or maculopapular eruption; most prominent on trunk and extremities
- Differential Diagnosis
  1. Rubeola (most often)
  2. Rubella
  3. Meningococcemia
  4. Pneumococcal bacteremia
- Diagnostic Tests/Findings: Progressive leukopenia as low as 2000 WBCs 3rd or 4th day of fever
- Management/Treatment
  1. Acetaminophen for fever and discomfort
  2. Educate parents concerning febrile convulsions
  3. Medical referral if fever persists or sign of meningeal irritation
  4. Parental reassurance that rash is a sign of recovery

Fifth Disease (Erythema Infectiosum)

- Definition: A moderately contagious, usually afebrile, exanthematous disease
- Etiology/Incidence
  1. Human parvovirus (B19)
  2. Most commonly seen in 5 to 14 year olds
  3. Usually seen in winter and spring
  4. Incubation period 7 to 18 days
  5. Transmitted by droplets via the respiratory tract
- Clinical Findings
  1. No prodromal symptoms
  2. Rash begins as fiery red rash on cheeks ("slapped cheek" appearance) spreading to upper arms and legs, trunk, hands and feet; rash begins to disappear becoming lacelike in appearance, then may reappear when skin is traumatized by pressure, sunlight, extremes of temperature; rash lasts from 2 to 39 days with a mean duration of 11 days
  3. Low grade fever may be present
  4. Can cause aplastic crises in patients with hemolytic diseases
- Differential Diagnosis
  1. Drug reactions
  2. Rubella, atypical measles
  3. Enteroviral diseases
  4. Systemic lupus erythematosus
- Diagnostic Tests/Findings: None
- Management/Treatment
  1. None indicated
  2. Reassure parents of benign nature of disease
  3. Most contagious before rash and unlikely to be infectious after rash develops

Herpes Infections

- Definition: Recurrent viral infection of the skin and mucous membrane characterized by clusters of vesicles filled with clear fluid
    1. Herpes Virus I—usually involves face and skin above the waist
        a. Gingivostomatitis
        b. Labialis ("cold sores")
        c. Ocular herpes
    2. Herpes Virus II—usually involves genitalia and skin below the waist (genital herpes) (see Genitourinary/Gynecologic disorders chapter)
    3. Neonatal Herpes—herpes in the newborn
- Etiology/Incidence
    1. Gingivostomatitis
        a. Most common form seen in children
        b. Peak incidence—1 to 4 years
    2. Labialis—common recurrence at same site (reactivation of latent virus)
    3. Ocular
        a. Common cause of corneal blindness
        b. Recurrence may be more severe
    4. Genital Herpes
        a. Incidence increasing due to increased sexual activity among adolescents
    5. Neonatal
        a. Transmission by HSV-2 in most cases, HSV-1 in 25%
        b. Greatest risk when mother has contracted herpes 2 to 4 weeks before delivery
        c. Premature infants affected 4 to 5 times as often as full-term infants
        d. 50% of HIV-affected babies demonstrate typical herpetic eruptions
        f. Overall risk 1 out of 20,000 live births
- Clinical Findings
    1. Gingivostomatitis

    a. Fever

    b. Irritability

    c. Poor feeding

    d. Tender, red, friable mucous membranes surrounding 2 to 3 mm white ulcerations 1 to 2 days later

    e. Severe halitosis

2. Herpes labialis (cold sores)—crusted vesicles on either the upper or lower lip

3. Ocular—manifestations may vary in severity from a superficial conjunctivitis to involvement of deeper layers of cornea

4. Genital

    a. Local pain, burning or paresthesia

    b. Fever

    c. Malaise

    d. Dysuria

    e. Inguinal lymphadenophy

    f. Vesicular lesions of the genital areas

5. Neonatal can manifest as

    a. Generalized systemic infection involving liver and other organs

    b. Localized CNS disease

    c. Localized infection of skin, eyes, and mouth (SEM)

    d. Ocular signs of conjunctivitis, keratitis, chorioretinitis

    e. Infections frequently severe with a high mortality rate and significant neurologic and/or ocular impairment, especially in the absence of antiviral therapy (AAP, 1994)

■ Differential Diagnosis

1. Type I

    a. Herpangina

    b. Coxsackie viruses

    c. Insect bites

    d. Conjunctivitis (bacterial)

  e. Impetigo

  f. Herpes roster

  g. Varicella

 2. Type 2

  a. Syphilis

  b. Sexually transmitted diseases

- Diagnostic Tests/Findings

 1. Tissue culture—viral detection

 2. Direct fluorescent antibody stain or enzyme immunoassay—detection of HSV antigens (specific, but less sensitive than culture)

- Management/Treatment

 1. Referral

 2. Acyclovir and vidarabine have been used primarily for potentially serious infections, such as those in neonates and immunocompromised children

 3. Genital infections—see chapter on Genitourinary/Gynecologic disorders

 4. Ocular involvement—referral to ophthalmologist; treatment with topical DNA inhibitors, e.g., 1% to 2% trifluridine, 1% iododeoxyuridine, 3% vidarabine (AAP, 1994)

 5. Gingivostomatitis

  a. Bland fluids, e.g., apple juice, liquid gelatin, lukewarm broth, popsicles

  b. Acetaminophen for fever and pain relief

  c. Use of local anesthetics (viscous lidocaine) discouraged

 6. Herpes labialis—antiviral therapy usually unwarranted

Diphtheria

- Definition: An acute contagious disease characterized by the formation of a fibrinous pseudomembrane, usually on the respiratory mucosa

- Etiology/Incidence

 1. *Corynebacterium diphtheriae*

2. Transmitted by direct contact with infected persons or contact with contaminated articles or carrier

3. Most common in autumn and winter

4. Prevented by immunization

- Clinical Findings

  1. Inflammation of the upper respiratory tract with mild sore throat

  2. Moderate fever, rapid pulse, severe prostration

  3. Membrane in throat white, in early stage of disease and progresses to dirty gray or gray-green

- Differential Diagnosis

  1. Upper respiratory infections

  2. Infectious mononucleosis

  3. Blood dyscrasias

  4. Croup, epiglottitis, bronchitis

  5. Foreign body aspiration

- Diagnostic Tests/Findings

  1. WBC—slight leukocytosis

  2. Löffler's culture positive for diphtheria bacilli

- Management/Treatment

  1. Hospitalization to include

  2. IV antitoxin (test for sensitivity to horse serum must be performed prior to administration)

  3. Antibiotics (erythromycin or procaine penicillin G)

  4. Bedrest 2 to 3 weeks to prevent myocarditis

  5. Adequate hydration

  6. Gag reflex and quality of voice check

  7. Care of exposed persons (see AAP Red Book)

Mumps (Epidemic parotitis)

- Definition: An acute contagious, generalized viral disease, usually causing painful enlargement of the salivary glands, most commonly the parotids

- Etiology/Incidence
    1. Caused by Paramyxovirus
    2. Transmitted by direct contact via respiratory route, airborne droplet and fomites contaminated with infected saliva
    3. Uncommon before 3 and after 40 years of age
    4. Preventable by vaccine

- Clinical Findings
    1. Primarily affects parotid glands and less often the sublingual and submaxillary glands, causing swelling
    2. Fever, pain around ear and malaise may precede parotid swelling
    3. Noticeable enlargement and tenderness of parotid gland follows
    4. Erythema of Stensen's duct

- Differential Diagnosis
    1. Mononucleosis
    2. Parotid gland tumor or obstruction produced by calculus in Stensen's duct
    3. Influenza
    4. Parotitis secondary to cytomegalovirus
    5. Suppurative parotitis

- Diagnostic Tests/Findings: Routine laboratory tests are nonspecific

- Management/Treatment
    1. Acetaminophen for pain and fever
    2. Educate parents concerning complications
        a. Pancreatitis
        b. Oophoritis
        c. Meningitis
        d. Orchitis
        e. Nerve deafness
    3. Adjust diet to child's tolerance
    4. Educate parents regarding child's return to school

Rubella (German measles)

- Definition: An acute contagious exanthematous viral disease; may result in abortion, stillbirth in infants born to mothers infected during early months of pregnancy

- Etiology/Incidence
  1. Caused by an RNA virus classified as a rubivirus
  2. Postnatal rubella transmitted mainly through direct or droplet contact from nasopharyngeal secretions
  3. Peak incidence late winter and early spring
  4. Preventable by active immunization (see Health Maintenance and Promotion chapter)

- Clinical Findings
  1. Prodrome, if present, lasts for only a few days and is characterized by slight malaise, low-grade fever and sometimes mild catarrhal symptoms
  2. Lymphadenopathy; most commonly involved are posterior auricular and suboccipital chains
  3. Erythematous, maculopapular discrete rash; starts on face and spreads rapidly downward over trunk and extremities; disappears by 3rd day
  4. Transient polyarthralgia and polyarthritis (adolescent females)
  5. A clinical diagnosis of rubella is subject to error without laboratory confirmation

- Differential Diagnosis
  1. Rubeola
  2. Rocky mountain spotted fever
  3. Scarlet fever
  4. Erythema infectiosum
  5. Drug rashes
  6. Infectious mononucleosis
  7. Adenovirus infections

- Diagnostic Tests/Findings
  1. HI test has been replaced more recently by more sensitive assays for

determining rubella immunity

    a. Latex agglutination

    b. Fluorescence immunoassay

    c. Passive agglutination

    d. Hemolysis-in-gel

    e. Enzyme immunoassay tests

  2. Rubella specific IgM antibody—presence indicates recent postnatal infection or congenital infection in newborn

- Management/Treatment

  1. Comfort measures

  2. Determine contacts who have not been immunized

  3. Medical referral for pregnant persons and persons with altered immunity who have been exposed

  4. Vaccine provides immunity (see Health Maintenance and Promotion chapter)

  5. Educate parents concerning possible complications of encephalitis and thrombocytopenia (rare)

Rubeola (10 day measles, red measles)

- Definition: An acute viral highly contagious disease
- Etiology/Incidence

  1. Caused by RNA virus, classified as a morbillivirus

  2. Transmitted by direct contact with infectious droplets or, less frequently by air-borne spread

  3. Peak incidence in unvaccinated populations occurs during winter and spring

  4. Preventable by active immunization (see Health Maintenance and Promotion chapter)

- Clinical Findings

  1. Prodrome

    a. Cold

    b. Hacking or barky cough

    c. Conjunctivitis with photophobia

    d. Fever—up to 105 °F

  2. Koplik's spots on buccal mucosa—usually appears 2 days before rash erupts; small irregular bright red spots with white speck centers

  3. Confluent maculopapular rash (lasts 5 days)

    a. Usually starts on upper lateral parts of neck, behind ears, along hairline, posterior cheeks

    b. Severity of disease correlated with severity of rash

    c. Desquamation of skin may occur

    d. Acute encephalitis major complication

    e. Respiratory complications common

■ Differential Diagnosis

  1. Roseola

  2. Rubella

  3. Infections due to echo-, coxsacki-, and adenoviruses

  4. Infectious mononucleosis

  5. Toxoplasmosis

  6. Meningococcemia

  7. Scarlet fever

  8. Rickettsial diseases

  9. Serum sickness

■ Diagnostic Tests/Findings

  1. Typically made from clinical pictures and history of exposure

  2. Serologic testing of measles specific IgM antibody titer at the acute and convalescent stages—reliability questionable

■ Management/Treatment

  1. Vitamin A in select cases (AAP, 1994)

  2. Acetaminophen for fever

  3. DO NOT GIVE ASPIRIN

  4. Medical referral for children who are at high risk or are not immunized

5. Report diagnosed cases to health authorities

6. Exclude child from school for 4 days after onset of rash

7. Tepid baths for fever control

8. Adequate fluid intake

9. Protect from strong light if photosensitive

10. Educate parents concerning complications

    a. Bronchopneumonia

    b. Otitis media

    c. Encephalitis

Poliomyelitis

- Definition: An acute viral paralytic disease with a broad spectrum of manifestations that range from subclinical to fatal bulbar disease

- Etiology/Incidence

  1. Causative agent—enterovirus, types 1, 2, and 3

  2. Transmitted by direct contact via fecal-oral and pharyngeal-oropharyngeal routes; perinatal transmission occurs

  3. More common in infants and young children, and occurs at an earlier age under conditions of poor hygiene (AAP, 1994)

  4. Rare in the U.S. at the present time

  5. Vaccine provides immunity (see Health Maintenance and Promotion chapter)

  6. Oral polio vaccine should not be given to those living in households with immunocompromised individuals, including HIV positive individuals, because these people can contract paralytic disease (AAP, 1994)

- Clinical Findings

  1. Three different forms

    a. Abortive (may last a few hours to a few days)

      (1) Fever, malaise

      (2) Sore throat, headache

      (3) Vomiting

(4)   Abdominal pain (unlocalized)

b. Nonparalytic

(1)   Symptoms same as abortive, but headache, nausea and vomiting are worse

(2)   Pain and stiffness in neck, back, legs

c. Paralytic

(1)   Same course as nonparalytic

(2)   Loss of selective tendon reflexes and asymmetric weakness or paralysis of muscle groups, depending on location of lesions

- Differential Diagnosis

    1. Infectious neuronitis (Guillain-Barre's syndrome)

    2. Brain abscess

    3. Peripheral neuritis

    4. Encephalitis

    5. Aseptic meningitis

- Diagnostic Tests/Findings

    1. Poliovirus can be isolated by tissue culture from feces, throat, urine and rarely cerebrospinal fluid

    2. Stool cultures from at least two specimens collected in first 15 days after onset of symptoms is diagnostic test of choice

- Management/Treatment

    1. No specific treatment—abortive or mild nonparalytic need only bed rest for several days

    2. Hospitalization and respiratory ventilation if respiratory paralysis

    3. Physical therapy after acute phase

    4. Sedatives to decrease anxiety

    5. Analgesics for pain

    6. Maintain bedrest

    7. Range of motion and moist hot packs to joints and muscles

    8. Educate families concerning

    a. Complications

        (1) Permanent paralysis

        (2) Respiratory arrest

        (3) Hypertension

        (4) Kidney stones from prolonged immobility

  9. Emotional support for family

Scarlet Fever (Scarlatina)

- Definition: An acute infection of the oropharynx caused by group A beta-hemolytic streptococci

- Etiology/Incidence

  1. Transmission results from person to person contact

  2. Occurs most frequently in children between 2 and 10 years of age

- Clinical Findings

  1. Acute onset with sore throat, chills, fever, headache, vomiting prior to onset of rash

  2. Rash—usually appears 24 to 48 hours after onset of infection; fine, erythematous maculopapular eruption which blanches on pressure with "sandpaper" texture; distribution of lesions begins on neck, forehead, cheeks, (circumoral pallor) and chest, then becomes generalized; desquamation occurs as rash fades

  3. "Beefy red" tonsils and pharynx

  4. "Coated" tongue appears "strawberry" in 50% of cases

  5. Transverse red streaks (pastia lines) usually in antecubital spaces

- Differential Diagnosis

  1. Kawasaki disease

  2. Rubella

  3. Drug reactions

  4. Toxic shock syndrome

  5. Enterovirus

- Diagnostic Tests/Findings

  1. Throat culture—positive for group A beta-hemolytic streptococcus

2. WBC—leukocytosis

■ Management/Treatment

1. Penicillin for 10 days or erythomycin for 10 days if allergic to penicillin

2. Generally noninfectious 48 hours after therapy initiated

3. Warm saline gargles; acetaminophen for fever and discomfort; encourage fluids

4. Educate parents concerning complications

   a. Otitis media

   b. Pyoderma

   c. Cervical adenitis

   d. Acute glomerulonephritis

   e. Rheumatic fever

5. Do not send child back to school until afebrile for 24 hours; follow-up throat culture after completion of antibiotic therapy

6. Notify other persons who have been exposed

Varicella-Zoster (Chicken pox)

■ Definition: An acute viral contagious disease

■ Etiology/Incidence

1. Caused by the varicella-zoster virus (VZV)

2. Transmission by direct contact with lesions or by air-borne droplets; most cases between 5- and 10-year-olds, but can occur at any age

3. Most prevalent in late winter and early spring

4. Contagious 1 to 2 days before rash and as long as 5 days after onset of lesions

5. Virus can cross placenta during 1st and early 2nd trimester of pregnancy to produce a congenital varicella syndrome

■ Clinical Findings

1. History of exposure 2 weeks before lesions appear or history of chickenpox in community

2. Usually begins with no prodrome or only anorexia, malaise and low-

grade fever

3. Individual lesions begin as faint erythematous macules that progress to papules, then vesicles within 12 to 24 hours; vesicles turn to pustules which develop moist crusts that dry and shed; crops of lesions continue to erupt for 3 to 4 days

4. At height of disease, lesions in all phases can be seen; total duration 7 to 10 days

5. Lesions can be severely pruritic; usually start on the trunk, spreads to face and centrifugally; vesicles may occur on mucous membranes of the mouth, conjunctiva, vagina, rectum

- Differential Diagnosis

  1. Hand-foot-and-mouth disease

  2. Insect bites

  3. Acute para psoriasis

  4. Herpes simplex

- Diagnostic Tests/Findings : None—routinely done

- Management/Treatment

  1. Relief of pruritis

      a. Wet dressings, soothing baths

      b. Calamine lotion, cetaphil lotion

      c. Antihistimines, e.g., diphenhydramine etc.

  2. Warm saline hydrogen peroxide gargle for oral lesions and compresses for genital lesions

  3. Acetaminophen for fever; avoid aspirin because of risk of Reye syndrome

  4. Infected lesions—oral and/or topical antibiotics

  5. Acyclovir—for severe cases with widespread disease or in immunocompromised individuals

  6. Passive prevention may be offered by giving varicella—a zoster immunoglobulin (VZIG) to susceptible individuals at high risk

  7. Medical referral for children with eczema or on immunosuppressive therapy

  8. Education

    a. CHILDREN WITH VIRAL INFECTIONS SHOULD NOT RECEIVE ASPIRIN OR OTHER SALICYLATES BECAUSE OF THE RISK OF REYE SYNDROME

    b. Keep nails trimmed

    c. Exclude child from school until lesions are crusted, usually 7 days

    d. Avoid contact with the elderly, pregnant women, neonates and immunocompromised children

    e. Lifetime immunity is generally conferred

    f. Education concerning complications

        (1) Secondary bacterial infection of lesions

        (2) Thrombocytopenia

        (3) Encephalitis, pneumonia

        (4) Reye syndrome—instruct parents to seek medical attention IMMEDIATELY if child appears to be recovering then develops repetitive vomiting

            (a) Lethargy and drowsiness are early symptoms

            (b) Within 24 to 48 hours agitation and disorientation follow

            (c) Periods of lethargy may alternate with combative behavior

            (d) Coma

Questions

Select the best answer

1. Severe acne may be treated with which of the following

   a. Systemic retinoid
   b. Hydrocortisone 1%
   c. Benadryl
   d. Nystatin cream

2. All of the following are possible contributing factors to the development of acne vulgaris except

   a. Environmental irritants
   b. Stress and hereditary factors
   c. "Fatty" foods
   d. Progesterone dominant anovulatory agents

3. Mary, an 8 month old infant, has an erythematous vesicular dermatitis on her face, scalp, and neck. Her mother says that she is always rubbing her rash. There is a strong family history of asthma and chronic skin rashes. The best assessment is

   a. Contact dermatitis
   b. Tinea
   c. Atopic dermatitis
   d. Scabies

4. Joseph has been diagnosed with cat scratch disease. In educating his parents about his condition you tell them

   a. Animals, usually cats or kittens, that transmit the disease are ill and must be destroyed.
   b. Skin tests will return to normal within 2 weeks after the onset of the disease.
   c. A white coating on the tongue and petechiae on the palate accompany the disease.
   d. Joseph's kitten is not ill, and therefore does not need to be destroyed

5. Atopic Dermatitis

   a. Is caused by emotional factors
   b. Affects approximately 50% of children
   c. Is treated with 5% hydrocortisone cream every 2 hours
   d. Is diagnosed by clinical manifestations and elevated IgE antibodies

6. A deep locally diffuse infection of the skin with regional lymphadenopathy, fever, and malaise and usually involving the extremities and face best describes

   a. Cellulitis
   b. Trauma
   c. Contact dermatitis
   d. Uticaria

7. Management of the above condition includes

   a. Cool, moist compresses to area to decrease pruritis
   b. Reporting of possible child abuse
   c. Rest, immobilization, antibiotics, and hot moist compresses
   d. Patch testing

8. Mrs. Smith's two children, Elizabeth and John, have intense pruritis of the hands and face. In questioning them further the PNP finds that the children were taken on a school field trip through the woods to identify flowers and trees. Three other students in the class have the same symptoms. The most likely diagnosis would be

   a. Scabies
   b. Contact dermatitis
   c. Lyme disease
   d. Eczema

9. Contributing factors to diaper rash include all the following except

   a. Friction
   b. Caregiver neglect
   c. Allergy
   d. Prolonged exposure to urine and feces

10. Beefy-red, shiny confluent erythema with satellite lesions in the inguinal creases and genital area is characteristic of

    a. Monilia diaper rash
    b. Chlamydia
    c. Contact diaper dermatitis
    d. Seborrheic diaper dermatitis

11. Mr. Green brings his son, Glen, to the PNP's office one cold winter morning. Glen complains of a mildly sore throat and "feeling hot." On physical examination the PNP discovers that Glen has a fever of 101.6 °F, rapid pulse, and a fibrinous grey-green pseudomembrane in his throat. The most likely diagnosis would be

    a. Streptococcal pharyngitis
    b. Epiglottitis
    c. Diptheria

    d. Mononucleosis

12. Seven-year-old Ashley, enters the PNP's office. She looks like someone has slapped her across both facial cheeks. Her cheeks appear bright red. She had a low grade fever yesterday, but not today. What is her probable diagnosis?

    a. Child abuse
    b. Fifth Disease
    c. Rubella
    d. Drug reaction

13. Julie has vesicular lesions which have eroded and crusted on her genitalia. She complained of itching and burning a few hours before the lesions appeared and painful urination. PNP management of this condition would include

    a. Tissue culture
    b. Remove crusts from lesions
    c. Permethrin 1%
    d. CBC

14. Mrs. Smith brings 4 year old Michael to your office one day, complaining of "sores" on his arms and legs. She states that he had lots of mosquito bites, scratched them, and now they look infected. Upon P.E., you note numerous honey colored crusted lesions with an erythematous base on both upper and lower extremities. You also note several pustular lesions with erythematous bases around the nose. There are no other positive findings on P.E. What is the probable diagnosis?

    a. Pediculosis
    b. Rubeola
    c. Scabies
    d. Impetigo

15. Which of the following are causes for impetigo?

    a. *H. influenzae* type b
    b. Group A ß hemolytic streptococcus and staphylococcus
    c. *Candida albicans*
    d. Cytomegalovirus

16. Mrs. McCaleb brings her 8-year-old son to your office. He has a "bull's eye" rash of various sizes on his armpits, thighs, and buttocks. You suspect Lyme Disease and tell the mother

    a. Ticks that live on dogs are carriers of the disease
    b. Her son's nails must be cut to prevent damage from scratching
    c. Remove the tick with your hands immediately
    d. Early intervention will lead to a better prognosis

17. Other symptoms the PNP might observe during early stages of Lyme Disease include all of the following except

    a. Fever
    b. Malaise
    c. Jaundice
    d. Sore throat

18. All of the following may be complications of mumps except

    a. Meningitis
    b. Pneumonia
    c. Orchitis
    d. Pancreatitis

19. Which of the following would you use in the education of the parents of a child who has been diagnosed with mumps

    a. Child may return to school after beginning antibiotic treatment
    b. Place child on NPO diet since child's throat may be painful
    c. Child should be placed on strict bedrest until fever decreases
    d. The disease is transmitted by direct contact via respiratory airborne droplets, and fomites contaminated with infected saliva

20. The three steps in management of controlling and managing pediculosis include all the following except

    a. Nit combing
    b. Application of a pediculicidal agent
    c. Treatment of all exposed persons
    d. Environmental measures

21. When applying a pediculicidal product one should remember to

    a. Cover the child's eyes
    b. Lean the child's head over the sink
    c. Avoid applying treatment in tub or shower
    d. All of the above

22. Mr. Jackson brings his 6-year-old son to the PNP. The child has a rash and is complaining of pruritis on the back, neck and extremities. Upon physical examination you find the child is afebrile and has scaly, papulovesicular lesions localized to the back in a "Christmas tree" configuration. What is the PNP's assessment?

    a. Pityriasis Rosea
    b. Roseola
    c. Contact dermatitis

d. Rubeola

23. Although the incidence of poliomyelitis has drastically decreased in the United States since the vaccine has been introduced, the PNP might suspect this disease if a child presented with all of the following except

a. Pain and stiffness in neck, back, and legs
b. Headache and asymetrical weakness of muscle groups
c. Abdominal edema, lymphadenopathy, and jaundice
d. Unlocalized abdominal pain, nausea, and vomiting

24. Which of the following best describes the rash of roseola?

a. Beefy red
b. Begins as a bright red eruption on cheek ("slapped cheeks") and spreads to upper arms and legs, trunk, hands and feet, and then becomes lace-like
c. Macular or maculopapular eruption most prominent on trunk and extremities usually appearing after temperature returns to normal
d. Fine pink maculopapular eruptions which start on face, spread rapidly downward toward trunk and disappear by the 3rd day

25. Complications of rubella include

a. Impetigo
b. Encephalitis and thrombocytopenia
c. Bronchitis and pneumonitis
d. Jaundice and subsequent liver failure

26. Mrs. Stanley brings 7-year-old Lauren to the PNP. After examining Lauren, the PNP finds the following: hacking cough, fever 104.8 °F, conjunctivitis, and red eruptions with white centers on the buccal mucosa and a confluent maculopapular rash on the upper neck and spreading downward. What is the PNP's assessment?

a. Rubella
b. Rubeola
c. Roseola
d. Fifth disease

27. Nancy Adam's physical examination is remarkable for an oral temperature of 102.8°F, a mucopurulent nasal discharge, conjunctivitis, and red eruptions with white centers on the buccal mucosa. These are characteristic of measles. What are these eruptions called?

a. Pastia's spots
b. Koplik's spots
c. Rubeola spots
d. Strawberry spots

28. Which of the following is characteristic of rubella?

    a. Vesicular, crusted lesions and high fever
    b. Posterior auricular lymphadenopathy and low grade fever
    c. Intense pruritis usually in finger webs, buttocks, thighs, and ankles
    d. "Sandpaper" textured, maculopapular rash which blanches with pressure

29. Seven year old Tommy has a scaly, papulovesicular rash between his fingers, on his ankles, and thighs. There are several excoriations in a linear pattern. Itching is intense, especially at night. The best assessment is

    a. Contact dermatitis
    b. Tinea
    c. Atopic dermatitis
    d. Scabies

30. All of the following are true regarding the rash of scarlet fever except

    a. The rash begins at the base of the neck and spreads to the cheek and chest, then becomes generalized
    b. The rash blanches on pressure and has a fine sandpaper-like texture
    c. Transverse red streaks may appear in antecubital spaces
    d. The rash is more prevalent on the extremities of the body

31. Other symptoms than the rash which may help the PNP arrive at an assessment of scarlet fever include

    a. "Slapped cheeks"
    b. Koplik's spots on the throat
    c. "Beefy red" tonsils and "strawberry" tongue
    d. Low grade fever and pruritis

32. Possible complications of scarlet fever include

    a. Otitis media and acute glomerulonephritis
    b. Meningitis and respiratory arrest
    c. Thrombocytopenia and anemia
    d. Pancreatitis and orchitis

33. Mrs. Jones' 3-month-old daughter has a moderate case of seborrheic dermatitis. Which of the following would you recommend to Mrs. Jones

    a. Permethrin 1% creme rinse for 10 minutes
    b. Application of calamine lotion t.i.d.
    c. Gentle scrubbing with an antiseborrheic shampoo
    d. Tinactin cream b.i.d.

34. All of the following are preventative measures against sunburn except

    a. Use of protective clothing and hats

    b. Use of petrolatum based lotions

    c. Use of sunscreen agents

    d. Avoidance of excessive overexposure to ultraviolet rays

35. Possible dangers of long-term overexposure to sunlight include

    a. Headaches and seizures

    b. Anemia and pruritis

    c. Hypopigmentation and gall bladder disease

    d. Premature aging of the skin and melanoma

36. Which best describes the diagnosis of Tinea capitis

    a. Circular erythematous patches with papular, scaly annular borders and clear centers on the body

    b. Inflamed scaly dry patches with broken hairs on the scalp

    c. Toe web lesions with erythema and scaling borders

    d. Scaly, pruritic erythematous lesions on inguinal creases and inner thighs

37. Differential diagnosis of Tinea capitis include

    a. Traction alopecia

    b. Alopecia areata

    c. Trichotillomania

    d. All of the above

38. John is being treated for chicken pox. His mother asks you when she might send him back to school. You explain to her that John can return to school when lesions are crusted which usually occurs at

    a. 15 days

    b. 7 days

    c. 5 days

    d. 2 days

39. Peter, age 3, is John's younger brother. If he gets the chicken pox, what should mom expect

    a. Peter may have no illness preceding chicken pox or mild symptoms such as loss of appetite and low-grade fever

    b. The rash will begin at the hairline

    c. Since he is younger, his symptoms may be more severe than the older child

    d. Giving Peter aspirin will alleviate all his symptoms

40. David, age 8 years, has a plantar wart on the bottom of his right foot. The PNP advises all of the following except

    a. Podophyllin is the best and most effective treatment

b. Repeated irritation may cause enlargement of warts
c. Salicylic acid paints usually effective
d. Wear proper fitting shoes to avoid pressure

Answer key

1.	a	21.	d
2.	c	22.	a
3.	c	23.	c
4.	d	24.	c
5.	d	25.	b
6.	a	26.	b
7.	c	27.	b
8.	b	28.	b
9.	c	29.	d
10.	a	30.	d
11.	c	31.	c
12.	b	32.	a
13.	a	33.	c
14.	d	34.	b
15.	b	35.	d
16.	d	36.	b
17.	c	37.	d
18.	b	38.	b
19.	d	39.	a
20.	c	40.	a

Bibliography

American Academy of Pediatrics. (1994). *Report of the committee on infectious diseases* (23rd ed.). Elk Grove Village, IL: American Academy of Pediatrics

Behrman, R. E., Kliegman, R. M., Nelson, W. E., & Vaughn, V. C. (Eds.). (1992). *Nelson textbook of pediatrics*. (14th ed.). Philadelphia: W. B. Saunders Co.

Bradford, B. J. (1991). Immunization: A 1991 update. *Journal of School Nursing, 7*(3), 28-37.

Chauvin, V. G. (1989). Common skin rashes in children and adolescents. *School Nurse. 5*(1), 23-38.

Cohen, B. (1992). Atopic dermatitis: Breaking the itch-scratch cycle. *Contemporary Pediatrics. 9*(8), 64-81.

Farrington, E. (1992). Acyclovir in the treatment of chickenpox. *Pediatric Nursing. 18*, 499-503.

Hoekelman, R. A., Friedman, S. B., Nelson, M. M., & Seidal, H. M. (Eds.). (1992). *Primary pediatric care*. (2nd ed.). St. Louis: Mosby Year Book.

Jacobs, R. F. (1991). Tick talk: Lyme disease. *Audio Digest Pediatrics. 37* (7).

Weston, W. T., & Lane, A. T. (1991). *Color textbook of pediatric dermatology*. St. Louis: Mosby Year Book.

Whaley, L. F., & Wong, D. L. (1991). *Nursing care of infants and children (4th ed.)* St. Louis: Mosby Yearbook.

Zitelli, B. J., & Davis, H. W. (Eds.) (1993). *Atlas of pediatric physical diagnosis*. London: Wolfe Publishing

Eye, Ear, Mouth Disorders

Carole Stone

Hordeolum (Stye)

- Definition: An acute purulent inflammation of sebaceous glands (meibomian or zeisian) of the eyelids
- Etiology/Incidence: Usually caused by infection with *Staphylococcus aureus*.
- Clinical Findings
    1. Initial sign is edema of the lid which may be diffuse; localization of redness on the lid margin follows
    2. Pain and tenderness, especially over affected gland
- Differential Diagnosis
    1. Chalazion
    2. Blepharitis
- Diagnostic Tests/Findings: none indicated; culture usually not necessary
- Management/Treatment
    1. Warm, moist compresses
    2. Topical antibiotic drops or ointment q.i.d. may be used to prevent complicating conjunctivitis and spread to other glands, but usually not necessary
    3. Instructions for compresses and instillation of eye drops/ointment; avoidance of squeezing stye; importance of hand washing

Chalazion

- Definition: Chronic inflammatory lipogranuloma of a meibomian gland in the upper or lower lid; usually involves the midportion of the tarsus
- Etiology/Incidence: Results from obstruction of the gland duct with secondary inflammation
- Clinical Findings
    1. Progressive, painless swelling of the lid; localized palpable mass
    2. Feeling of irritation of the eye
    3. A large chalazion may press on cornea causing astigmatism and distortion of vision
- Differential Diagnosis—other disorders of the lid

1. Hordeolum
2. Blepharitis

- Diagnostic Tests/Findings: None indicated
- Management/Treatment
  1. Small chalazions may resolve spontaneously
  2. Large, recurrent or secondarily infected should be treated with local antibacterial drops or ointments q.i.d.
  3. Surgical removal indicated for nonresponse to conservative treatment

Blepharitis

- Definition
  1. A chronic inflammation of the lid margin that begins in early childhood and frequently continues throughout life
  2. May produce secondary conjunctivitis, recurrent chalazion, loss of lashes and thickening of lid margins
  3. Types
     a. Simple squamous—characterized by hypertrophy and desquamation of the epidermis near lid margin
     b. Ulcerated—arises from acute and chronic suppurative inflammation of the follicles of the lashes and meibomian and/or zeisian glands
- Etiology/Incidence
  1. *Staphylococcus aureus* is usually the causative agent in the ulcerated type
  2. *Staphylococcus epidermidis, and Propionibacterium acnes* also frequently isolated
  3. Seborrheic dermatitis is usually associated with the simple squamous type
- Clinical Findings
  1. Erythema and scaling of the lid margins with simple squamous type; seborrheic dermatitis often found in scalp
  2. Frequent rubbing and irritation of the eye
  3. Erythema and bleeding of eyelid margins with formation of small

ulcers found in ulcerated type

- Differential Diagnosis— other disorders of the lid
  1. Chalazion
  2. Hordeolum
- Diagnostic Tests/Findings: None indicated
- Management/Treatment
  1. Goal is control; complete cure difficult
  2. Warm, moist compresses to lid margins
  3. Mechanical scrubbing of lid margin with dilute baby shampoo; usually daily, using a cotton-tip applicator; or soft cloth
  4. Topical antibiotic ointment massaged into lid margin (erythromycin or bacitracin drugs of choice 1 to 2 times per day)
  5. Treat seborrheic dermatitis simultaneously
  6. Precise instruction on treatment; tendency for chronicity should be emphasized; permanent loss of eyelashes possible in severe cases
  7. Steroid ointments discouraged

Dacryostenosis

- Definition
  1. Obstruction of the nasolacrimal duct; the most common abnormality of the infant lacrimal apparatus
  2. Can be unilateral or bilateral
- Etiology/Incidence
  1. Usually caused by incomplete canalization of the nasolacrimal duct
  2. May also be acquired following trauma or chronic conjunctivitis
- Clinical Findings
  1. History of persistent tearing and crusting of lashes
  2. Tearing; wet look in the eye
  3. Expression of mucopurulent discharge from lacrimal sac
  4. May be associated conjunctivitis
  5. Redness and swelling over lacrimal sac or duct usually indicative of associated dacryocystitis

■ Differential Diagnosis: Must differentiate from conjunctivitis due to other causes

■ Management/Treatment

    1. Massage of the lacrimal sac and nasolacrimal duct from brow downward several times a day

    2. For conjunctivitis or significant discharge, administration of antibiotic drops or ointment four times per day (10% sodium sulfacetamide or erythromycin ointment)

    3. Surgical probing of the duct may be necessary for persistent obstruction and recurrent purulent drainage beyond six months; referral to ophthalmologist for evaluation and treatment

    4. Education for massaging nasolacrimal duct and instilling eye medications

    5. Presence of dacrocystitis requires systemic antibiotics and referral to an ophthalmologist

Conjunctivitis of the Newborn (Ophthalmia Neonatorum)

■ Definition: Inflammation and/or infection of the conjunctiva of the newborn

■ Etiology/Incidence

    1. Chemical conjunctivitis—due to irritation from instillation of silver nitrate or erythromycin used for prophylaxis

    2. Gonococcal conjunctivitis—purulent infection with *Neisseria gonorrhoeae* obtained from perinatal transmission. Occurs in approximately 0.6% of newborns; treatment with erythromycin ophthalmic ointment, topical silver nitrate and tetracycline are considered equally effective for prophylaxis of ocular gonorrheal infection (AAP, 1994)

    3. Inclusion conjunctivitis—infection with *Chlamydia trachomatis* obtained from perinatal transmission at birth; the most common infectious agent causing ophthalmia neonatorum; may be self-limited with spontaneous resolution; recommended prophylaxis for prevention of gonococcal ophthalmia will not reliably prevent neonatal chlamydia conjunctivitis (AAP, 1994)

    4. Other bacterial conjunctivitis—pathogens including *Haemophilus influenzae, Staphylococcus aureus,* and Enterococci may be responsible

after the first week of life

- Clinical Findings

    1. Chemical conjunctivitis—typically mild; begins several hours after instillation and lasts no more than 24 to 36 hours

    2. Gonococcal conjunctivitis—acute presentation 2 to 4 days after birth with marked purulent discharge, chemosis and marked lid edema; look for central nervous system findings

    3. Chlamydia conjunctivitis—clinical presentation varies but usually presents 5 to 12 days after birth with mild mucopurulent discharge and moderate lid edema, erythema and chemosis; look for evidence of pneumonia

    4. Other bacterial conjunctivitis—usually presents on the 5th day with lid edema, chemosis and purulent discharge

- Differential Diagnosis—must differentiate based on history, clinical presentation and laboratory tests

- Diagnostic Tests/Findings

    1. Obtain conjunctival scrapings with a blunt spatula for Gram stain and Giemsa stain; the presence of intracellular gram negative diplococci is indicative of infection with gonococci; the presence of basophilic intracytoplasmic inclusions in the conjunctival epithelial cells is indicative of infection with chlamydia

    2. Cultures—will be positive for specific organism

- Management/Treatment

    1. Chemical conjunctivitis—No treatment necessary; explanation to parents important; mothers should be allowed to hold and nurse infant before instillation of prophylaxis whenever possible

    2. Gonococcal conjunctivitis—ceftriaxone (25 to 50 mg/kg/day, IV or IM not to exceed 125 mg) given once; cefotaxime (50 to 100 mg/kg/day, IV or IM in 2 divided doses) for 7 days is an alternative; topical treatment alone is inadequate and unnecessary when systemic therapy is given (AAP, 1994)

    3. Chylamydia conjunctivitis—oral erythromycin (50 mg/kg/day in 4 divided doses) for 14 days; oral sulfonamides may be used after immediate neonatal period for infants who do not tolerate erythromycin; topical treatment ineffective and unnecessary (AAP, 1994)

4. Bacterial conjunctivitis—depends on organisms; erythromycin ointment q.i.d.-gram positive organisms; gentamicin ophthalmic solution q.i.d. for gram negative organisms; warm, moist compresses may help; stress handwashing

Childhood Conjunctivitis

- Definition: Inflammation and/or infection of the conjunctiva in childhood
- Etiology/Incidence
  1. Very common in children throughout the world
  2. Epidemics occur in school-age children and in day care
  3. Bacterial conjunctivitis—the most common infectious agents include *Staphylococcus aureus, Haemophilus influenzae* and *Streptococcus pneumoniae*
  4. Viral conjunctivitis accounts for most infections in older children; usually caused by adenovirus; the two most common types are pharyngoconjunctival and epidemic keratoconjunctivitis
  5. Allergic conjunctivitis; usually part of a more diffuse allergic process, i.e., hay fever
  6. Herpes Simplex Keratoconjunctivitis; usually occurs as a unilateral acute conjunctivitis with regional lymphadenitis in children 10 years or younger; primary infection is usually not serious, but the recurrent infection which develops in 26% of cases involves the corneal epithelium, which can result in corneal scarring and visual loss
- Clinical Findings
  1. Itchy, irritated sensation
  2. Watery discharge (viral or allergic)
  3. Purulent discharge (most often bacterial)
  4. Sticky eyelids on awakening
  5. Swelling of lids
  6. Erythema of conjunctiva
  7. Photophobia may be present
  8. May be associated otitis media (indicates bacterial infection with *Haemophilus influenzae*)
  9. Preauricular adenopathy (usually associated with viral agents)

10. May have associated pharyngitis and fever

11. Cobblestone papillae beneath upper lid (vernal conjunctivitis)

12. Stringy, thick mucoid discharge (allergic, especially vernal type)

13. Primary skin lesion of single or grouped vesicles or crusted ulcers (primary herpes infection)

■ Differential Diagnosis: Focus should be on determining the probable cause and type of conjunctivitis based on history; geographic area; time of year; signs and symptoms; physical findings

■ Diagnostic Tests/Findings: Cultures usually not necessary unless severe or unresponsive to treatment

■ Management/Treatment

1. Bacterial—treated according to etiologic agent; empirical treatment with topical ophthalmic antibiotic or sulfacetamide, e.g., tobramycin, erythromycin, polymyxin B + trimethoprim

2. Viral—no specific treatment, but broad spectrum topical antibiotics often used to prevent secondary infection

3. Allergic—elimination of allergies; cold compresses; systemic antihistamines; sometimes weak corticosteroid eyedrops during acute phase; refer to ophthalmologist if persistent or if vernal conjunctivitis present

4. Herpes—referral to ophthalmologist usually necessary; **any child with a history of a herpes ocular infection who presents with a red eye should be referred immediately;** treatment includes both topical and systemic medications; DNA inhibitors such as trifluridine, iododeoxyuridine and vidarabine are used; oral acyclovir is the preferred systemic medication

5. Referral indicated for any conjunctivitis that is

   a. Unresponsive to treatment

   b. Associated with corneal involvement

   c. Orbital cellulitis

   d. Hyperacute conjunctivitis

   e. Associated with loss of vision, photophobia, pain

6. Proper hygiene, especially hand washing, should be emphasized to control spread of infection

Keratitis

- Definition: Inflammation and/or infection of the cornea; can be caused by bacteria, fungi, viruses or parasites

- Etiology/Incidence

  1. Xerophthalmia—vitamin A deficiency found in malnourished children or anomalies associated with malabsorption of vitamin A

  2. Bacterial ulcers—following trauma by a foreign body or injuries infected by bacteria; ulcers lead to pus in the anterior chamber, corneal destruction and loss of eye if not treated intensively; *Staphylococcus aureus* the most common cause; also streptococcus, pseudomonas and other pathogens may be involved

  3. Allergic reaction to certain proteins (tuberculosis, bacterial or fungal)

  4. Interstitial keratitis—associated with congenital or acquired syphilis or may follow herpes zoster, mumps or TB

  5. Viral keratitis—lesions due to herpes simplex

  6. Mycotic ulcers—usually associated with penetration of the cornea with vegetable material (e.g., a stick); similar lesions may be located elsewhere on face, nose or mouth

  7. U.R.I. may accompany ocular signs

- Clinical Findings—recurrent viral infection may occur and cause corneal scarring and visual loss

  1. Pain

  2. Photophobia

  3. Tearing

  4. Blurred vision

  5. Iritis is usually associated (cilliary flush)

  6. Corneal epithelial ulceration with mucopurulent exudate

  7. Other signs and symptoms specific to type/etiology

- Diagnostic Tests/Findings: Other lab test specific to suspected etiology usually done by ophthalmologist

- Management/Treatment

  1. **Refer to ophthalmologist immediately for definitive diagnosis and**

treatment

2. Corneal involvement can lead to iritis and blindness

3. Contact lens wear is a significant risk factor; appropriate education emphasized

Orbital/Periorbital Cellulitis

- Definition

  1. Inflammation/infection of soft tissues surrounding eye may be secondary to sinusitis or may be secondary to complications of trauma and septicemia

  2. **This is a serious condition that requires prompt assessment, referral and treatment**

- Etiology

  1. Paranasal sinusitis most common cause of bacterial orbital cellulitis in children; ethmoiditis most frequent source under 10

  3. Most common organisms are

     a. *Staphylococcus aureus*

     b. *Streptococcus pyogenes*

     c. *Haemophilus influenzae*

  2. Routes of infection

     a. Direct inoculation from trauma

     b. Extension from adjacent structure

     c. Metastatic spread from other parts of body

- Clinical Findings

  1. Erythema and swelling of eyelids

  2. Orbital pain, headache and tenderness on palpation

  3. Conjunctival and orbital tissues are not involved in periorbital cellulitis

  4. Enlargement of preauricular nodes may be present

  5. Conjunctival chemosis, proptosis and decreased ocular movements, rhinorrhea, and fever (102 °F-104 °F) are present with orbital cellulitis

- Differential Diagnosis

  1. Need to distinguish between orbital (inflammation within the true

orbit) and periorbital (occurring in front of the orbital septum) cellulitis

   2. Allergic reaction

   3. Trauma

- Diagnostic Tests/Findings:

   1. Sinus roentgenograms

   2. Orbital sonography

   3. CT Scan

   4. CBC

   5. Blood and eye cultures

- Management/Treatment

   1. **Refer to ophthalmologist if suspected, immediately**

   2. Specific systemic antibiotic therapy indicated

   3. Hospitalization may be necessary

   4. Complications may include loss of vision, meningitis, cerebral abscess

Cataract

- Definition: Opacity of the lens or capsule which may be present at birth or develop in childhood; may be bilateral; congenital cataracts can be classified according to their location and morphology

   1. Polar—opacity of anterior and posterior poles involving capsule and lens

   2. Zonular—opacity of an entire layer of the lens leaving other parts normal

   3. Total—opacity involving the entire lens

   4. Membranous—opacity of entire lens which is thick and fibrotic

- Etiology/Incidence

   1. Congenital—maternal rubella during first trimester

     a. Uncommon

     b. Frequently, there is a positive family history

     c. Chance of appearance in subsequent siblings is approximately 1:40

   2. Acquired cataracts

    a. Trauma—penetrating wounds or blunt trauma to eyeball

    b. Systemic disease—diabetes, hypoparathyroidism, galactosemia, Down Syndrome

    c. Poisoning—ingestion of naphthalene or diphenyl

    d. Complications of other eye diseases, e.g., glaucoma, uveitis, etc

    e. Long term use of corticosteroids

- Clinical Findings

    1. Opacity of lens on examination

    2. Absent red reflex

    3. Strabismus—may be first indication in child

    4. Diminished vision

    5. Nystagmus with severe decreased visual acuity

    6. No pain

    7. Other physical findings such as failure to thrive (FTT), other congenital anomalies

- Management/Treatment

    1. Referral to ophthalmologist when suspected, for diagnosis and treatment

    2. Surgical measures indicated

    3. Search for etiology should be made

    4. Complete physical examination with lab tests necessary to determine whether cataract is an isolated disorder or part of systemic disorder

Glaucoma

- Definition: Increased intraocular pressure involving one or both eyes which causes optic nerve damage and loss of vision

- Etiology/Incidence

    1. May be congenital (children under 3 years of age); autosomal recessive trait; congenital glaucoma accounts for approximately 5% of blindness in schools for the blind

    2. Over 60% diagnosed in first 6 months of life

    3. Bilateral in 75% of cases

4. May follow injury or eye disease

5. Complication of corticosteroid therapy

- Clinical Findings

    1. Photophobia; watering of eyes

    2. Persistent pain (sometimes)

    3. Decreased vision (peripheral vision affected first)

    4. Enlarged eye with increased corneal diameter; corneal edema

    5. Dilated pupil; thin, bluish sclera

    6. Large eyeball, firm to pressure

    7. Increased cupping of optic nerve

    8. Marked difference between normal and affected eye

    9. A systemic disorder frequently co-exists (e.g., cardiac anomalies, pyloric stenosis, deafness, etc.)

- Management/Treatment

    1. Immediate referral to ophthalmologist for diagnosis and treatment

    2. Anti-glaucoma drops; surgery indicated to relieve intraocular pressure

    3. Enucleation sometimes necessary

    4. Disease usually slowly progressive; blindness occurs without treatment

Myopia (Nearsightedness)

- Definition: The refractive error that occurs when light is focused anterior to the retina

- Etiology/Incidence

    1. Usually results from excessive length of the eyeball

    2. May also be caused by increased refractive power in the cornea or lens

    3. Often hereditary

    4. Frequently associated with prematurity

    5. Myopia tends to be progressive with age; usually first appearing around 8 years of age

- Clinical Findings

    1. Poor vision for distant objects

    2.   Squinting

    3.   Difficulty reading blackboard

    4.   Learning difficulties

    5.   Vision/screen abnormal

■ Management/Treatment

    1.   Refer to ophthalmologist or optometrist if suspected for definitive diagnosis and correction of refractive error

    2.   Education—importance of early detection and follow-up of abnormal vision screen; importance of wearing glasses once diagnosed

Hyperopia (Farsightedness)

■ Definition: The refractive error that occurs when light is focused behind the retina

■ Etiology/Incidence

    1.   Familial pattern

    2.   Usually results when eyeball is too short

    3.   May also be due to reduced refractive power of the cornea or lens

    4.   Some degree of hyperopia is normal in young children before puberty

■ Clinical Findings

    1.   May be asymptomatic

    2.   Headache and eye strain during close work in older children

    3.   Strabismus often seen when hyperopia is significant

    4.   Vision screening abnormal

■ Management/Treatment

    1.   Referral to ophthalmologist or optometrist, if suspected

    2.   Some improvement expected as child grows

    3.   Optical correction necessary with marked hyperopia or associated strabismus

Astigmatism

■ Definition: The refractive error that occurs from an irregularity in the shape of the cornea, or lens.

- Etiology/Incidence
    1. Largely familial; involves developmental variations in the curvature of the cornea
- Clinical Findings
    1. Often associated with other refractive errors
    2. Headache, fatigue, eye pain; frowning; reading difficulties
- Differential Diagnosis: Other refractive errors
- Management/Treatment
    1. Refer to ophthalmologist or optometrist if suspected, for diagnosis and treatment
    2. Eye glasses may be required for close or continuous work, depending on presence of other refractive errors

Strabismus

- Definition—ocular deviation with failure of eyes to maintain parallelism
    1. Intermittent alternating strabismus may be normal in the first six months of life
    2. Because of the inability to maintain parallelism, the image of the deviating eye is suppressed, with subsequent loss of vision on that side (amblyopia) which may be permanent if not treated
- Etiology/Incidence
    1. Often cannot be determined
    2. Congenital or hereditary pattern more common than acquired
    3. Occurs in 2 to 3% of children
- Clinical Findings—age dependent
    1. Squinting; decreased vision
    2. School problems
    3. Deviation of eye—noticed by parents
    4. Intermittent, alternating or continuous, esotropia or exotropia
    5. Abnormal Hirschberg and/or cover test
    6. Abnormal vision screen
- Management/Treatment

1. Immediate referral to ophthalmologist for any children over 6 months if suspected by history and physical examination and/or vision screen

2. Immediate referral to ophthalmologist for any children under 6 months if strabismus is fixed or continuous

3. Dependent on cause and associated pathology and refractive errors

4. May involve patching, corrective lens and surgery

Ocular Trauma

General

- Definition/Incidence/Etiology

    1. Ocular trauma is a frequent occurrence in pediatric injuries and a common cause of visual loss

    2. The National Society to Prevent Blindness estimates that ⅓ of eye loss in the child under 10 years is due to trauma

    3. Ocular trauma in sports is common (hockey, archery, darts, BB guns most common and serious)

    4. Other injuries result from bicycling, motorcycling, racquet sports, baseball, boxing and basketball

    5. Incidence higher in school age child

- Clinical Findings

    1. Detailed history of circumstances and agent involved very important; evaluate ocular mobility after perforation has been ruled out

    2. Minor signs of external trauma may hide severe intraocular injury

    3. Measure visual acuity of each eye separately; grossly estimate visual fields

    4. Examine lids and adnexa carefully; determine extent and depth of injury including lacrimal system

    5. Palpate orbital rim for crepitus (orbital or nasal fracture); x-ray with suspected orbital facture

    6. Examine pupils, size, shape, reaction to light

    7. Examine conjunctivae for lacerations, foreign body or underlying scleral perforation

8. Examine cornea under magnification if possible with Wood's Lamp or Slit Lamp; use fluorescein paper to stain cornea and Wood's Lamp to detect abrasions; evaluate anterior chamber for iritis, pus, blood

9. Observe for quivering of iris (iridodonesis), associated with dislocated lens

10. Topical anesthetic if needed for ease of examination

11. Evaluate immunization status

    a. Consider tetanus immunization and

    b. Rabies prophylaxis if appropriate

- Management/Treatment

1. Ocular injuries requiring immediate medical attention include

    a. Chemical burns to the eye (represents emergency)

    b. Severe lid lacerations

    c. Lacerations of the globe

    d. Hyphemas (blood in the anterior chamber)

    e. Intraocular foreign bodies or penetrating injury

    f. Blow-out fractures

2. Refer immediately to ophthalmology if positive findings so indicate

3. Place a protective shield over affected eye; avoiding any pressure to globe

4. Always be alert to the possibility of child abuse

5. Photograph injuries, when possible

6. Injury prevention—primary and secondary for all children and families; age appropriate (especially use of protective eyewear in sports)

Corneal Abrasion

- Definition: Scattered fine pinpoint loss of epithelium from corneal surface of one or both eyes

- Etiology/Incidence

1. Caused by foreign bodies located in upper lid; by abrasion from toy or fingernail; contact lenses; ultraviolet light exposure

    2.   Extremely common in pediatric age group

- Clinical Findings
  1. Photophobia
  2. Pain
  3. Lacrimation

- Management/Treatment
  1. Topical anesthetic may be required for evaluation *only*
  2. Remove foreign body with cotton tip applicator or irrigation with normal saline
  3. Fluorescein stain to detect corneal abrasions; examine with Wood's Lamp; green stain appears on epithelial defect
  4. Place eye shield to protect until evaluated
  5. May need referral to ophthalmologist

Chemical Burns

- Definition/Etiology
  1. **True ocular emergency—can result in significant visual loss and possible loss of eye**
  2. Common household agents often cause chemical injuries to eye; alkali burns usually more damaging than acid

- Management/Treatment—*EMERGENCY*
  1. Copious irrigation with water, 0.9% sodium chloride, or other bland fluids for 30 minutes; refer to ophthalmologist immediately
  2. In hospital, lid should be held apart with retractor and irrigation should continue 20 to 30 minutes with normal saline connected to IV tubing
  3. Topical anesthetic may ease pain and discomfort; sedation and analgesics may be necessary

Hyphema

- Definition/Etiology/Incidence
  1. Accumulation of blood in the anterior chamber; produced by rupture of iris or ciliary body blood vessels due to blunt or perforating injuries
  2. Most fill less than ⅓ of chamber and usually last 5 to 6 days

- Clinical Findings
  1. History of injury
  2. Blood in anterior chamber
  3. Drowsiness—unknown reason, but often occurs
- Management/Treatment
  1. Refer to ophthalmologist
  2. Bedrest with head elevated 30 to 40 degrees to promote resorption of blood; hospitalization often necessary; monocular eye patch for 5 days; no aspirin

Ocular Tumors

Retinoblastoma

- Definition: Malignant tumor that arises from immature retina
- Etiology/Incidence
  1. The most common intraocular malignancy of childhood; occur once in 17,000 to 34,000 live births; similar for black and white children
  2. Average age of diagnosis 18 months
  3. No sex preference or race predilection
  4. Positive family history in 6%; autosomal dominant transmission
  5. Specific chromosomal abnormality has been demonstrated in approximately 5% of patients; most occur as a spontaneous mutation
  6. Tumor occurs in both eyes—25 to 30%
- Clinical Findings
  1. Vary depending on stage of tumor
  2. Most common presenting sign is leukokoria ("white pupil") yellowish-white pupillary reflex
  3. Loss of vision; poor vision; strabismus (fixed in 20% of cases)
  4. Red, painful eye
  5. Ocular inflammation
  6. Heterochromia iridis
  7. Hyphema

8. Nystagmus

9. White spots on iris

- Differential Diagnosis: Misdiagnosis occurs in about 20% of cases

    1. Inflammatory disease of eye

    2. Glaucoma; retinal detachment; cataract

    3. Trauma

    4. Blind eye

- Management/Treatment

    1. Immediate referral to ophthalmology, if suspected and prompt referral for other ophthalmological disorders that could present as symptoms of retinoblastoma (e.g., strabismus)

    2. Primary treatment involves enucleation and irradiation

    3. Genetic counseling

    4. The prognosis depends on the extent of disease at the time of diagnosis

Common Problems of the Ear

Hearing Loss

- Definition

    1. Sensorineural loss—damage to the inner ear structures, e.g., cochlea, and or auditory nerve; is irreversible and can range from mild to total

    2. Conductive loss—interference with transmission of sound through external auditory canal to middle ear and/or problems in the middle ear, e.g., cerumen, serous otitis media

    3. Hearing loss

        a. Mild—26 to 40dB

        b. Moderate—41 to 55dB

        c. Severe—71 to 90dB

        d. Profound—91dB and above

- Etiology/Incidence: 0.5 to 1/1000 in newborns; 1.5 to 2/1000 < 6 years

    Types

    1. Congenital

    a. Sensorineural (moderate to profound loss)

        (1) Hereditary—recessive Y-linked or dominant

        (2) Asphyxia

        (3) Erythroblastosis

        (4) Maternal rubella and other viruses

    b. Conductive (moderate loss)

        (1) Congenital atresia, stenosis or other deformities of ossicles

  2. Acquired

    a. Sensorineural (mild to profound loss)

        (1) Labyrinthitis

        (2) Measles

        (3) Meningitis

        (4) Mumps

        (5) Tumors

        (6) Trauma (may also be conductive or mixed)

    b. Conductive (mild to moderate loss)

        (1) Cerumen

        (2) Foreign bodies

        (3) Perforated tympanic membrane

        (4) Otitis media with middle effusion (most frequent case)

        (5) Cholesteatoma

■ Clinical Findings

  1. Behavioral

    a. Zero to 4 months—failure to respond to voice or noise

    b. Four months to 1 year—failure to localize a source of sound; lack of response to the spoken word

    c. One to 2 years—failure to have varied vocalizations of consonants and vowels; failure to develop age appropriate language

    d. Two years+—retarded speech/language development, educational problems, behavior problems

2. Physical Findings

   a. May reveal abnormalities of external ear canal and tympanic membrane, presence of middle ear fluid, evidence of obstructive adenoids

   b. Abnormalities of tuning fork Weber and Rinne tests

   c. Other evidence of congenital malformations

■ Management/Treatment

1. Hearing loss must be detected as early as possible so that intervention can be instituted immediately. It is now possible to test infants as young as 3 months

2. Referral for full audiological testing and language evaluation as soon as deficit strongly suspected or when middle ear effusion persists > 3 months or with recurrent otitis media

3. Prevention

   a. Early and periodic hearing and language screening

   b. Prompt identification and treatment of middle ear disease or obstruction

   c. Avoidance of persistent loud noise

Otitis externa ("Swimmer's ear")

■ Definition: Inflammation and or infection of external ear canal

■ Etiology/Incidence

1. Predisposing factors that disrupt normal protective mechanisms and increase vulnerability to inflammation and infection with pathogens

   a. Humidity

   b. High temperature

   c. Allergy

   d. Stress

   e. Excessive wetness (swimming, bathing or increased environmental humidity)

   f. Loss of protective cerumen and chronic irritation usually due to excessive moisture in canal

   g. Excessive dryness (eczema)

h. Trauma (foreign body or digital irritation)

2. Most common organisms are *Pseudomonas aeruginosa*, *Enterobacter aerogenes*, *Proteus mirabilis*, *Klebsiella pneumoniae*, *Staphylococcus epidermis*, and fungi, e.g., *Candida*, Aspergillus (Behrman, 1992)

3. More common in summer months

■ Clinical Findings

1. Pruritus of ear canal may be an early symptom

2. Prominent ear pain, tenderness more pronounced with pressure and/or manipulation of the pinna

3. Edema and erythema of external canal with white or green discharge

4. Signs of infection beyond skin of ear canal (cellulitis of pinnae, fever, adenopathy)

5. Often a history of frequent swimming

■ Differential Diagnosis

1. Foreign bodies

2. Furunculosis

3. Otitis media

4. Mastoiditis

■ Management/Treatment/Nursing Considerations

1. Remove debris by gentle irrigation with warm water or saline or 2% acetic acid

2. Topical antibiotic containing neomycin, polymyxin and corticosteroid Otic drops (Cortisporin Otic), 3 to 4 drops for 7 days

3. Insertion of gauze wick in ear canal for first 24 to 48 hours may facilitate distribution of medication when edema and inflammation are severe

4. Analgesic for pain when severe

5. Prevention: Instillation of white vinegar and rubbing alcohol (50/50) in both ear canals at the end of each swim; recommended for frequent infections; avoidance of vigorous ear cleaning

6. Re-examine 5 to 10 days after treatment especially if unable to visualize the tympanic membrane due to swelling

Otitis media (O.M.)

- Definition: Acute or chronic inflammation and/or infection of the mucoperiosteal lining of middle ear cleft (eustachian tube, tympanic cavity, mastoid antrum, mastoid air cell system). Common terms include:

  1. Acute purulent otitis media (acute suppurative otitis media)
  2. Chronic purulent otitis media (chronic suppurative otitis media)
  3. Acute serous otitis media (acute otitis media with effusion [O.M.E.])
  4. Chronic serous otitis media (Chronic otitis media with effusion)

- Etiology/Incidence

  1. Very common childhood disease, especially prevalent under 2 years of age
  2. Children who have early O.M. onset are at high risk for recurrent O.M. and chronic O.M.E.
  3. More common in winter/spring
  4. More common in boys
  5. Whites, American Indians, and Eskimos more common than Blacks
  6. Predisposing factors
     a. Developmental considerations—eustachian tube of young child shorter, wider, and straighter than when fully matured; thus organisms from nasopharynx reach middle ear more easily
     b. May be familial predisposition
     c. Often occurs with or follows upper respiratory infection
     d. Bottle feeding in supine position predisposing factor
     e. Certain congenital defects (e.g., cleft palate)
     f. Allergy
     g. Parental smoking
     h. Children in group Day Care Centers
  7. Organisms frequently involved
     a. *Streptococcus pneumoniae* (most common bacteria)
     b. *Haemophilus influenzae*

    c. *Moraxella catarrhalis*

    d. Beta-hemolytic group A streptococcus

    e. Other organisms (*Staphylococcus aureus* and *Pseudomonas aeruginosa* more common in chronic otitis media)

    f. Viral (influenza, coxsackie, RSV less common)

    g. *Escherichia coli* and *Staphylococcus aureus* more common organisms in neonate

- Clinical Findings—classical presentation often not seen

  1. Vary with age and progression

    a. Fever varies greatly

    b. Ear ache; ear fullness, discomfort; tinnitus

    c. Malaise; irritability; poor feeding/appetite (especially in infants)

    d. Nausea and vomiting

    e. Nasal congestion

    f. Tugging on the ear

    g. Serosanguinous or bloody discharge indicative of ruptured tympanic membrane

    h. Conductive hearing loss

  2. Examination of middle ear—findings depend on progression and stage of otitis media

    a. Acute otitis media—tympanic membrane usually erythematous, opaque and may be bulging; pus may be evident; the light reflex is distorted or absent and the landmarks are indistinct or absent; pneumatic otoscopy reveals hypo or absent mobility; purulent drainage may indicate perforation

    b. Serous otitis media (otitis media with effusion)—tympanic membrane may be opaque or translucent with presence of air bubbles or air-fluid level; the membrane may be retracted due to negative pressure; mobility is always impaired or absent; land marks may be absent or prominent if retracted; the light reflex may be diffuse or absent

- Diagnostic Tests/Findings: Choice depends on toxicity, age of child, and stage of middle ear disease

  1. Pneumatic otoscopy (mobility always impaired)

2. Tympanometry Type B or Flat tympanogram 90% diagnostic (measures compliance)

3. Audiometric tests may be indicated for children > 3 years

4. Myringotomy or tympanocentesis and culture is considered the "gold standard" usually done by otolaryngologist for persistent problem

5. Language screen as indicated

- Management/Treatment

    1. Oral antibiotic therapy; choice based on suspected organisms and presence of beta-lactamase producing resistent organisms (See Table 1)

    2. Maintenance of hydration

    3. Management of pain, discomfort, and fever

        a. Analgesics; acetaminophen

        b. Local anesthetic drops (should never be used if perforation is suspected)

    4. Use of decongestants have not proven to be helpful

    5. Education

        a. Importance of follow-up; all children should be re-examined in 10 to 12 days or sooner if no response to treatment

        b. Importance of taking all medicine as prescribed

    6. Hospitalization may be necessary for neonate or young infant

    7. Complications

        a. Mastoiditis

        b. Sepsis in young infant

        c. Hearing loss

        d. Language impairment/delay

    8. Prevention

        a. Proper feeding techniques for infants; breast feeding shown to be protective

        b. Avoid vigorous nose blowing

        c. Antibiotic prophylaxis used in select cases of frequent and recurrent otitis media ($\geq$ 3 in 6 months); amoxicillin and sulfasoxazole are drugs of choice with one-half the therapeutic dose given daily

9. Referral to otolaryngologist

   a. Persistent/acute O.M. unresponsive to treatment

   b. Frequent recurrent O.M. (3 in 6 months)

   c. Persistent/chronic O.M.E. > 12 weeks

   d. Evidence of hearing loss and/or language delay

Table 1

Antibiotics Frequently Prescribed for Otitis Media	
Drug	**Dosage (Given for 10 days)**
Amoxicillin	40mg/kg/day in 3 doses q8h (most often 1st line drug)
Ampicillin	100mg/kg/day in 4 doses q6h
Amoxicillin-clavulanate	40mg/kg/day in 3 doses (with food) q8h
Erythromycin-sulfisoxazole	50mg/kg/day of erythromycin; 150 mg/kg/day of sulfasoxazole divided in 3 to 4 doses— q6-8h
Cefaclor	40mg/kg/day divided in 3 doses q8h
Trimethoprim-sulfamethoxazole	8mg/kg/day trimethoprim/ 40mg/kg/day sulfamethoxazole in 2 doses q12h
Cefixime	8mg/kg/day once daily or divided q12h
Cefprozil	15mg/kg/day in divided doses q12h
Loracarbef	30mg/kg/day in divided doses q12h

Mastoiditis

- Definition: Inflammation of the mastoid antrum and aircell with associated bone necrosis—usually a complication of otitis media
- Etiology/Incidence
  1. Rare since the advent of antibiotic therapy for O.M.
  2. Usually a history of recent or recurrent otitis media
  3. Frequent organisms
     a. *Streptococcus pneumoniae*
     b. Group A streptococcus
     c. *Staphylococcus aureus*
     d. *Haemophilus influenzae*
     e. *Pseudomonas* (chronic mastoiditis)
     f. *Mycobacterium tuberculosis* (rare, but should be considered)
- Clinical Findings
  1. Usually appear after episode of A.O.M.
     a. Pain behind ear and/or protrusion of pinna
     b. Low grade fever/irritability
     c. Mastoid tenderness, redness and swelling
     d. Continuous purulent discharge continuing after rupture of T.M. with A.O.M.
     e. Evidence of acute purulent O.M. on examination
- Diagnostic Tests/Findings
  1. CBC—WBC elevated
  2. PPD if high risk for tuberculosis
  3. Radiography of mastoids
  4. Myringotomy to define organism
- Management/Treatment
  1. Refer to ENT immediately
  2. IV antibiotics and possible surgery to drain middle ear indicated

3. Complications include meningitis and brain abscess

4. Prevention—early and proper treatment of otitis media

Mouth

Herpangina

- Definition: A common acute febrile viral illness characterized by oropharyngeal papulovesicular lesions (See Table 2)

- Etiology/Incidence

    1. Coxsackievirus, group A (most common)

    2. Echoviruses

    3. Affects children of any age—most common reported age 1 to 4

    4. Common in summer and fall/epidemic form

    5. Occurs in temperate climates

- Clinical Findings

    1. Sudden onset of fever with range of normal to 106 °F

    2. Headache

    3. Characteristic discrete vesicles or ulcers (or both) (one to two or several), most commonly on anterior tonsillar pillars, soft palate, uvula and pharyngeal wall; occasionally on tip of tongue

    4. Significant oral discomfort; drooling

- Differential Diagnosis: Mainly other diseases with exanthems

    1. Herpes stomatitis (Herpes simplex type 1)

    2. Aphthous stomatitis

    3. Steven-Johnson syndrome

    4. Epstein-Barr pharyngitis

    5. Kawasaki disease

    6. Streptococcal pharyngitis

    7. Adenovirus pharyngitis

- Diagnostic Tests/Findings: Of little value; not necessary; diagnosis made on clinical grounds

- Management/Treatment
    1. Antipyretic therapy; acetaminophen in appropriate doses
    2. Local analgesics sometimes helpful—2% viscous lidocaine, must be used with caution; may be harmful
    3. Adequate hydration
    4. Observation for more serious illness, especially in infant and young child
    5. Proper hand washing, personal hygiene and diaper handling to limit spread of disease

Hand, Foot, and Mouth Disease

- Definition: Common acute viral disease similar to that of herpangina with a vesicular exanthem distributed over buccal mucosa and palate, with similar lesions on the hands and feet and occasionally in the diaper area.
- Etiology/Incidence
    1. Coxsackie virus A16-most common
    2. Enterovirus 17
    3. Most cases < 10 years of age
    4. Summer and fall pattern
- Clinical Findings
    1. Papulovesicular lesions, shallow ulcers hard palate, buccal mucosa, tonsils and tongue
    2. Vesicular lesions on arms, legs, palms, soles and occasionally buttocks
- Differential Diagnosis
    1. Same as for herpangina
    2. Other dermatologic infections
    3. Other exanthems
- Diagnostic Tests/Findings: Unnecessary
- Management/Treatment: Same as herpangina; see Table 2

Thrush (Candidiasis)

- Definition: Common opportunistic fungal infection of the oral cavity
- Etiology/Incidence
    1. *Candida albicans*
    2. More common in neonate and infant than in other age groups
    3. Transmission—during vaginal delivery
    4. Predisposing factors
        a. Antibiotic therapy
        b. Steroid therapy
        c. Compromised immune system
- Clinical Findings
    1. Characteristic white plaques that do not scrape off easily
    2. Found on the buccal mucosa, tongue, pharynx or tonsils
    3. Raw erythematous surface when wiped off
- Diagnostic Tests/Findings: Systemic workup including immune workup if persistent or refractory to treatment
- Management/Treatment
    1. Antifungal therapy; nystatin oral suspension, 100,000 units applied to oral mucosa, four times a day for 10 days
    2. Careful instructions for proper administration and follow-up
    3. If infant breast feeding consider examining and treating mother for candidiasis of breast (cross-infection)
    4. Check diaper area for concurrent diaper rash

Table 2

Common Infectious Exanthems of the Mouth

Disease	Etiology	Exanthem	Associated S&S
Herpangina	Coxsackie group A	1-5 vesicles or ulcers on tonsils palate, uvula & anterior pillars	Fever Dysphagia
Hand Foot Mouth disease	Coxsackie A 5, A 10 A 16	1-several ulcers on tongue buccal mucosa +/ or tonsils	Fever Vesicles on palms & soles
Aphthous stomatitis	Unknown	1-3 ulcers inside lips, buccal mucosa or lateral aspect of tongue	No fever
Herpetic-gingivostomatitis	Herpes Simplex Type 1	1-several vesicles or ulcers coalesce lips, gingivae, tongue buccal mucosa/pharynx	Fever Very painful Adenopathy
Thrush	*Candida albicans*	White plaques tongue, buccal mucosa	Usually no fever

Dental Caries

- Definition: An infectious disease of the primary or permanent teeth causing decay and tooth destruction and may lead to premature loss of teeth and gum disease—occurrence varies widely for different populations

- Etiology/Incidence

  1. Baby bottle tooth decay (nursing caries) caused by infant or child sleeping with a bottle containing milk, juice, or anything except water—produces rapid decay; usually occurs between 1 and 2 years; occurs in approximately 15% of children and approximately 50% of some native american population

  2. Breast fed infants who sleep at the breast are at risk for caries—no data on prevalence

  3. Dental caries of the grooves of the molar teeth account for more dental caries in children

4. *Streptococcus mutans* organism responsible for infection

■ Clinical Findings

1. White spots on teeth appear first (decalcification of enamel)

2. Early cavity—light brown color progresses to dark brown of chronic caries and tooth destruction (caries can progress to tooth destruction in 1-2 months)

■ Diagnostic Tests/Findings: History and careful examination

■ Management/Treatment

1. Prevention—key

a. Proper feeding practices and nutrition

b. Proper and timely weaning from bottle and breast

c. Early brushing or wiping teeth soon as they appear

d. Discourage coating pacifiers with sweet substances

e. Proper brushing and flossing practices for older child

f. Fluoride supplement

g. Early dental visits (See Health Maintenance and Promotion chapter)

2. Refer to pediatric dentist as soon as detected

Questions

Select the best answer

1. During examination of a 6-year-old child, the nurse practitioner notes an opacity of the lens on the left eye. The right eye appears to have a normal red reflex. The following statements are true about cataracts, except

   a. Frequently there is a possible family history
   b. Cataract may be a complication of long-term use of corticosteroids
   c. Strabismus may be the first indication of cataract in a child
   d. The child will usually complain of constant pain and discomfort in the affected eye

2. During a "well child" examination, a mother complains that her 3-year-old child does not seem to hear well. Each of the following conditions may be associated with acquired conductive hearing loss, except

   a. Foreign bodies
   b. Otitis media
   c. Impacted cerumen
   d. History of measles

3. A 15-month-old boy has had repeated episodes of acute otitis media. The parents are concerned about the effects this may have on his future school performance. In responding to the parents' concerns, each of the following statements about otitis media might be made, except

   a. The incidence of otitis media is highest during the first 2 years of life
   b. Bilateral otitis media with effusion may produce a temporary hearing deficit
   c. The presence of a hearing deficit may interfere with the acquisition of language skills
   d. There is a correlation between the number of days a child has otitis media with effusion and later measures of IQ

4. The most common organisms responsible for the majority of otitis media include all of the following, except

   a. *Streptococcus pneumoniae*
   b. *Haemophilus influenzea*
   c. *Moraxella catarrhalis*
   d. *Mycoplasma pneumoniae*

5. Ocular injuries that require immediate referral to the ophthalmologist include all

of the following, except

    a. Chemical burns to eye
    b. Severe lid lacerations
    c. Hyphemas
    d. Corneal abrasions

6. A 2-week-old infant comes for a scheduled "well" baby check-up. On examination of the eye, you note a mucopurulent drainage from the left eye. There is moderate lid edema and the conjunctivae are erythematous bilaterally with moderate chemosis. In considering the kind of conjunctivitis presenting in this infant, your differential would include all of the following, except

    a. Gonococcal conjunctivitis
    b. Chlamydia conjunctivitis
    c. Chemical conjunctivitis
    d. Bacterial conjunctivitis

7. Prophylactic treatment of the newborn with instillation of erythromycin 1% ophthalmic ointment should be effective in preventing

    a. Gonococcal conjunctivitis
    b. Chlamydia conjunctivitis only
    c. Chemical conjunctivitis
    d. Gonococcal Chemical and chlamydia conjunctivitis as well as chlamydia pneumonia

8. The drug of choice for the treatment of gonococcal conjunctivitis in the newborn is

    a. Systemic and topical Penicillin G 50,000 U/kg/day for 7 to 10 days
    b. Ceftriaxone 25 to 50mg/kg/day given once
    c. Sodium sulfacetamide 10% ophthalmic solution q.i.d. for 21 days
    d. Erythromycin 50mg/kg/day for 14 days

9. Stringy thick mucoid discharge and a cobblestone appearance of inner aspect upper lid is most likely indicative of

    a. Chemical conjunctivitis
    b. Bacterial conjunctivitis
    c. Vernal conjunctivitis
    d. Herpes simplex keratoconjunctivitis

10. When assessing a child who presents with a tender erythematous mass in the upper eyelid margin, the nurse practitioner should consider the following to be true about lesions in the eyelids except

    a. A Hordeolum may begin with diffuse edema of the eyelid
    b. Hordeolum involves the sebaceous gland in the lid margin

c. Chalazions must always be referred for surgical removal

d. The most frequent organism found to cause hordeolum is Staphylococcus aureus

11. A 4-year-old-boy presents with a small lump in the lower eyelid It has been there for some time according to his mother and does not seem to bother the child. The vision screen is normal. The most likely diagnosis to consider would be

a. Hordeolum
b. Blepharitis
c. Chalazion
d. Slow progressing tumor of the eyelid

12. When advising a family about the management of blepharitis the nurse practitioner should advise the child and parent that

a. The eyelids should be left alone to heal on their own
b. Referral to an allergist for testing and possible allergy shots will be indicated
c. Application of steroid ophthalmic ointment once daily will help control symptoms
d. The goal in management should be to control symptoms, using warm, moist compresses and gentle scrubbing of the lid margins with baby shampoo daily.

13. Clinical findings commonly associated with dacryostenosis include all of the following except

a. Persistent tearing of one or both eyes
b. Crusting of the eyelashes
c. Erythema and swelling over the lacrimal sac
d. Mild to moderate erythema of the conjunctivae

14. Which of the following statements is true about dacryostenosis?

a. Administration of antibiotic ophthalmic drops is always indicated for an infant with dacryostenosis.
b. Surgical probing of the lacrimal duct may be indicated in an infant who has persistent dacryostenosis beyond 6 months
c. 25% of infants who have dacryostenosis go on to develop dacryocystitis
d. Dacryostenosis is usually associated with poor hygiene

15. While examining a 9-month-old-child during a well child visit, you notice that the child's right eye appears considerably larger than the left. The mother comments that the child rubs the eye frequently because it waters and appears to bother her. In considering the possible causes of these symptoms, all of the following clinical findings would alert you to the diagnosis of glaucoma except

a. An increased corneal diameter in the affected eye
b. A dilated pupil in the affected eye

c. A large eyeball that is firm to pressure
d. Erythema of the bulbar conjunctiva

16. The following statements are true about glaucoma except

a. Most cases of glaucoma in children are diagnosed in the first 6 months of life
b. Glaucoma may follow injury to the eye
c. Most cases of glaucoma in children involve only one eye
d. Congenital glaucoma is an autosomal recessive trait

17. The primary management of this child would be

a. Instillation of anti-glaucoma drops and a follow-up visit in two weeks
b. Explanation to the mother that the child will probably develop blindness
c. Immediate referral to an ophthalmologist for diagnosis and treatment
d. Observation and instructions for mother to return if symptoms worsen

18. The refractive error that occurs when light is focused behind the retina is known as

a. Astigmatism
b. Myopia
c. Hyperopia
d. Anistropia

19. All of the following clinical findings may be seen in children with strabismus except

a. Squinting
b. Deviation of the eye
c. School problems
d Excessive tearing

20. In assessing a child who presents with ocular trauma, the nurse practitioner should

a. Refer the child immediately to the ophthalmologist
b. Administer a DT booster and initiate rabies prophylaxis
c. Obtain a detailed history of the circumstances and agent(s) involved in the injury
d. Proceed immediately with a careful examination of the eye

21. A mother calls your office and reports that her 15 month old child appears to have gotten a household disinfectant in his eyes. The child is crying hard and rubbing his eyes. In addition to calling 911 you instruct her to

a. Put patches over both eyes and wait for the rescue squad
b. Put patches over eyes and go immediately to the emergency room
c. Immediately flush the eyes with water and continue flushing until the rescue squad arrives
d. Administer acetaminophen for the pain and bring the child to the office for evaluation

22. A 2-year-old-child is noted to have leukokoria in one eye on physical examination. All of the following causes should be considered in the differential diagnosis except

    a. Glaucoma
    b. Retinoblastoma
    c. Strabismus
    d. Cataract

23. When counseling a parent about measures to take to prevent the recurrence of otitis media, the following would be considered potential aggravating factors except

    a. Taking a bottle to bed at night
    b. Presence of cigarette smoke
    c. Day care
    d. Sleeping in parent's bed

24. Indications for referral of a child with otitis media to an otolaryngologist for evaluation and treatment would include all of the following except

    a. Evidence of hearing loss or language delay
    b. Persistent chronic middle ear effusion lasting more than 12 weeks that is unresponsive to treatment
    c. Recurrent otitis media involving 2 to 3 infections in the past 12 months
    d. A persistent acute purulent otitis media that is unresponsive to treatment with 3 courses of antibiotics

25. The most appropriate first line antibiotic to be used in the treatment of acute otitis media is

    a. Erythromycin-sulfisoxazole
    b. Cefaclor
    c. Amoxicillin
    d. Augmentin

26. In considering the diagnosis of Herpangina for a child who presents with lesions in the mouth, the following clinical findings would support this diagnosis except

    a. Vesicles and/or ulcers present primarily in the posterior oral cavity (tonsils, uvula, anterior pillars
    b. Fever
    c. Blisters on lips and gingivae and tongue
    d. Mild to moderate dysphagia

27· The presence of white plaques on the buccal mucosa and tongue that do not scrape off indicates an infection with

    a. Coxsackievirus group A
    b. *Streptococcus pyogenes*

c. *Candida albicans*
d. Epstein Barr Virus

28. When counseling parents about the prevention of early dental caries in the primary teeth, which of the following considerations is most important?

a. Early and regular dental visits
b. Avoidance of sleeping with a bottle or at breast and timely weaning from bottle and breast
c. Frequent brushing of infant's teeth
d. Early fluoride supplements

29. Organisms most often involved in the cause of otitis externa include all of the following except

a. *Staphylococcus epidermis*
b. *Mycoplasma pneumoniae*
c. *Pseudomonas aeruginosa*
d. *Proteus mirabilis*

Answer Key:

1.	d	15.	d
2.	d	16.	c
3.	d	17.	c
4.	d	18.	c
5.	d	19.	d
6.	c	20.	c
7.	a	21.	c
8.	b	22.	c
9.	c	23.	d
10.	c	24.	c
11.	c	25.	c
12.	d	26.	c
13.	c	27.	c
14.	b	28.	b
		29.	b

Bibliography

American Academy of Pediatrics (1994). *Report of the committee on infectious diseases* (23rd ed.). Elk Grove Village IL: American Academy of Pediatrics.

Barfa, M., & Baum, J. (1992). Ocular infections. *Infectious Disease Clinics of North America, 6*(4), 769-815, 925-952.

Behrman, R. E., Kliegman, R. M., Nelson, W. E., & Vaugh, V. C. (Eds.). (1992). *Nelson textbook of pediatrics* (14th ed.). Philadelphia: W. B. Saunders.

Bluestone, C. (1989). Modern management of Otitis Media. *The Pediatric Clinics of North America, 36*(6), 1371-1385.

Bluestone, C., & Klein, J. (1988). *Otitis media in infants and children*. Philadelphia: W. B. Saunders.

Dysor, A. T., et al. (1989). Speech characteristics of children after otitis media. *Journal of Pediatric Health Care, 1*(5), 26-265.

Goycoolea, M. (Ed.). (1992). Otitis media—The pathogenesis approach. *The Otolaryngologic Clinics of North America, 24*(4), 757-979.

Josell, S., & Abrams, R. (1991). Pediatric oral health. *The Pediatric Clinics of North America, 38*(5), 1049-1342.

Klein, B., & Scars, M. (1992). Pediatric ocular injuries. *Pediatrics in Review, 13*(1), 422-428.

Klein, J. (1994). Preventing recurrent otitis; what role for antibiotics? *Contemporarty Pediatrics 11*, 44-60.

Malinow, I., & Powell, K. (1993). *Periorbital cellulitis*. Pediatric Annal, 22, 241-246.

Nelson, L. B. (1993). Pediatric ophthalmology. *Pediatric Clinics of North America, 40*(4), 698-891.

Northern, J. L. (1987). Advanced techniques for measuring middle ear function. *Pediatrics 61*, 761.

Rice, D. H. (Ed.). (1993). Inflammatory diseases and the sinuses. *The Otolaryngologic Clinics of North America, 26*(4), 507-700.

Wright, P., Sell, S., McConnell, K., Sitten, A., Thompson, J., Vaughan, W., & Bess, F. (1988). Impact of recurrent otitis media on middle ear function, hearing, and language. *The Journal of Pediatrics, 113*, 581-587.

Respiratory Disorders

Carole Stone

Acute Nasopharyngitis (Common Cold)

- Definition: Acute communicable viral infection involving the upper respiratory tract characterized by nasal stuffiness, sneezing, coryza, throat irritation, and no or minimal fever

- Etiology/Incidence

  1. Susceptibility varies among individuals but is universal; usually 5 to 8 infections per year; highest during first 2 years

  2. Peak occurrence in fall, winter spring

  3. Transmission by contact with nasal secretions or airborne in close contact

  4. Causative Organisms: More than 200 different viral organisms

     a. Rhinoviruses (most common)

     b. Other common agents include Parainfluenza viruses, Respiratory syncytial virus, Corona virus, Adenovirus, Enterovirus, Influenza virus, Reovirus, Mycoplasma pneumonia, Other organisms (> 100 viral types)

- Clinical Findings—may be more severe in young child than in older children; duration of illness 4 to 7 days

  1. Infants

     a. Irritability

     b. Restlessness

     c. Nasal obstruction

     d. Coryza

     e. Occasional vomiting and diarrhea

     f. Fever (34 °C to 39 °C; 100.4 °F to 102.2 °F)

  2. Older children

     a. Nasal discharge, sneezing, nasal congestion

     b. Sore throat, malaise, headache, cough, chills, low-grade fever, muscle aches

  3. Physical Findings

     a. Nasal discharge serous to purulent

    b. Moist, boggy sometimes erythematous nasal mucosa

    c. May have mild erythema of oropharynx with mild erythema of tympanic membrane in early stages (mobility and landmarks all normal)

- Differential Diagnosis

    1. Allergic rhinitis

    2. Sinusitis

    3. Pharyngitis

    4. Early signs of other illnesses

- Diagnostic Tests/Findings: Usually unnecessary

- Management/Treatment

    1. Symptomatic and supportive care

        a. Analgesics—acetaminophen in age-appropriate doses only if indicated by discomfort and/or significant fever

        b. Relief of nasal obstruction

            (1) Saline nose drops

            (2) Gentle aspiration with nasal bulb syringe

            (3) Cool mist humidification

            (4) Discourage use of decongestants and antihistamines, especially in young infants

            (5) No role for antibiotics; role of vitamin C inconclusive

        c. Consider secondary bacterial infection for prolonged signs and symptoms

        d. Encourage fluids to liquefy secretions

    2. Prevention

        a. Isolation impractical; limited to child with high susceptibility to complications (semi-isolation from crowds and other persons)

        b. Hand washing; use of tissues and proper nasal toilet

        c. Proper cleansing of toys, play areas, and other contaminated objects

    3. Complications

        a. Otitis media, most common in younger child

b. Cervical adenitis

c. Sinusitis, laryngitis, adenoiditis, pharyngitis

d. Pneumonia

e. Bacterial infections of lower respiratory tract

Allergic Rhinitis

- Definition: An IgE mediated allergic disease of the nose which produces an inflammation of the nasal mucosa following an immediate hypersensitivity response in a child who has been sensitized to inhaled allergens or irritants

- Etiology/Incidence—specific IgE is fixed to the basophils in the nasal secretions and to the mast cells of the nasal mucosa

  1. The most common cause of nasal congestion in childhood affecting approximately 10% of children and 15% of adolescents; may be episodic or perennial

     a. Seasonal—usually inhaled pollens

     b. Perennial—house dust mite, molds, animal danders (most common allergens)

- Clinical Findings

  1. Signs/symptoms—vary from season to season

     a. Paroxysms of sneezing

     b. Itching of nose, eyes, conjunctiva, palate and pharynx

     c. Rhinorrhea watery, profuse

     d. Nasal congestion/obstruction; mouth breathing and snoring at night

     e. General malaise, fatigue, irritability, loss of appetite

     f. May be associated signs of allergic conjunctivitis, sinusitis, and/or serous otitis media; atopic dermatitis

  2. Physical findings

     a. Allergic "shiners"

     b. Hypertrophy of gingival mucosa

     c. Allergic "salute"

     d. Gaping expression ("allergic gape")

     e. Hypertrophied lymphoid tissue

     f. Edema of nasal mucous membranes

     g. Boggy, blue-grey, edematous nasal mucosa with watery or mucoid discharge

     h. Halitosis

■ Differential Diagnosis

   1. Acute or chronic sinusitis; viral or bacterial U.R.I.

   2. Congenital lesions/anatomic obstruction; nasal polyps

   3. Vasomotor rhinitis

   4. Rhinitis medicamentosa

   5. Chronic cocaine use

■ Diagnostic Tests/Findings

   1. Examination of nasal mucosa for eosinophils (10 to 100% may be found)

   2. Blood eosinophils level and total IgE (may be elevated or normal)

■ Management/Treatment: Individualized—referral to allergist may be necessary

   1. Identification and avoidance of specific allergens and irritants when possible

   2. Air conditioning units and air-purifying units

   3. Drug therapy—highly individualized

     a. Antihistamine Newer H_1 receptor antagonists (terfenadine, astemizole, loratadine) do not cause as much sedation as older drugs (chlorpheniramine)

     b. Oral decongestant sympathomimetic (phenylpropanolamine, pseudoephedrine); short term relief

     c. Topical sympathomimetics used only in severe nasal congestion for brief period (2 to 3 days); may cause rebound congestion

     d. Cromolyn sodium nasal solution 3 to 6 times day; prevents hypersensitivity response; does not prevent nasal congestion

     e. Topical corticosteroids, such as beclomethasone, flunisolide highly effective; may reduce or eliminate need for other medications; should start about 1 to 2 weeks before pollen season

   4. Immunotherapy—time-consuming and expensive; saved for difficult cases

Epistaxis

- **Definition**: Nasal bleeding which is spontaneous or triggered by some minor external trauma or irritation
- **Etiology**
  1. The most common cause is mucosal irritation due to nose picking, sneezing and blowing, often in the presence of an inflamed and friable nasal mucosa
  2. Mucosa drying most often in winter secondary to drying of the air from central heating systems
  3. Trauma due to falls or blows
  4. Infection (especially with group A beta-hemolytic streptococcus or coagulase positive staphylococcus)
  5. Foreign bodies
  6. Other causes—rare but should be considered with profuse or recurrent bleeding that is difficult to stop
     a. Bleeding disorders, e.g., hemophilia, aplastic anemia, leukemia, idiopathic thrombocytopenia
     b. Vascular abnormalities, e.g., hereditary hemorrhagic telangiectasis and juvenile nasopharyngeal angiofibroma
     c. Hypertension
- **Clinical Findings**
  1. History should include
     a. Whether episode is acute or recurrent; unilateral or bilateral
     b. Duration of bleed and approximate volume of blood loss (number of handkerchiefs or tissues soaked); mild bleeding that is controlled by application of pressure is more suggestive of irritation or infection
     c. Recent URI; allergic rhinitis; other allergies
     d. Medications such as ASA or NSAID
     e. Other signs and symptoms of underlying disease
  2. Physical Findings
     a. Inspection of the nose for points of hemorrhage, signs of

obstruction, lesions or foreign bodies; (gentle cleansing of clots and discharge may be necessary for proper visualization)

b. Dilated septal vessels of Kiesselbach's plexus most frequent site (bleeding usually triggered by mucosal irritation or infection)

c. Excoriation and erythema of nasal septum with purulent nasal discharge (usually indicates infection)

d. Exam of the oropharynx for posterior flow of blood

e. Vital signs including blood pressure

- Diagnostic Tests/Findings

    1. Nasal culture if infection suspected

    2. CBC, platelets, PT, PTT; coagulation profile as indicated by history and clinical findings

- Management/Treatment

    1. Most stop spontaneously within a few minutes

    2. Local compression of the nares; position in upright position with head tilted forward

    3. Humidification

    4. Local nasal phenylephrine HCL drops 0.125-0.25% sometimes helpful

    5. Topical antibiotic ointment and oral antibiotics may be indicated if infection is suggested

    6. Referral to otolaryngologist for persistent, profuse bleeding or recurrent bleeding unresponsive to treatment

Sinusitis

- Definition: Purulent infection of mucosal lining in one or more of paranasal sinuses occurring most often after a cold or following allergic inflammatory disease; trapped secretions with ciliary damage occurs; may be acute or chronic

- Etiology/Incidence

    1. Common organisms

        a. *Haemophilus influenzae* and *Streptococcus pneumonia* (two most common, especially in acute)

        b. *Moraxella catarrhalis*

        c. Group A beta hemolytic Streptococcus and *Staphylococcus aureus*

Pediatric Nurse Practitioner

(especially in chronic)

2. May be associated with septal deviation or adenoid hypertrophy (chronic)

3. More common in allergic than nonallergic children

4. Most common in winter months after a respiratory illness; may be associated with swimming

5. Boys affected more than girls

- Clinical Findings

    1. Young child—vague

        a. Persistent rhinorrhea (beyond 7 to 10 days); usually purulent, can be watery

        b. Cough, especially at night

        c. Occasional periorbital edema

    2. Older child

        a. Persistent rhinorrhea or cold symptoms beyond 7 to 10 days

        b. Postnasal drip, headache, facial pain, halitosis, cough

    3. Physical Findings

        a. Mucopurulent discharge from nose and/or posterior pharynx

        b. Erythema of nasal mucosa; possible erythema of throat

        c. Tenderness over involved sinus; pain with percussion; erythema/edema in area of affected sinus

        d. Otitis media with effusion may be present especially in younger child

- Differential Diagnosis

    1. Foreign bodies, allergic rhinitis, common cold, purulent rhinitis

    2. Dental infections

- Diagnostic Tests/Findings

    1. Nasal cultures to determine organism—sometimes done but may not accurately reflect causative organism

    2. May find eosinophils in nasal secretions (suggests allergy)

    3. Roentgenography often used, but may be misinterpreted

- Management/Treatment

1. Antibiotic therapy—important to penetrate sinuses; usually given minimum of 2 weeks; often continued for 21 days

    a. Amoxicillin 40 mg/k/d in 3 divided doses (appropriate for most uncomplicated acute sinusitis cases)

    b. Alternative choices for chronic sinusitis or sinusitis unresponsive to initial treatment

        (1) Trimethoprim/sulfamethoxazole 8 and 40 mg/kg/day respectively in 2 divided doses

        (2) Erythromycin/sulfisoxazole 50 and 150 mg/kg/day respectively in 4 divided doses

        (3) Cefaclor 40 mg/kg/day in 3 divided doses

        (4) Amoxicillin—potassium clavulanate—40 mg/kg/day in 3 divided doses

2. Vasoconstrictive nose drops—sometimes prescribed on a selective basis, for short-term use, 2 to 3 days only

3. Decongestants/antihistamines limited usefulness except in children with associated allergies

4. Humidification

5. Analgesics for discomfort (acetaminophen)

6. Local steroids (beclomethasone nasal spray) may be helpful to control inflammation

7. Prevention

    a. Not usually preventable

    b. Sometimes elimination of swimming advised; use of nose plugs

    c. Management of allergies

8. Refer to pediatrician or subspecialist for chronic sinusitis. Functional endonasal sinus surgery may be considered for severe cases

9. Observe for complications

    a. Periorbital cellulitis

    b. Subperiosteal abscess

Pharyngitis

- Definition—Acute inflammation and infection of the pharynx including tonsillitis, pharyngotonsillitis and nasopharyngitis
- Etiology/Incidence
  1. Causative organisms
     a. Viruses predominant in all age groups (80 to 90%)
     b. Adenovirus (most common in young child)
     c. Influenza virus, serotypes A and B
     d. Parainfluenza virus
     e. Epstein-Barr virus
     f. Enteroviruses
     g. *Mycoplasma pneumoniae*
     h. Less common bacteria
        (1) Streptococcus pyogenes (Group A beta hemolytic) *primary cause of bacterial infection*
        (2) *Haemophilus influenzae*
        (3) *Neisseria meningitides*
        (4) *Corynebacterium haemolyticum*
  2. Transmission by close contact with affected individuals
  3. Depends on age, season, exposure, and environment
  4. Bacterial infection more common in cold weather; infection with enteroviruses more common in summer and fall
- Clinical Findings
  1. Vary depending on pathogen; much overlapping of signs and symptoms; almost impossible to make diagnosis based on clinical findings alone
     a. Sudden or gradual onset
     b. Sore throat—pain on swallowing
     c. Fever—can be as high as 104 °F
     d. Headache, malaise, anorexia
     e. Occasionally nausea, vomiting and abdominal pain

    2.   Physical Findings

       a. Erythema of throat on inspection, sometimes with ulcerative petechial lesions and exudate

       b. Tonsils may be enlarged and infected and may be covered with exudate

       c. May be erythema of nasal mucous membranes with mucus discharge

       d. Enlargement and possible tenderness of cervical nodes

- Differential Diagnosis

    1.   Major differential streptococcal vs. non-streptococcal pharyngitis

    2.   Peritonsillar abscess

    3.   Retropharyngeal abscess

    4.   Infectious mononucleosis

    5.   Diptheria if membranous exudate present

- Diagnostic Tests/Findings

    1.   Throat culture or rapid identification test (or both) to rule out group A beta hemolytic streptococcus

    2.   Other studies, depending on history, age and suspected diagnosis (i.e., STD, tests to rule out mononucleosis, diphtheria)

    3.   WBC usually elevated with bacterial infection

- Management/Treatment

    1.   Usually supportive and symptomatic care for nonbacterial illness

       a. Acetaminophen

       b. Hydration

       c. Throat lozenges, mouthwashes

       d. Avoid decongestants, and antihistamines

    2.   Oral antibiotic therapy for bacterial disease

       a. Penicillin drug of choice for Group A beta hemolytic streptococcus pharyngitis 125 to 250 mg t.i.d. for 10 days; erythromycin for penicillin allergies

       b. If increased frequency of therapeutic failures reported, may try cephalosprins, macrolides or clindamycin as second line therapy

3. Education

   a. Instruct parents to seek follow-up if signs and symptoms persist

   b. Stress importance of taking all medicine as prescribed for streptococcal pharyngitis

4. Complications

   a. Acute rheumatic fever—sequelae of untreated group A beta-hemolytic streptococcal pharyngitis

   b. Glomerulonephritis may be sequelae of nephritogenic strain of group A beta hemolytic streptoccal infection; not related to treatment

   c. Others—depends on organisms

Retropharyngeal abscess

- Definition: Accumulation of pus between anterior border of cervical vertebrae and posterior pharyngeal wall

- Etiology: More common in young children than other age groups; usually secondary to suppurative adenitis of retropharyngeal nodes which atrophy in adolescence; may be a complication of bacterial pharyngitis

   1. Mixed organisms found

      a. Group A hemolytic streptococcus (most common)

      b. Anaerobic organisms

      c. *Staphylococcus aureus*

- Clinical Findings

   1. Signs/symptoms—usually a history of acute pharyngitis and may still have persistent signs and symptoms

      a. Abrupt onset of high fever

      b. Airway stridor

      c. Severe throat pain with dysphagia, drooling

      d. Tachypnea, dyspnea, stridor

      e. Hyperextension of head, stiff neck

   2. Physical findings

      a. Toxic appearing child; child may hold head in hyperextension

b. Noisy, gurgling respirations

c. Swelling or bulging of the posterior pharyngeal wall; sometimes bulging of the soft palate/marked erythema; may not always be visible on inspection

- Differential Diagnosis
    1. Epiglottitis
    2. Acute pharyngitis
    3. Peritonsillar abscess
    4. Acute infectious mononucleosis
    5. Meningitis

- Diagnostic Tests/Findings
    1. Lateral neck radiography
    2. Complete blood cell count (CBC)—elevated WBC
    3. Computed tomography (CT) scan

- Management/Treatment
    1. **Emergency attention necessary/immediate referral to ENT**
    2. Hospitalization necessary
    3. Surgical intervention (incision and drainage) necessary
    4. Intravenous (IV) antibiotics (penicillin)
    5. Careful cardiorespiratory monitoring; child is at risk for airway obstruction
    6. Preparation for resuscitation and intubation—protocol should be established

Peritonsillar Abscess

- Definition: Accumulation of purulent material within tonsillar fossa.
- Etiology/Incidence:
    1. Group A ß-hemolytic streptococci; anaerobic microorganisms
    2. *Staphylococcus aureus*
    3. May follow any virulent tonsillitis
    4. Rare in young children

   5.   More common in preadolescent or adolescent patients
- Clinical Findings
   1.   Severe pain on swallowing
   2.   History of sore throat
   3.   Trismus
   4.   Toxic and febrile
   5.   Difficulty speaking, muffled voice; drooling
   6.   Enlargement of tonsils (greater on one side); marked erythema; fetid breath; displaced uvula
   7.   May be febrile and appear toxic
- Differential Diagnosis
   1.   Epiglottitis
   2.   Retropharyngeal abscess
- Diagnostic Tests—CBC—expect increased WBC
- Management/Treatment
   1.   Refer to ENT
   2.   Hospitalization may be necessary
   3.   Surgical intervention often necessary (I&D)
   4.   IV antibiotics

Cervical Lymphadenitis

- Definition: Inflammation of one or more lymph nodes in the neck
- Etiology/Incidence
   1.   Occurs in all age groups; higher in preschool period; no sex preference
   2.   Often secondary to pharyngitis/tonsillitis
   3.   May also occur secondary to dental abscess, facial impetigo, otitis externa
   4.   Organisms
        a.   *Staphylococcus aureus,* group A streptococcus
        b.   *Mycobacterium tuberculosis*
        c.   Other organisms

- Clinical Findings

  1. Fever

  2. Enlarged lymph node or nodes (usually unilateral and isolated) (> 2 to 6 cm); tenderness on palpation; erythema may be present

- Differential Diagnosis

  1. Non-specific lymphadenopathy due to U.R.I.s (usually bilateral, less tender and no erythema)

  2. Infectious mononucleosis

  3. Mumps

  4. Diphtheria

  5. Cat scratch fever

  6. Tuberculosis

- Diagnostic Tests/Findings

  1. CBC—elevated WBC

  2. Mantoux test

  3. Throat culture

  4. Other tests depending on suspected differential diagnosis; consultation or referral to physician or subspecialist may be necessary; especially if fluctuation noted

- Management/Treatment

  1. Antibiotics—dicloxacillin may be drug of choice for 10 days

  2. Surgical aspiration may be needed

  3. OR conservative observation

Epiglottitis (Supraglottitis)

- Definition: A severe, rapidly progressive infection of the epiglottis and surrounding tissues; leads to airway obstruction

- Etiology/Incidence

  1. *Haemophilus influenzae* type b (almost always)

  2. Age range—2 to 7 years; peak incidence about 3½ years; can occur from infancy to adulthood

  3. Marked variability in seasonal incidence

4. Male/female ratio approximately 3:2

5. Decreasing with use of HIB vaccine

■ Clinical Findings

1. Onset usually acute; sore throat, hoarseness and frequently high fever develop abruptly in a previously well child or sudden onset of respiratory distress may develop within 12 hours of initial symptoms

2. Dysphagia and respiratory distress characterized by drooling

3. Retractions—suprasternal and subcostal; inspiratory stridor

4. Choking sensation; muffled voice; usually won't talk

5. Restlessness, irritability; anxious, apprehensive, frightened appearance

6. Hyperextension of neck, leaning forward and chin thrust out

7. With early toxicity may demonstrate signs of shock, cyanosis, prostration, and loss of consciousness

■ Differential Diagnosis (See Table 1)

1. Croup syndrome; acute laryngeal edema; foreign body

2. Diphtheria; pertussis

3. Retropharyngeal abscess; bacterial tracheitis

■ Diagnostic Tests/Findings—often deferred to minimize distress

1. CBC—expect highly elevated WBC

2. Blood cultures—usually positive for *Haemophilus influenzae* type b in 50% of cases

3. X-rays—lateral neck shows a thickened mass in the area of the epiglottis

■ Management/Treatment

1. **Constitutes a true emergency—if epiglottitis is suspected no attempt should be made to visualize epiglottis**

2. Advance planning imperative; nurse practitioner should be fully aware of protocol for suspected epiglottitis—establishing airway primary goal of management

3. Laboratory tests, x-rays, and extensive history may be deferred if epiglottitis highly suspected

4. Resuscitation equipment readied

5. Skilled personnel prepared for airway stabilization and ventilation support (anesthesiologist and otolaryngologist)

6. Child must be kept calm, preferably in parent's arms; staff must accompany child to radiology department

7. Nasotracheal or endotracheal intubation or elective tracheotomy usually performed after diagnosis

8. IV antibiotic therapy (Ampicillin and ceftriaxone often initial choice until results of sensitivities available)

   a. Cephalosporins (2nd and 3rd generation) or

   b. Ampicillin and ceftriaxone

9. Rifampin prophylaxis (AAP, 1994)

   a. Index patient (patient with disease); should be initiated during hospitalization, usually just before discharge

   b. All household contacts irrespective of age in those households with at least one unvaccinated contact less than 4 years of age

   c. Partially immunized or unvaccinated children

10. Prevention—*Haemophilus influenzae* type b vaccine

Table 1
Upper Airway Obstructive Disorders

	Epiglottitis	**Viral Croup Syndrome**	**Bacterial tracheitis**
Causative Organism	Haemophilus Influenzae type b	Viruses primarily Para influenza viruses, Respiratory syncytial virus,	*S. aureus* predom
Common Age	2-7 yrs; most common > 2	3 months - 3 yrs	Same as croup
Season	Marked variability	Peak incidence late fall, winter	Fall/ winter
Onset	Rapid; acutely ill	Gradual—preceded by rhinitis and cough for several days; spasmodic croup usually more abrupt onset, especially at night	Preceded by croup like illness, followed by sudden acute illness
Fever	Sudden elevation, usually high > 39.4 °C (105 °F)	Variable 37.8-40 °C (100.2 °F-104 °F), usually mild	Mild followed by acute increase
Dysphagia	Marked; drooling	None	None
Sore throat	Marked	Mild; none	None to minimal
Cough	Usually none	"Barky" cough	"Barky" cough
WBC	Usually high > 18,800	Usually normal	Usually elevated
Diagnosis	"Cherry red" epiglottis on direct visualization or thickened mass on lateral neck x-ray	Clinical Presentation; "steeple sign" on lateral neck x-ray	Tracheal cultures positive; lateral neck x-ray shows subglottic narrowing with membranous tracheal exudate

Viral Croup Syndrome

- Definition: Inflammation of larynx, trachea, and bronchial tubes that takes different progressive forms presenting a syndrome of laryngeal obstruction (edema of the subglottic region leads to narrowing of the airway). May be divided into types

    1. Acute laryngotracheitis

2. Laryngotracheobronchitis

3. Spasmodic croup (more abrupt onset, milder course)

- Etiology/Incidence

    1. Most commonly caused by a viral infection in the subglottic area of the larynx transmitted via droplets from nasal secretions or close airborne contact

    2. Most cases involve children age 3 months to 3 years

    3. More common in boys

    4. Peak incidence late fall, early winter

        a. Parainfluenza virus, (type I most common pathogen)

        b. Influenza virus A and respiratory syncytial virus (RSV), adenoviruses, rhinovirus (less common pathogens)

- Clinical Findings—initial U.R.I. precedes progression

    1. Croupy (barky) cough (often occurring at night)

    2. Inspiratory stridor

    3. Hoarseness

    4. Coryza

    5. Fever (can be slightly elevated or as high as 104 °F)

    6. Minimal to marked respiratory distress

        a. Nasal flaring

        b. Inspiratory stridor

        c. Intercostal, suprasternal, infrasternal retractions

        d. Respiratory rate slightly increased

    8. Lungs usually clear to auscultation

    9. Inflamed pharynx (may or may not be present)

- Diagnostic Tests/Findings—depends on severity of signs/symptoms

    1. WBC normal or mildly elevated

    2. AP and lateral neck x-ray (narrowed subglottic region with "steeple sign" in 40 to 50% of cases)

    3. Chest x-ray sometimes indicated to rule out lower respiratory infection

- Differential Diagnosis (see Table 1)

1. Epiglottitis
2. Aspiration of foreign body
3. Retropharyngeal abscess
4. Peritonsillar abscess
5. Bacterial tracheitis
6. Acquired or congenital subglottic stenosis
7. Infectious mononucleosis
8. Diphtheria

- Management/Treatment—varies with severity

1. Humidified air (mist therapy) considered cornerstone of treatment although unclear whether this is effective; bathroom steam, humidifier, cool night air
2. O_2 therapy added if hypoxemia present
3. Use of corticosteroids controversial, but sometimes used
4. Nebulized racemic epinephrine by means of IPPB in select cases. (requires hospitalization)
5. Observation and careful instruction for follow-up; parent should be aware of signs of increasing respiratory distress and/or dehydration

Bacterial Tracheitis

- Definition: Also known as pseudomembranous croup or membranous laryngotracheitis. An acute infection of the larynx, trachea and sometimes bronchi characterized by a thick, obstructive exudate capable of causing life-threatening airway obstruction

- Etiology/Incidence—believed to be a secondary bacterial infection complicating a viral disease

1. *Staphylococcus aureus* (most common)
2. Group A ß-hemolytic streptococci; *Haemophilus influenza* type b
3. *Pneumoniae*
4. *Moraxella Catarrhalis*

- Clinical Findings

1. History of croup-like illness with gradual progression of mild airway

symptoms followed by high fever and toxicity

    2.   Inspiratory stridor

    3.   Barking Cough

- Differential Diagnosis

    1.   Croup

    2.   Epiglottitis

    3.   Acute Infectious mononucleosis

    4.   Retropharyngeal abscess

    5.   Peritonsillar abscess

    6.   Diphtheria

    7.   Foreign body aspiration

- Diagnostic Test/Findings

    1.   AP and lateral neck radiograph—clouding of the tracheal air column

    2.   Chest radiograph—pneumonia infiltrates in 50% of children

    3.   CBC—elevated WBC

    4.   Tracheal culture—usually positive for bacteria

    5.   Blood culture—usually negative

- Management/Treatment

    1.   Early intervention crucial—referral to pediatrician or ENT necessary

    2.   Artificial airway established and removal of membranous exudate

    3.   Antibiotic therapy usually includes

        a. Nafcillin and cefuroxime

        b. Cefotaxime

    4.   Hydration

    5.   Humidification

Foreign Body Aspiration

- Definition: Aspiration of foreign body into laryngotracheal area and/or main stem bronchus
- Etiology/Incidence

1. Children between 7 months and 4 years are at high risk for aspiration of small objects, including seeds, nuts, toy parts, buttons, pebbles, grapes

2. This diagnosis should be highly suspected in all cases of acute wheezing, unexplained cough and radiographic findings of atelectasis and infiltrates in this age group

- Clinical Findings

1. Signs and symptoms depend on degree of obstruction and nature of the foreign body

2. History of swallowing or playing with a small object followed by sudden onset of cough, choking or gagging or wheezing; there may be a period of no symptoms following initial episode

3. Laryngeal foreign bodies may completely obstruct airways and may elicit stridor, high pitched wheezing, cough or aphonia and cyanosis

4. Tracheal foreign bodies usually elicit cough, some stridor or wheezing and may produce "slap" sound

5. Bronchial foreign bodies usually cause wheezing or coughing and are frequently misdiagnosed as asthma; may present with decreased vocal fremitis, impaired or hyperresonant percussion note, and diminished breath sounds distal to foreign body

- Differential Diagnosis

1. Croup

2. Asthma

3. Bronchitis

4. Other upper and lower airway disease

- Diagnostic Tests/Findings

1. Upper airway foreign bodies may be visualized on standard roentgenography

2. Bronchial foreign bodies may be identified with inspiratory-expiratory roentgenograms or video fluoroscopy

3. Bronchoscopy is usually required for definitive diagnosis of foreign bodies in the larynx and trachea

- Management/Treatment

1. Rarely coughed up spontaneously

2. Removed by means of direct laryngoscopy or bronchoscopy

3. Establish airway if child is in obvious distress

4. CPR; back blows, Heimlich maneuver

5. Prevention is most important aspect; age appropriate anticipatory guidance, including siblings

Pertussis (Whooping Cough)

■ Definition: Highly contagious bacterial infection of respiratory tract characterized by prolonged and protracted episodes of cough, usually ending in an inspiratory "whoop."

■ Etiology/Incidence

1. *Bordetella pertussis*

2. Transmission—aerosol droplets from respiratory tract of infected persons; indirect contact with freshly contaminated articles

3. Cases—50% occur in children younger than 1 year; 75% occur in children younger than 5 years

4. Incubation period 7 to 10 days, usually 10

5. Communicability—greatest in catarrhal stage

■ Clinical Findings

1. Catarrhal stage—initial sign and symptoms (continue for 1 to 2 weeks)

    a. Mild cough, coryza, lacrimation

    b. Low-grade fever

2. Paroxysmal phase

    a. Increased, severe paroxysmal cough interspersed with characteristic inspiratory whoops; may persist for weeks

    b. May vomit with episodes of cough

    c. Cough triggered by feeding, crying, or activity

3. Life-threatening effects of the toxin include thrombocytopenia and neurologic problems, including paralysis

■ Differential Diagnosis

1. Pneumonia (bacterial, viral, chlamydial)

2. Acute bronchitis

3. Tuberculosis

4. Cystic fibrosis

5. Foreign body

- Diagnostic Tests/Findings

  1. Chest radiographs—may reveal thickened bronchi and evidence of atelectasis and bronchopneumonia

  2. CBC—marked leukocytosis

  3. Cultures—posterior nasopharyngeal mucosa with direct fluorescent antibody stain (DFA) (expect positive findings in initial stage of illness); almost always negative after 4 to 5 weeks of symptoms

- Management/Treatment

  1. Referral to pediatrician necessary if suspected

  2. Hospitalization with strict respiratory isolation necessary; supportive care

  3. Antibiotic therapy—usually erythromycin (40 to 50 mg/kg/day)

  4. Prevention

     a. Proper immunization with pertussis vaccine is primary prevention (see Health Maintenance and Promotion chapter)

     b. Household and other close contacts—children younger than 7 years who are unimmunized or who have received fewer than 4 doses of pertussis vaccine (DTP or DTaP) should have pertussis immunization initiated or continued according to the recommended schedule

     c. Third dose received 6 months or more before exposure should be given a fourth dose at this time

     d. Those who have received at least 4 doses should receive a booster dose of DTaP or DTP unless a dose has been given within last 3 years or they are over 6 years old

     e. Erythromycin (40 to 50 mg/kg/day orally in 4 divided doses) for all household contacts and other close contacts *irrespective of vaccination status* (AAP, 1994)

        *Refer to *Red Book* (American Academy of Pediatrics, (1994) or Centers for Disease Control and Prevention guidelines for further measures and information on cases of exposed persons

Lower Respiratory Disorders

Acute Bronchitis (Tracheobronchitis)

- Definition: Inflammation of larger airway passages (trachea and bronchi); usually associated with an upper respiratory infection
- Etiology/Incidence
    1. Viral agents usual cause, although *M. pneumoniae* common cause in children older than 6 years
    2. More common in fall than other seasons; peaks in winter
    3. Boys affected more frequently than girls
- Differential Diagnosis
    1. Asthmatic bronchitis
    2. Asthma
    3. Pneumonia
    4. Pertussis
    5. Chronic sinusitis
    6. Cystic Fibrosis
- Clinical Findings
    1. Usually preceded by upper respiratory infection
    2. Physical findings vary with patient and stage of disease
    3. Initially afebrile or low-grade fever
    4. Rhinitis (usually precedes cough)
    5. Prominent progressive cough; initially harsh, brassy; later, loose and productive
    6. Older child may have purulent sputum
    7. Younger child may have gagging and vomiting
    8. As disease progresses, rales and rhonchi may be heard on auscultation
- Diagnostic studies
    1. CBC—expect negative findings
    2. Chest radiography—expect negative findings
- Management/Treatment

1. Primarily supportive

   a. Analgesics; acetaminophen in appropriate doses

   b. Antitussive medicine (dextromethorphan hydrobromide) in select cases of repeated coughing bouts with exhaustion and insomnia; use with caution, especially if cough is productive

   c. Encourage fluids to hydrate and decrease viscosity

   d. Humidity and mist therapy may be helpful

2. Education

   a. Avoid antihistamines and decongestants; proper hygiene in handling secretions; antibiotics usually not necessary

   b. Follow-up important if recurrent or persistent symptoms

Bronchiolitis

- Definition: Acute viral infection of lower respiratory tract that predominantly presents in infancy. Characterized by obstruction of the bronchioles, edema, secretions and wheezing

- Etiology/Incidence

  1. Respiratory syncytial virus (RSV) is most frequent causative organism followed by parainfluenza viruses, types 1 and 3, adenoviruses and rhinoviruses

  2. *Mycoplasma pneumoniae, Chlamydia pneumoniae* may also be etiologic agents

  3. Occurs primarily in winter and spring during first 2 years of life with peak incidence at 2 to 6 months of age

  4. Boys affected more frequently than girls

  5. May indicate early manifestation of hyperactive airway disease (asthma)

- Clinical Findings

  1. Begins with cough, rhinorrhea, nasal congestion, slight fever over 2 to 5 days

  2. Followed by wheezing, increased respiratory rate, dyspnea

  3. Grunting, nasal flaring, tachycardia, retractions of chest wall may develop as disease progresses

  4. Irritability; poor feeding; vomiting

5. Harsh rhonchi and fine, inconsistent rales and intermittent diffuse wheezing on auscultation

6. Abdominal distention

■ Differential Diagnosis

1. Bronchial asthma

2. Aspiration pneumonia

3. Gastoesophageal reflux (GER)

■ Diagnostic Tests/Findings

1. CBC—usually negative findings

2. Chest radiography usually shows hyperinflation and an increased anteroposterior diameter

3. ABGs may be indicated if cyanosis present

4. Identification of organism in nasopharyngeal secretions by immunofluorescence

■ Management/Treatment

1. Careful observation for increased hypoxemia, respiratory failure, dehydration

2. Elevated position to facilitate breathing

3. Cool mist humidification at home may be helpful

4. Hydration important but observe for and avoid over hydration; encourage small amounts of fluids at frequent intervals

5. Hospitalization and oxygen therapy may be necessary in young infant and in severe cases of hypoxemia

   a. Ribavirin by means of nebulizer may be used for children infected with respiratory syncytial virus, especially in children at high risk from chronic cardiopulmonary disease

6. Important to evaluate family's ability to observe and care for child at home; follow-up is crucial

9. Complications

   a. Dehydration

   b. Respiratory failure

   c. Bacterial superinfection

        d. Apnea

Pneumonia

- Definition: Inflammation of lungs caused by bacterial, viral, or other nonbacterial pathogens and aspiration of foreign substances

  1. Occurs in all seasons; winter and spring predominate
  2. Boys affected more frequently than girls
  3. Incidence increases with environmental crowding
  4. Transmission: droplet spread; close contact; newborn-transplacental or aspiration during delivery and nursing contact
  5. Children with chronic heart and lung disease are at high risk

- Etiology

  1. Viruses predominate (except in newborn)

     a. Respiratory syncytial virus (RSV) (most common in children younger than 5 years)

     b. Parainfluenza viruses 1, 2, and 3

     c. Influenza virus, serotypes A and B

     d. Adenoviruses

     e. Measles virus, varicella zoster virus and rubella virus

     f. Epstein-Barr virus

  2. Mycoplasma pneumonia (more common in children older than 5 years)

  3. Bacterial causes

     a. *Streptococcus pneumonia*—primary cause in all age groups (except newborn)

     b. Group B streptococcus—major causative organism in newborn

     c. *Staphylococcus aureus*—more common in infants

     d. *Haemophilus influenzae type b*

     e. Group A streptococcus—more common in children older than 5 years

     f. *Pneumocystic carinii* (opportunistic infection)—in patients with immunodeficiency disease or immunosuppression

- Clinical Findings

1. Clinical differentiation between viral and bacterial forms is difficult

2. Clinical signs and symptoms vary with pathogen, age, and systemic reaction to the infection

3. Onset may be more sudden and child may be more toxic with greater respiratory distress in bacterial infection, as compared with viral infection

4. Coryza, cough, congestion

5. Decrease in appetite

6. Tachypnea out of proportion to fever

7. Fever and chills

8. Respiratory distress (increased respiratory rate and heart rate, flaring of nares, shallow breathing, retractions, grunting)

9. Decreased breath sounds and/or rales

10. Irritability

11. Vomiting

12. Cyanosis may occur

13. Chest pain

14. Abdominal distention

15. Headache, malaise

16. Young infants—clinical manifestations may be nonspecific

    a. Apnea spells may occur

    b. Poor feeding and irritability

- Differential Diagnosis

    1. Asthma

    2. Foreign body aspiration

    3. Bronchopulmonary dysplasia (BPD)

    4. Cystic Fibrosis (CF)

    5. AIDS

- Diagnostic Tests/Findings

    1. Depends on signs and symptoms

        a. CBC—expect increased WBC; more likely with bacterial disease

      b. Sedimentation rate—elevated

      c. C-reactive protein—elevated

      d. Blood cultures—may be positive for specific organism

      e. Tracheal aspirate

      f. Chest radiographs—may find patchy infiltrates, atelectasis, pleural effusion

      g. Cold agglutination titer—titers greater than 1:16 considered diagnostic

- Management/Treatment

   1. Optimal treatment depends on detection of pathogen, which is often not possible

   2. Antibiotic therapy if bacterial disease is suspected or cannot be ruled out; antibiotic chosen should cover most common bacterial pathogens (e.g., amoxicillin or erythromycin)

   3. Close monitoring of vital signs

   4. Adequate hydration important (increased loss of fluids because of fever, anorexia, and increased respiratory effort)

   5. Humidification and cool mist

   6. Oxygen therapy for dyspnea or cyanosis

   7. Analgesic and antipyretic therapy as needed; acetaminophen in appropriate doses; minimal use so cause of discomfort can be monitored

   8. Proper toilet of mouth and secretions

   9. Important to evaluate family's compliance and ability to observe and care for child

  10. Hospitalization may be necessary in young infants or with evidence of moderate to severe respiratory distress or dehydration or inability of parents to care for child properly

  11. Importance of follow-up in 24 to 48 hours must be stressed

  12. Education

      a. Careful instructions to parents to detect signs and symptoms of upper respiratory distress or deterioration

      b. May instruct parents in chest physiotherapy, postural drainage

13. Prevention

   a. Annual influenza vaccine with split—product vaccines recommended for high-risk children

Asthma

■ Definition: A diffuse, obstructive,inflammatory reversible airway disease characterized by hyperresponsiveness of the trachea and bronchi to a variety of stimuli that can be allergenic and non-allergenic and manifested by widespread reversible narrowing of the airways. The obstruction is a result of inflammation of the airways with edema of the mucous membranes, increased secretions and spasm of the smooth muscle

■ Etiology/Incidence

1. Cause unknown—multifactorial genetic predisposition likely (strong family history)

2. Factors that precipitate asthma

   a. Viral infection, e.g., RSV, PAV, and rhinovirus

   b. Allergens—less contributory in infant and young child; larger role in older child

      (1) Inhalants—dust mite, mold, pollens, animal saliva/danders, feathers, fungi, air pollution, tobacco smoke, wood burning stoves and noxious fumes from aerosolized chemicals

      (2) Ingested allergens such as milk, eggs, nuts, grains, chocolate, soybean or castor bean proteins

   c. Environmental and physical factors

      (1) Cold air

      (2) Vigorous exercise

      (3) Abrupt changes in climate

      (4) Heat and/or humidity

   d. Gastroesophageal reflux

   e. Emotional factors—considered less a major factor; more likely that asthma itself precipitates stress and emotional factors

   f. Medications such as aspirin, nonsteroidal anti-inflammatory agents

3. The most common chronic illness in children; prevalence varies greatly

within the U.S. with 10 to 12% of children being affected at some time

4. Most common onset first few years of life—with majority onset (80%) by age 5 years

5. Leading cause of hospitalization among children in U.S. and the major cause of school absenteeism

6. A significant number of children experience remission during puberty, but few actually "outgrow" the disease entirely

■ Clinical Findings—vary with age and stimulating factors

1. Onset may be

   a. Acute or immediate, occurring within minutes of exposure

   b. Delayed and insidious, occurring hours following exposure

2. History

   a. Positive family history of allergic/atopic disease or asthma

   b. Bronchiolitis in infancy

   c. Atopic dermatitis; allergic rhinitis; cough, especially at night; frequent URIs

3. Specific/may be progressive signs and symptoms

   a. Cough, dyspnea, shortness of breath; wheezing

   b. Restlessness, fatigue, irritability

   c. Noisy, rattly breathing; rapid breathing, mouth breathing; retractions, nasal flaring; cyanosis

4. Physical Findings—vary with age, severity of attack, and presence of other allergic disease

   a. General

      (1) Atopic stigmata (allergic shiners, crease and/or salute)

      (2) Hyperarched palate; geographic tongue; cobblestone appearance of posterior pharynx; dry mucous membranes

      (3) Presence of chronic or serous otitis media

      (4) Conjunctival changes

      (5) Pale, bluish grey, and/or boggy nasal mucous membranes

      (6) Clear mucoid discharge from nose

      (7) Signs of URI may be present (purulent nasal discharge,

infected pharynx, fever)

    (8)   Atopic skin changes

    (9)   Barrel chest (chronic recurrent asthma); tachycardia

  b. Respiratory findings:

    (1)   High-pitched rhonchi and/or wheezing on expiration throughout chest

    (2)   Increased prolongation of expiration with pallor and difficulty speaking as obstruction becomes more severe

    (3)   Hyperresonance on percussion

    (5)   Suprasternal and intercostal retractions; increasing use of accessory muscles

  c. In severe attack

    (1)   Decreased breath sounds with little or no wheezing; marked dyspnea

    (2)   Hypotension, pulsus paradoxus; increased tachycardia; increased cyanosis

    (3)   Drowsiness, coma

■ Differential Diagnosis—detailed history extremely important to rule out other causes of wheezing

  1. Bronchiolitis (difficult to differentiate from asthma in infant)

  2. Congenital malformations of respiratory, cardiovascular or gastrointestinal systems

  3. Foreign bodies in airway or esophagus

  4. Hypersensitivity pneumonitis

  5. Tuberculosis

  6. Foreign body aspiration

  7. Cystic Fibrosis

  8. Gastroesophageal reflux disease

  9. Immunodeficiency syndrome

  10. Bronchopulmonary dysplasia

■ Diagnostic Tests/Findings

  1. CBC usually normal; may be increased WBC with infection; increased

hematocrit with dehydration

2. Nasal cytology from nasal smear—eosinophils > 10% significant

3. Pulmonary function tests more valuable in older child (over 6 years)

   a. Aerosol bronchodilator response—increase of at least 10% in peak expiratory flow rate (PFR) or forced expiratory volume in 1 sec (FEV_1) following administration of aerosol therapy strongly suggestive of asthma

   b. Vital capacity (VC)—FEV and peak flow are decreased; residual volume and functional residual capacity (FRC) are increased, PCO_2 decreased; with more severe or prolonged attack, PCO_2 increased, PO_2 decreased

4. Pulse oximeter to measure hypoxemia

5. Blood gases and pH as indicated by hypoxemia

6. Chest radiograph (routine chest radiograph with each attack not warranted); bilateral hyperinflation, bronchial thickening and peribronchial infiltration and areas of densities may be present

7. Sinus radiograph if indicated; may show sinusitis

8. Serum IgE on individual basis—elevation may indicate atopy

9. Skin testing—indicated when asthma is thought to be exacerbated by identifiable and available allergens; careful interpretation and correlation with other evaluation methods is necessary

10. Specific IgE testing on select cases

11. Diagnostic tests for CF, GER, immunodeficiency as indicated

- Complications

   1. Pulmonary atelectasis; pneumomediastinum

   2. Pneumothorax

   3. Decreased growth

   4. Respiratory failure

   5. Psychologic problems

- Managment/Treatment

   1. General

      a. Management should be highly individualized and is determined by age of child, severity of disease, resources available, and self-care capabilities of the family

 b. Children with asthma should be co-managed under the supervision of the pediatrician or sub-specialist; a consistent primary care provider is very important in reducing morbidity

 c. Asthma and Allergy Foundation of America

2. The goals of treatment should include:

 a. Reversal and control of symptoms using the least amount of medications

 b. Prevention of acute episodes requiring hospitalization and emergency room treatment

 c. Increased knowledge, understanding and self-care management of the disease

 d. Prevention of physical and psychosocial consequences of the disease

 e. Normalization of daily life and activities to optimum capacity

3. Specific therapies

 a. Avoidance of contact with known or suspected allergens and irritants is the foundation of therapy; this requires detailed history, environmental assessment and control, possible skin testing, and dietary challenge testing

 b. Pharmacotherapy

  (1) ß-Adrenergic agonists—second generation sympathomimetic agents (albuterol, metaproterenol, terbutaline); most widely used group of bronchodilators used for acute asthma attacks; effectively reverse bronchoconstriction caused by hyperactive airway; no anti-inflammatory effects; may produce an increase in bronchial re-activity and increased bronchial obstruction

  (2) ß-Adrenergic agonists—first generation sympathomimetic agents (Epinephrine, Susphrine) for parenteral use; occasionally used in acute attacks to reverse bronchoconstriction; shorter duration of action, more side effects than second generation agents; use declining throughout U.S.

  (3) Theophylline preparations (quick release and sustained released) long-term bronchodilators; major use in daily

continuous prophylaxis against attacks triggered by both allergic and non-allergic factors; use and compliance often limited by side-effects; indicated for moderate to severe chronic asthma

(4) Cromolyn sodium—prophylactic drug; used to control inflammatory response; inhibits both early and late phase response; prevents bronchospasm mediated by allergens and non-allergenic agents; prevents asthma caused by exercise; often combined with bronchodilators in the management of acute and chronic asthma

(5) Corticosteroid (inhaled, oral, parenteral)—controls anti-inflammatory response produced by asthma triggers; have been very valuable in treatment of severe, acute and chronic, moderate to severe asthma; significant side-effects with long-term use of systemic steroids; inhaled steroids relatively safe for long-term use; becoming an important drug in management of moderate and severe asthma

(6) Antibiotics indicated only when evidence of bacterial infection exists

c. Peak Flow monitoring to determine severity of attack and guide selection of drug therapy

d. Adequate hydration and nutrition both in acute and chronic phase of disease

e. Fitness and exercise strongly encouraged; may use guidance of physical therapist

f. Specific ongoing child/family education; self-care programs should be recommended; nurse practitioners may have a key role in this component of management

g. Immunotherapy may be beneficial

4. Management of types of asthma (management should be based on current guidelines from National Asthma Education Program)

a. ACUTE ATTACK: Child may be managed initially at home, depending on severity, provided family has knowledge and experience with treatment; previous instruction necessary and continued guidance must be available; referral to emergency room or office necessary for progressive symptoms; careful follow-up essential; one or more of a combination of the following medications are used; inhalation therapy has become the preferred mode for first line treatment

(1) Aerosolized and/or oral beta-adrenergic agonist agents; frequency determined by severity and response to therapy

(2) Epinephrine followed by susphrine may be used in office or emergency room—use has declined dramatically

(3) Theophylline short-acting loading dose (theophylline level may be necessary for child who has previously received theophylline)—use declining throughout U.S.

(4) O_2 therapy as indicated

(5) Corticosteroid therapy if no response to nebulized beta-adrenergic agonists

b. MILD ASTHMA (occasional attacks)—once every 2 to 3 months that respond to mild treatment at home or in the office. Intermittent therapy may be appropriate with inhaled beta-adrenergic agonsist agents or a combination of inhaled and/or oral beta-adrenergic agonist agents and short acting theophylline

c. CHRONIC ASTHMA (moderate and severe asthma)—frequent attacks and emergency room visits and/or hospitalization; frequent school absenteeism, restriction of normal activities, growth interference; daily medication necessary—a combination of bronchodilators (beta-adrenergic agonist agents and theophylline), cromolyn sodium and inhaled corticosteroids may be used, individually tailored to child's needs; if severe, chronic asthma—oral steroid therapy may be added to bronchodilators and used for longer duration

d. EXERCISE INDUCED ASTHMA: Prevented by administration of medicine before exercise; inhaled medications 15 minutes before exercise. (cromolyn sodium, and/or beta-adrenergic agonists); oral bronchodilators 30 to 60 minutes before exercise (not as effective as inhaled medications); daily theophylline sometimes added

e. STATUS ASTHMATICUS (Intractable asthma)—requires hospitalization and should be considered a medical emergency

Cystic Fibrosis (CF)

- Definition: A generalized disease which can affect any organ of the body but most often includes the triad of chronic progressive obstructive pulmonary disease, pancreatic exocrine deficiency and sweat electrolyte elevation

- Etiology/Incidence
    1. CF gene location chromosome 7
    2. Autosomal recessive genetic disorder
    3. The pulmonary and pancreatic disease results from excessive and abnormally thick secretions which obstruct tubes, ducts and airways
    4. Most common, lethal genetic disorder affecting Caucasians, approximately 1:2500; approximately 5% of Caucasians in the U.S. are carriers of gene; incidence in U.S. Blacks approximately 1:17,000

- Clinical Findings
    1. Signs/symptoms
        a. Respiratory tract
            (1) Chronic cough
            (2) Wheezing
            (3) Recurrent upper and lower respiratory infections—sinusitis or bronchopneumonia, bronchiectasis, atelectasis
        b. Gastrointestinal tract
            (1) Meconium ileus or plug syndrome; gastroesophageal reflux, intussusception, malabsorption symptoms
            (2) Frequent, bulky, greasy stools; poor weight gain
    2. Physical examination
        a. Respiratory tract
            (1) Barrel chest deformity
            (2) Use of accessory muscles in respiration
            (3) Digital clubbing
            (4) Cyanosis
            (5) Nasal polyps
        b. Gastrointestinal tract
            (1) Thin extremities
            (2) Failure to thrive/growth retardation
            (3) Protroburent abdomen

(4)   Nutritional deficiency

■ Differential Diagnosis

1.   Upper and lower respiratory tract allergy

2.   Asthma

3.   Gastrointestinal tract allergy

4.   Other chronic pulmonary conditions

■ Diagnostic Tests/Findings

1.   Sweat test—pilocarpine iontophoresis and quantitative analysis of sweat sodium and chloride confirms or rules out disease; concentrations > 60 mEq/L diagnostic of CF

2.   Chest x-ray—hyperinflation found early; subsequent changes include bronchial thickening, infiltrates, patchy atelectasis, bronchiectasis

3.   Pulmonary function tests—not reliable until 4 to 6 years; usually will show typical pattern of obstructive pulmonary disease

4.   Other tests as indicated by disease involvement (pancreatic enzyme assays and GI series)

■ Management/Treatment

1.   Referral to appropriate sub-specialist; long-term management necessary

a.   Vigorous and regular chest physical therapy

b.   Antibiotics

c.   Bronchodilators

d.   Possible anti-inflammatory agents including corticosteroids

e.   Nutritional replacement and supportive therapy

2.   Treatment involves treating and preventing pulmonary infection and treating nutritional deficiencies which include pancreatic extract preparations

3.   Prospects for gene therapy being explored

4.   Cystic Fibrosis Foundation

5.   Stress importance of routine health maintenance; may need psychological help

Tuberculosis (TB)

- Definition: A chronic infectious disease affecting 1 billion people world wide. The disease can be pulmonary, extrapulmonary or disseminated; the primary complex being in the lungs in 95% cases
- Etiology/Incidence
  1. *Mycobacterium tuberculosis*
  2. Transmission from person to person through inhalation of contaminated droplets
  3. In U.S. approximately 23,000 cases/year (approximately 5 to 6% represent children); rate increasing since 1985
  4. Children of all ages susceptible; infants and postpubertal adolescents at highest risk
  5. Higher among minority groups, especially in urban areas, homeless and institutionalized population
  6. High risk factors
     a. Poverty and overcrowding
     b. Immunodeficiency, especially HIV infection
     c. Malnutrition
     d. Immunosuppression related to viral infection or drugs
- Clinical Findings
  1. Most infected chldren are asymptomatic when tuberculin reaction is found to be positive (AAP, 1994)
  2. Broad range of variability in signs and symptoms
  3. History of possible contact helpful
  4. Early symptoms and signs occurring 1 to 6 months after initial infection include one or more of the following
     a. Infrequent cough
     b. Lymphadenopathy of hilar, mediastinal, cervical or other nodes
     c. Low-grade fever, night sweats
     d. Weight loss or FTT, fatigue
  5. Other clinical manifestations that can occur later include tuberculosis of the middle ear and mastoid, bones, joints and skin (AAP, 1994)

■ Differential Diagnosis

   1. Other pulmonary infections of lung especially fungus disease

   2. Persistent bronchopneumonia

   3. Cystic fibrosis

   4. AIDS

   5. Aspiration of foreign bodies

■ Diagnostic Tests/Findings

   1. Tuberculin skin test is only practical tool for diagnosing infection in asymptomatic individuals (AAP, 1994)

      a. In most children a positive reaction can appear as early as 3 to 6 weeks or as long as 3 months following the initial infection

      b. Types

         (1) Mantoux test

            (a) Considered "gold standard"

            (b) Uses a standard antigen (5 tuberculin units of purified protein derivative [PPD] administered intradermally)

         (2) Multiple puncture tests (MPT)

            (a) Antigens are either PPD or old tuberculin (OT)

            (b) Problems limit usefulness—exact dose introduced into skin cannot be standardized; need for subsequent Mantoux test leads to booster phenomenon (increased reaction to a skin test); variable and high rates of false-positive and false-negative results compared to Mantoux test

      c. Recommendations for skin testing

         (1) Routine annual skin testing with Mantoux tests—children at high risk (see AAP, 1994)

         (2) No routine annual testing in children with no risk factors in low-prevalence communities

         (3) Periodic Mantoux tests at 1, 4 to 6 and 11 to 16 years of age recommended for children with no risk factors but who reside in high-prevalence regions or with incomplete or unreliable history for risk factors

   2. BCG vaccination

       a. Previous vaccination is never a contraindication to tuberculin testing

       b. No method available to differentiate between reaction due to BCG vaccination or natural infection (AAP, 1994)

   3. Chest x-ray—pulmonary infiltrates, pleural effusion, hilar adenopathy); used chiefly as a supplement to other diagnostic methods; may be normal

   4. Sputum or gastric aspirate—presence of acid-fast bacilli for microbial confirmation

■ Management/Treatment

   1. Refer to pediatrician or subspecialist if diagnosis is made or highly suspected

   2. Treatment should be carefully supervised (refer to most current edition of AAP Red Book for specific protocols)

   3. Chemotherapeutic agents—currently used for initial therapy

       a. Isoniazid (INH)

       b. Rifampin

       c. Pyrazinamide

       d. Ethambutol

       e. Streptomycin

   4. Anticipatory guidance in taking medications crucial

   5. Strong emphasis on education and prevention; elimination of high risk factors; compliance with treatment regimes

   6. Mandatory reporting of all cases to public health authorities

Bronchopulmonary Dysplasia (BPD)

- Definition: A chronic respiratory disorder of prematurely born infants that results from the complication of Acute Respiratory Distress Syndrome and its treatment during the first week of life; usually involving mechanical ventilation and oxygen therapy; is associated with persistent chronic respiratory distress beyond the first month of life

- Etiology/Incidence

  1. Exact cause remains controversial and incompletely understood. Predisposing factors include

     a. Immaturity

     b. Lung injury secondary to oxygen toxicity

     c. Abnormal lung mechanics due to immaturity, surfactant deficiency, atelectasis

     d. Cyclic increase in demands for ventilation and oxygen which cause further lung injury

     e. Excessive fluid administration

     f. Patent ductus arteriosus

     g. Pulmonary interstitial emphysema, pneumothorax

     h. Infection

  2. Estimated incidence between 10 and 40% depending on how BPD is defined

- Clinical Findings

  1. Clinical findings and course of illness variable depending on extent of damage to lung and stage of disease

     a. Mild—respiratory symptoms requiring oxygen for a few months

     b. Severe—respiratory disease requiring tracheostomy and mechanical ventilation and oxygen for the first 2 years of life

     c. Frequent—respiratory exacerbations requiring frequent outpatient care and frequent and prolonged hospitalizations

     d. Gradual—improvement with degree of sequelae depending on the severity of the disease

- Differential Diagnosis

  1. Neonatal Period

a. Meconium aspiration

b. Congenital infections

c. Recurrent aspiration

d. Cystic Fibrosis

e. Congenital heart disease

f. Cystic adenomatoid malformation

g. Idiopathic pulmonary fibrosis

h. Pulmonary lymphangiectasia

2. Older child—all other forms of chronic lung disease including

a. Severe asthma

b. Cystic fibrosis

c. Immune deficiency related disease

- Diagnostic Tests/Findings

1. Extensive work-ups involved in the neonatal intensive care period in conjunction with neonatologist

2. Additional tests dependent on ongoing problems and complications

- Management/Treatment

1. Depending on severity of disease, primary management by neonatologist and subspecialist in the neonatal and early infant period; continued management by pediatrician and subspecialist often necessary; management requires multidisicplinary and collaborative care

a. Beta-adrenergic agonists, theophylline, corticosteroids inhaled/oral, and cromolyn are common agents used to manage the bronchial hyperactivity and inflammation

b. Intermittent or long-term diuretic therapy may be indicated for recurrent pulmonary edema and sodium and water retention

c. Oxygen therapy and hypoxia monitoring and management

d. Monitoring and management of nutritional problems including hypercaloric formulas and gastrostomies

e. Administration of influenza vaccine recommended

f. Monitoring and intervention for developmental issues, speech and physical therapy

g. Frequent and ongoing reassessment and support

h. Assessment and intervention for family stress and fatigue involved with home management

Sudden Infant Death Syndrome (SIDS)

■ Definition: "The sudden death of an infant under 1 year of age which remains unexplained after a thorough case investigation, including performance of a complete autopsy, examination of death scene and review of clinical history." (National Institute of Child Health and Human Development [NICHD], 1991)

■ Etiology/Incidence

1. Accounts for approximately 90% post neonatal mortality in the U.S. (> 5000 deaths per year)

2. Etiology remains unknown

3. Predisposing factors in infant

   a. Low birth weight—prematurity, IUGR; risk increases proportionate to decrease in birth weight below 2500 g

   b. Males at higher risk

   c. American Indians and Blacks at higher risk than whites, Asians, and Hispanics

   d. Occurrence greater in cold weather months

   e. Infants who sleep in prone position

   f. Infants who do not breast feed

4. Maternal risk factors

   a. Cigarette smoking and other drugs

   b. Lack of prenatal care

   c. Lower socioeconomic class

   d. Unmarried mother

   e. Young maternal age (teenagers at time of 1st birth)

   f. Shorter intervals between pregnancies

5. Peak age 2 to 3 months

- Clinical Findings
  1. Autopsy—SIDS
     a. Apparently well developed, well nourished infant
     b. Small amount mucus, watery or bloody fluid at nares of nose
     c. Cyanosis of lip and nail beds
  2. Apparent life-threatening event (ALTE)—an episode which is frightening to the observer and includes a combination of
     a. Apnea
     b. Limpness
     c. Cyanosis
     d. Choking/gagging
- Differential Diagnosis
  1. Sepsis/meningitis
  2. Seizure disorders and other neurologic abnormalities
  3. Cardiac anomalies and arrythmias
  4. Vascular ring
  5. Severe GER with reflux
  6. Trauma/battered child
  7. Metabolic disease
  8. Sickle cell disease
- Diagnostic Tests/Findings
  1. Pneumocardiogram
  2. Polysomnogram
  3. Complete work up to rule out other causes of apnea or ALTE
- Management/Treatment
  1. Referral to appropriate center a previous ALTE or sibling of a SIDS
     a. Home monitoring—to alert parent and caretakers to impending life threatening events
     b. Possible drug therapy
     c. Comprehensive parent education including CPR

2. National Sudden Infant Death Syndrome Foundation for information, support groups and counseling

3. Ongoing support for families and siblings of an infant who dies from SIDS

Questions

Select the best answer.

1. A mother brings her 7-month-old boy to the clinic with complaints of nasal congestion, poor feeding and irritability. On examination you find bilateral, intermittent rales and expiratory wheezing. The respiratory rate is increased and the temperature is 101 °F. Your differential diagnosis would most likely include all of the following, except

   a. Pneumonia
   b. Bronchiolitis
   c. Asthma
   d. U.R.I. rhinitis

2. After careful evaluation, you decide on a diagnosis of bronchiolitis. The following statements are true about bronchiolitis except

   a. Occurs during first 2 years of life
   b. The most common causative organism is respiratory syncytial virus
   c. The WBC is usually markedly elevated
   d. A chest x-ray will show characteristic hyperinflation

3. The treatment for bronchiolitis includes all of the following, except

   a. Careful observation for increased respiratory distress and monitoring of fluid intake.
   b. Cool mist therapy
   c. Possible administration of bronchodilators and steroids
   d. Possible hospitalization and use of ribavarin via nebulizer for severe attack

4. A 6-year-old child presents with abrupt onset of high fever, stridor, drooling, tachypnea and severe throat pain. The least likely diagnosis the nurse practitioner would consider is

   a. Epiglottitis
   b. Peritonsillar abscess
   c. Retropharyngeal abscess
   d. Bronchiolitis

5. In evaluating this child, the most helpful information in the history that would lead to a diagnosis of retropharyngeal abscess would be

   a. A recent history of acute pharyngitis
   b. History of incomplete immunization status
   c. History of allergic disease

d. Child goes to a day care center

6. In considering a diagnosis of epiglottitis, the following statements are true, except

a. It is most common in children older than 2 years
b. It is almost always caused by *Haemophilus influenzae*
c. The WBC will be markedly elevated
d. Fever usually variable and mild

7. A 4-year-old child comes to the clinic with complaints of cough and wheezing. In evaluating this child, the most appropriate first step would be to

a. Give a therapeutic trial of ß-adrenergic-agonist medication
b. Do skin testing
c. Order a roentgenogram of the chest, and CBC
d. Obtain a careful history, including history of allergy

8. On physical examination, the most significant physical finding in making the diagnosis of asthma would be

a. Dark circles under the eyes
b. Bluish, boggy, nasal turbinates
c. Expiratory wheezing
d. Inspiratory rhonchi

9. After the diagnosis is established, appropriate management of this patient might include each of the following, except

a. Pharmacologic treatment
b. Referral to a pediatric allergist
c. Reassurance to the parents that he will outgrow it
d. Education involving the nature of the disease, and identification and avoidance of allergens

10. The most common etiologic agent in pneumonia in young children after the newborn period is:

a. *Streptococcus pneumonia*
b. *Haemophilus influenzae b*
c. Respiratory syncytial virus
d. *Mycoplasma pneumoniae*

11. Which of the following statements is true about aspiration of foreign bodies in children?

a. Children under 6 months are at the highest risk for aspiration of foreign bodies
b. The diagnosis should be highly suspected when a young child presents with sudden onset of acute wheezing and unexplained cough
c. A period of no wheezing or symptoms following an initial episode of cough,

choking or wheezing rules out the possibility of aspiration of a foreign body

    d. Upper airway foreign bodies cannot be visualized on standard roentgenography

12. The clinical findings for pertussis would most likely include

    a. An initial stage of upper respiratory catarrhal symptoms for 1 to 2 weeks, followed by markedly increasing paroxysmal cough persisting for several weeks

    b. Sudden onset of conjunctivitis, paroxysmal cough, high fever and vomiting

    c. Sudden onset of high fever, vomiting and conjunctivitis, followed by gradual development of "whoopy" cough that persists for several weeks

    d. Onset of "whoopy cough," fever, rhinorrhea subsiding within 1 to 2 weeks

13. The recommended treatment for a child with suspected pertussis is

    a. Ampicillin 100 mg/kg/day divided every 4 hours for 14 days

    b. Amoxicillin 50 mg/kg/day divided every 4 hours for 14 days

    c. Ceftriaxone 150 mg/kg/day IV for 7 days

    d. Erythromycin 40-50 mg/kg/day divided in 4 doses for 14 days

14. A 7-year-old child presents with a history of a mild respiratory infection with a dry cough for the past week, complicated by the more recent development of a loose productive cough. The child is afebrile and appears nontoxic and is eating and drinking without difficulty. Diffuse rhonchi are evident on auscultation, especially on expiration. There is no history of allergies. The most likely diagnosis would be

    a. Acute asthma

    b. Bronchiolitis

    c. Acute bronchitis

    d. Pneumonia

15. The most appropriate treatment for this child would be

    a. Antibiotic therapy with Amoxicillin 40mg/kg/day divided in 3 doses for 10 days

    b. Supportive care including increased fluids, rest, and humidity

    c. Expectorants every 4 to 6 hours during the day and a cough suppressant at night

    d. Beta-adrenergic agonist inhaler 2 puffs every 6 hours

16. When assessing a one-year-old child for the possibility of cystic fibrosis which of the following clinical findings would be *least* significant?

    a. A history of recurrent pneumonia including 3 episodes in the past year

    b. A decline in weight and height on the growth curve

    c. Presence of coarse rhonchi and scattered respiratory wheezing on auscultation of the chest

    d. Hypoactive abdominal sounds on auscultation

17. When considering a diagnosis of pneumonia in a young child, which of the clinical

findings would be most suggestive of the diagnosis?

   a. Headache, malaise, congestion, scattered rhonchi
   b. Fever, tachypnea, rales on auscultation
   c. Fever, vomiting, coryza and cough
   d. Irritability, fever and decreased appetite

18. The following statements are true about pneumonia except

   a. Bacteria predominate as the cause except in the newborn
   b. Children with chronic heart and lung disease are at higher risk
   c. Optimal treatment depends on detection of pathogen which is often not possible
   d. Prevention includes recommendation of annual influenza vaccine for high risk children

19. Diagnostic tests that might be most helpful in supporting diagnosis of pneumonia would include

   a. CBC, chest x-ray and lumbar puncture
   b. Chest x-ray, sedimentation rate
   c. CBC, chest x-ray, cold agglutinins
   d. CBC, electrolytes

20. The treatment of a 4-year-old-child with suspected bacterial pneumonia might include all of the following except

   a. Adequate hydration
   b. Antibiotic therapy
   c. Inhaled corticosteroids to decrease inflammation
   d. Close follow-up

21. The most accurate means for identifying children infected with tuberculosis is

   a. Tine Test (multiple puncture test)
   b. Chest x-ray
   c. Mantoux test
   d. All of the above

22. Clinical findings that might be consistent with tuberculosis in a young child include all of the following except

   a. No symptoms other than a positive skin test
   b. Fatigue, weight loss
   c. Sudden onset of high fever and cough
   d. Lymphadenopathy and low grade fever

23. Chemotherapeutic agents currently in use for the treatment of uncomplicated pulmonary tuberculosis include all of the following except

   a. Isoniazid

   b. Rifampin
   c. Ribavirin
   d. Pyrazinamide

24. Predisposing neonatal risk factors for SIDS include all of the following except

   a. Low-birth-weight
   b. Female infant
   c. Sleeping in prone position
   d. Black race

25. Maternal risk factors that may predispose an infant to SIDS include all of the following except

   a. Cigarette smoking
   b. Lack of prenatal care
   c. Short intervals between pregnancies
   d. Older maternal age (> 35 years)

26. You are counseling an adolescent mother of a child who describes a recent ALTE (Apparent Life Threatening Event) that brought the child to the emergency room 3 days ago. You would

   a. Refer the mother and infant to an appropriate medical center for full evaluation and consideration of home monitoring
   b. Reassure and counsel the mother to return if such an event occurs again
   c. Get a complete workup including CBC, electrolytes and sonogram of the infant
   d. Initiate a trial therapy with theophylline

27. Events that are most often involved with the onset of bronchopulmonary dysplasia include

   a. Premature birth, respiratory distress syndrome, and long-term mechanical ventilation and oxygen therapy
   b. IUGR, congenital infection and long-term hospitalization
   c. Long-term hospitalization and premature birth
   d. Inborn errors of metabolism and family history of asthma

28. Of the following, the most common cause of epistaxis is

   a. Polyps in the nose
   b. Sinusitis
   c. Mucosal trauma or irritation from nose picking
   d. Bleeding disorders

Answer Key

1.	d	15.	b
2.	c	16.	d
3.	c	17.	b
4.	d	18.	a
5.	a	19.	c
6.	d	20.	c
7.	d	21.	c
8.	c	22.	c
9.	c	23.	c
10.	c	24.	b
11.	b	25.	d
12.	a	26.	a
13.	d	27.	a
14.	c	28.	c

Bibliography

American Academy of Pediatrics. (1994). *Report of the committee on infectious diseases* (23rd ed.). Elk Grove Village, IL: American Academy of Pediatrics.

Behrman, R. E., Kliegman, R. M., Nelson, W. E., & Vaughn, V. C. (Eds.). (1992). *Nelson textbook of pediatrics* (14th ed.). Philadelphia: W. B. Saunders.

Evans, D., & Mellins, R. B. (1991). Educational programs for children with asthma. *Pediatrician*, 18, 317-323.

Hen, J. (Ed.). (1992). Asthma and allergy. *Pediatric Annals* 21 (9).

Hersch, G., & Rachelefsky, G. (1989). Sinusitis: Early recognition, aggressive treatment. *Contemporary Pediatrics, 6*, 22.

Hunt, C. (1992). Apnea and SIDS. *Clinics in Perinatology*, 19 (4).

Lafer, R., & Younis, R. (1992). The current management of sinusitis in children. *Clinical Pediatrics, 31*, 30-36.

National Heart, Lung, and Blood Institute National Asthma Education Program Expert Panel Report. (1991). Guidelines for the diagnosis and management of asthma. *Journal of Allergy and Clinical Immunology*, 88, 425-534.

Pichichero, M. (Ed.). (1992). Streptococcal infections. *Pediatric Annals*. 21.

Saipe, C. (1990). Respiratory emergencies in children. *Pediatric Annals, 19*, 637-646.

Shapiro, G. (1992). Childhood Asthma: Update. *Pediatrics in Review*, 12(11), 403-411.

Shaw, K. (1991). Outpatient assessment of infants with bronchiolitis. *American Journal of Diseases of Children, 145*, 151-

Skolnik, N. S. (1989). Treatment of croup: A critical review. *American Journal of Diseases of Children, 143*, 1045-1049.

Szilagyi, P. (1990). What can we do about the common cold. *Contemporary Pediatrics*, 7(2), 23-32.

Starke, G., Jacobs, R., & Jereb, J. (1992). Resurgence of tuberculosis in children. *Journal of Pediatrics*, 120, 839-855.

Stempel, D., & Szefler, S. (1992). Asthma. *The Pediatric Clinics of North America,* 39 (6).

Stiehm, S. (1991). Allergic rhinitis: Always in season. *Contemporary Pediatrics,* 8(4),

88-108.

Traver, G. A., & Martinez, M. (1988). Asthma update. Part I. Mechanisms, pathophysiology, and diagnosis. *Journal of Pediatric Health Care, 2,* 221-226.

Traver, G. A., & Martinez, M. (1988). Asthma update. Part II. Treatment. *Journal of Pediatric Health Care, 2,* 227-233.

U.S. DHHS. (1991 June). *Executive Summary: Guidelines for the diagnosis and management of asthma. National Asthma Education Program Expert Panel Report.* Washington, D. C.: Government Printing Office.

Cardiovascular Disorders

Carole Stone

Innocent or Functional Heart Murmurs

- Definition
    1. A murmur present in a healthy child that is not associated with cardiovascular disease
    2. Considered a normal heart sound of the developing child
- Etiology/Incidence
    1. Turbulence of blood flowing through the normal heart (usually at the origin of the great arteries) which causes vibrations that are transmitted to the chest wall
    2. Almost one out of three children will have an innocent murmur during childhood
    3. Over 30% of children will have an innocent murmur on routine examination; incidence increases under high cardiac output circumstances, e.g., fever, infection, anxiety, exercise
    4. Heard most frequently from 3 to 7 years of age
- Clinical Findings
    1. Asymptomatic
    2. Characteristics of an Innocent heart murmur
        a. Seldom loud I-III/VI
        b. Never associated with a thrill
        c. Always systolic
        d. Completely normal physical examination with normal S_1, S_2
- Differential Diagnosis
    1. Heart murmur—associated with congenital heart disease (CHD) must be ruled out
    2. See Table 1 for types of Innocent Heart Murmurs
- Diagnostic Tests/Findings
    1. Electrocardiogram (ECG)—normal
    2. Chest radiograph—normal
- Management/Treatment
    1. Reassure parents that these are normal heart sounds
    2. Experienced listener will be able to ascertain whether murmur is Innocent or not without extensive diagnostic evaluation
    3. Refer to cardiologist if

a. Characteristics of murmur are not within normal limits
b. Positive family history for CHD
c. Child is symptomatic

Table 1
Innocent Heart Murmurs

Type	Age Incidence	Location	Quality Grade Timing in Cycle	Comments
Newborn Murmur	Very common heard in 1st few days of life. Transient PDA or tricuspid regurgitation	LSB or 2nd LIS usually no radiation	Soft—I-III/VI vibratory; early systolic	Usually disappears within 24-48 hrs Any murmur persisting after 48 hrs or first appearing on day 3 should not be considered innocent until evaluated further
Pulmonary Flow murmur of newborn	Very common, especially in SGA & premature infants	ULSB transmitted to axillae and back	I-II/VI SEM	May last up to 6 mos
Still Murmur	Most common murmur of early childhood; 3 to 6 yrs, adolescence	Mid to LLSB may radiate through precordial area	Musical I-III/VI, or vibratory SEM	Loudest in supine position; diminishes or disappears with change in position or during valsalva maneuver
Pulmonary Ejection Flow Murmur	May be heard throughout childhood 8-14 yrs	ULSB, pulmonic area; radiates to lungs	Soft I-III/VI short, early to mid SEM; may have ejection click	Increases in supine position; decreases on standing Differential PS, ASD
Venous Hum	Very common; 3 to 6 yrs	UL & RSB supra and infra-clavicular areas	Blowing I-III/VI continuous musical hum; continuous; may increase in diastole and with inspiration	Always disappears in supine position or when jugular vein is compressed
Carotid Bruit	More common in older child	Right supra-clavicular areas and over carotids	Harsh II-III/VI SEM	Increased with light pressure on carotid; Differential AS
Hemic Murmur	Associated with anemia, fever or increased cardiac output states	Aortic & Pulmonic area	High Pitched I-II/VI SEM	Disappears with normalization of cardiac output

LSB—Left sternal border
ASD—Atrial septal defect
RSB—Right sternal border

PS—Pulmonary stenosis
ULSB—Upper left sternal border
VSD—Ventricular septal defect

LLSB—Lower left sternal border
SEM—Systolic ejection murmur
LIS—Left interspace

Congenital Heart Disease (CHD)

■ Definition: A group of cardiovascular malformations that results from abnormal structural development of the heart and/or vessels in utero

■ Etiology/Incidence

1. Primary genetic defect/chromosomal abnormality < 8%

2. Multifactorial inheritance patterns; probably genetic predisposition interacting with an environmental trigger

3. Almost 50% have VSD or PS; another 1/3 will have ASD or AS; the remainder will have a wide variety and type

4. Approximately 8/1000 live births; approximately 25 to 35,000 children per year born in the U.S.

5. Perinatal risk factors associated with CHD

   a. Rubella exposure especially 1st trimester

   b. Maternal drug therapy, e.g., anticonvulsants, hormones, lithium, dextroamphetamines, thalidomide

   c. Maternal alcohol ingestion (FAS)

   d. Maternal diabetes and insulin therapy

   e. Exposure to radiation

   f. Maternal age over 40 years

■ Clinical Findings—Most CHD is well tolerated in fetal life until maternal circulation is eliminated and the infant's own cardiovascular system is independently sustained. The impact of the abnormal heart then becomes apparent clinically. As the infant's cardiovascular system continues to change after birth, an additional hemo-dynamic effect is produced on the cardiac lesion producing characteristic signs and symptoms

1. History

   a. Maternal history of illness in the first trimester such as bleeding, anemia, excessive vomiting, rubella; medication, drug/alcohol consumption

   b. Family history of heart disease in a first degree relative

2. Signs/symptoms

   a. Poor weight gain

    b. History of feeding problems

    c. Fainting spells or black outs or sighing attacks (in infants)

    d. Difficulty swallowing with frequent reflux

    e. Difficulty breathing (dyspnea or stridor tachypnea)

    f. Cyanosis (intermittent or continuous)

    g. Exercise intolerance; child assumes a squatting position when fatigued

3. Physical findings

    a. Growth failure: below or falling off normal growth curve

    b. General appearance may be restless, agitated or lethargic

    c. Color may be dusky, pale or cyanotic

    d. Diaphoresis

    e. Tachypnea

    f. Persistent tachycardia

        (1)   > 200 newborns

        (2)   > 150 infants

        (3)   > 120 older children

    g. Bradycardia, irregular heart rate

    h. Abnormal pulses—unequal, bounding, wide pulse pressure, decreased pulses (femoral and/or dorsalis pedis)

    i. Venous pulsations or distention

    j. Prominence of precordial chest wall:

        (1)   Increased precordial activity

        (2)   Diffuse PMI

        (3)   Presence of thrill

        (4)   Right ventricular lift

        (5)   Left sided heave

    k. Abnormal heart sounds:

        (1)   Abnormal splitting or intensity of S_2 (widened or fixed)

        (2)   Presence of ejection clicks

        (3)   Presence of S_3 (can be functional but often associated with abnormality)

        (4)   Presence of S_4 (not normally heard)

        (5)   Murmurs (most common cardiovascular finding); varies in location, radiation, relation to cardiac cycle, intensity, quality and changes with position

    l.   Pulmonary rales; hepatomegaly; peripheral edema

- Differential Diagnosis

    1.   Need to differentiate from other causes of CHF when present, especially during infancy when non-cardiovascular causes are more important

        a. Respiratory diseases; acidosis

        b. Acquired myocardial disease

        c. Dysrhythmias

        d. Rheumatic fever

        e. CNS disease

        f. Anemia

        g. Sepsis

        h. Hypoglycemia

    2.   Specific heart lesions (see Tables 2 and 3)

- Diagnostic Tests/Findings

    1.   Chest radiography provides structural and functional data, evaluates heart size, presence of pulmonary vascular markings

    2.   EKG—evaluates heart rate, rhythm disturbance, ventricular or atrial enlargement, myocardial ischemia

    3.   Hematologic data—arterial blood gases and pH; (hypoxemia and acidosis), Hgb and Hct (polycythemia)

    4.   Echocardiogram—diagnostic for many lesions; determines spatial relationships of chambers, vessels and evaluates septal integrity

    5.   Cardiac catheterization/angiography— major tools in diagnosing specific CHD lesions; blood samples and pressures and O_2 saturation are measured

    6.   Exercise Testing—some symptoms of specific abnormalities only

appear after exercise; determines degree of functional impairment caused by lesion

7. Phonocardiography—records heart sounds and murmurs

■   Management/Treatment

1. Specific treatment and management will be done by the cardiologist. Referral should be made as soon as possible based on history and physical examination. Surgical repair will be the treatment of choice for most cardiac lesions

2. The primary care provider should continue to be involved to

    a. Assist in coordination of care

    b. Monitor and offer guidance in maintaining nutritional status; a high protein and high vitamin diet

    c. Prevent common childhood illnesses

        (1) Avoid exposure

        (2) Active immunizations

        (3) Passive immunization when exposed

        (4) Prophylactic antibiotics for procedures (See Table 4)

    d. Monitor growth and development carefully; allow for maximum independence and autonomy

    e. Offer guidance and teaching to parents related to specific CHD and management

Table 2
Congenital Heart Disease With Cyanosis
(Dominant R to L Shunt)

Name	Description	Clinical Features
Tetralogy of Fallot (TOF)	Consists of 1. Pulmonary stenosis 2. VSD 3. Dextroposition of the aorta 4. RV hypertrophy Accounts for 6% of CHD	Cyanosis may not be present at birth; increases as child grows; dyspnea on exertion, growth delay; loud III-V/VI SEM, harsh, radiates, single S_2; occasional ejection click
Pulmonary Atresia With VSD	Extreme form of TOF; pulmonary valve is atretic or absent; pulmonary trunk is hypoplastic 1% CHD	Similar to TOF with earlier manifestations; cyanosis within 1st few days of birth; soft, systolic murmur; ejection click after S_1 single S_2; continuous PDA, murmur over entire myocardium; signs of CHF may be present
Pulmonary Atresia with intact ventricular septum	Uncommon—absent pulmonary valve; main pulmonary artery is hypoplastic 1% CHD	Cyanosis within a few days of birth; severe and progressive respiratory distress; may be no murmur or soft blowing systolic continuous murmur at ULSB; single S_2; death if not treated
Tricuspid Atresia	Relatively rare; approx. 1% of CHD; complete atresia of tricuspid valve resulting in no direct communication between R atrium and R ventricle; entire systemic venous return enters L heart through foramen ovale	Marked cyanosis may be present at birth; polycythemia; easy fatigability; Hypoxic episodes; II-III/VI pansystolic murmurs along LSB—S_2 single
Transposition of the Great Vessels (TGA)	Consists of 2 parallel circuits; arota arises from R ventricle and pulmonary artery arises from L ventricle; systemic veins return to R atrium and pulmonary veins to L atrium; survival depends on patent foramen ovale or ductus arteriosus, or VSD; assorted intracardiac abnormalities present in most cases (VSD, PDA, PS, PDA) present; accounts for majority of deaths of infants less than 1 yr with CHD; accounts for approximately 5% of CHD	Varies in relationship to associated defects; In most cases, cyanosis at birth or shortly after CHF; growth failure after neonatal period; feeding difficulties; cyanotic episodes, frequent respiratory infections S_1 single; murmur not always present; systolic murmur present with VSD, PS
Total Anomalous Pulmonary Venous Return With Or Without Obstruction (TAPVR)	Abnormal development of the pulmonary veins resulting in partial or complete drainage into the systemic venous circulation; abnormal point of entry may be the R atrium, SVC, IVC, coronary sinus, or below diaphragm (portal vein) 1% CHD	Depends on type—may have cyanosis at birth with S/S of CHF, II-V/VI SEM in pulmonic area radiating through lung fields— early to mid-diastolic murmur at LLSB; precordial bulge; S_2 wide split and fixed

Table 2 (Continued)
Congenital Heart Disease With Cyanosis
(Dominant R to L Shunt)

Name	Description	Clinical Features
Truncus Arteriosus (TA)	1-2% of CHD; a single arterial trunk arises from the ventricular part of the heart supplying the systemic, pulmonary and coronary circulation. VSD is always present. The number of valve leaflets varies and the valve may be abnormal.	Varies with age and degree of pulmonary blood flow; may present with CHF S_1 loud, S_2 loud & single; systolic ejection murmur sometimes with thrill at LSB; frequently a systolic ejection click present
Hypoplastic Left Heart Syndrome	A related group of anomalies which include underdevelopment of the left side of heart. The left ventricle is small and non-functional, & mitral and/or aortic atresia present. Subsequent severe obstruction to filling or emptying the L ventricle. Male predominance. Accounts for almost 25% of deaths from CHD in the first month of life.	Cyanosis soon after birth; CHF within 1st week of life; Non-descriptive systolic murmur; Invariably fatal within first year of life without surgical intervention in the neonatal period (staged reconstructive surgery or cardiac transplantation)
Dextrocardia	A right sided heart with or without situs inversus; heart may have other associated defects	Apical pulse & heart sounds on R side of chest X-ray shows cardiac silhouette on R side; inverted p-wave

Table 3
Congenital Heart Disease With Little or No Cyanosis

Name	Description	Clinical Features
Ventricular Septal Defect (VSD)	Most common cardiac abnormality; Accounts for 25% of CHD; Defect in the membranous (majority) or the muscular portion of the ventricular septum; 50% will close spontaneously; magnitude of the L to R shunt is determined by the size of the defect and the degree of pulmonary vascular resistance	Varies w/size of defect and the pulmonary blood flow and pressure; Small defect, most common asymptomatic, acyanotic murmur II-IV/VI; loud pansystolic LSB, may have thrill, may not be audible 1st 2-3 days of life. Large Defects; dyspnea, feeding difficulties, poor growth, diaphoresis, CHF; Murmur IV-V/VI pansystolic; maximal at LLSB; radiates throughout precordium
Atrial Septal Defect (ASD)	Very common—approximately 10% of CHD; more common in girls; Types: 1. Foramen secundum defect (high in atrial septum) 2. Foramen primum (low in atrial septum) Often with deformity of mitral or tricuspid valve and with persistent A-V canal. 3. Lutembacher's syndrome with ASD with mitral stenosis	Often asymptomatic; linear growth retardation; fatigability; precordial bulge due to large R ventricle; Murmur II-IV/VI blowing to harsh systolic ejection at 2nd LIS and may radiate to apex or back; Widely split & fixed S_2; sometimes diastolic murmur; X-ray may show RVH
Patent Ductus Arteriosis (PDA)	Common abnormality; approx. 12% of CHD; persistence in extra-uterine life of the ductus arteriosis which joins the pulmonary artery to the aorta; Common following rubella exposure; 2:1 female, preemie PDA 20-60%	Asymptomatic with small PDA; large PDA results in bounding pulses, widened pulse pressure; normal S_1; narrow split S_2 Murmur machinery like continuous, maximal at 2nd ICS at LSB and under L clavicle; radiates over lung fields; Diastolic flow murmur may be heard at apex
Coarctation of the Aorta	Common cardiac abnormality; accounts for about 6% of CHD; Constriction of varying length in the aorta; usually occurs in thoracic portion of the Ductus Ateriosis; most infants will have associated defects (PDA, VSD, bicuspid aortic valve); 3:1 male; Murmur blowing, systolic, radiating from sternum to axillae, back and neck.	Commonest cause of CHF from 1 wk to 1 mo/age; Infant CHF, unequal pulses (diminished or absent in lower extremities; BP higher in arms than legs; heart sounds may be normal; II/VI SEM at URSB & LSB radiating to L axillae and L interscapular area of back. Older child numbness of legs, headaches, epistaxis, decreased exercise tolerance, fatigue; femoral & dorsalis pulses weak or absent or delayed; BP higher in upper extremities
Aortic Stenosis	Accounts for approximately 5% of CHD; most common is valvular aortic stenosis (75%) 3:1 males; Obstruction to the outflow from the L ventricle as a result of constriction at or near the aortic valve	Depends on severity of obstruction. Infants CHF w/severe obstruction; most are asymptomatic until adults II-IV/VI harsh SEM at 2nd & 3rd ICS radiating down SB to apex and to neck with prominent thrill at suprasternal notch; diastolic murmur may also be audible

Table 3 (continued)
Congenital Heart Disease With Little or No Cyanosis

Name	Description	Clinical Features
Pulmonary Valve Stenosis (PS) With Intact Ventricular Septum	Accounts for approx. 8% of CHD The most common form of R ventricular outflow obstruction due to deformity of the pulmonic valve. Obstruction occurs during systole. The cusps are thickened.	Usually asymptomatic during infancy; Dyspnea, fatigue develops later; Risk of CHF; Murmur loud III-V/VI SEM ULSB; often with thrill, radiating to back, systolic ejection click ULSB; S_2 may be widely split
Mitral Valve Prolapse (MVP)	Syndrome resulting from abnormal mitral valve mechanism that causes billowing of one or both mitral leaflets into the L atrium at the end of systole; More common in females (2-20%); May be at risk to develop endocarditis; Antibiotic Rx for procedures	Often not recognized until adolescence. Usually asymptomatic; may have chest pain, palpitations, dizziness Murmur mid-late SEM at apex; May be preceded by click; heard best in standing or squatting position; at times only click is audible; EKG and chest x-ray normal
Vascular Rings	Vascular anomalies that may compress the traches include: double aortic arch, R aortic with R brachiel arch, anomalous innominate artery and anomalous left carotid artery	Usually asymptomatic; constriction may cause vomiting, dysphagia, stridor and predispose to recurrent respiratory infections; child may hold head in hyperextension

Table 4
Recommended Antiobiotics for Prevention of Bacterial Endocarditis

Dental, Oral, Respiratory Tract Procedures

AMOXICILLIN 50mg/kg PO	One hour before procedure and ½ the initial dose 6 hrs after first dose
AMPICILLIN 50 mg/kg IV or IM	Thirty minutes before procedure and ½ the dose 6 hours after the first dose

Penicillin-Allergic Patients

ERYTHROMYCIN 20 mg/kg	Two hours before procedure and ½ initial dose 6 hours after first dose
CLINDAMYCIN 10 mg/kg PO	One hour before procedure and ½ dose 6 hours after first dose
CLINDAMYCIN 10 mg/kg IV	30 min before procedure and ½ initial dose 6 hours after first dose
VANCOMYCIN 20 mg/kg IV	One hour before procedure, given over one hour. No repeat necessary.

Genitourinary and Gastrointestinal Procedures

AMPICILLIN 50 mg/kg IV *and*	Thirty minutes before procedure
GENTAMYCIN 2 mg/kg IV	Thirty minutes before procedure
AMOXICILLIN 50 mg/kg PO	Six hours after IV dose of Ampicillin and Gentamycin

Rheumatic Fever (RF)

- Definition—A diffuse inflammatory systemic disease of the connective tissue that is a delayed sequela to an upper respiratory infection with group A beta-hemolytic streptococci. It involves primarily the heart, blood vessels, joints, central nervous system, and subcutaneous tissues. Diagnosis is based upon evidence of the streptococcal infection and *Jones Criteria* (Dajani, Ayoub & Biermanm, 1992), which requires the presence of two major manifestations or one major and two minor manifestations (see Table 5)

Table 5
Jones Criteria Revised For Diagnosis of Rheumatic Fever

Major Criteria	Minor Criteria
Carditis	Fever
Polyarthritis	Arthralgia
Chorea	History of RF or RF heart disease
Erythema marginatum	Elevated ESR
Subcutaneous nodules	Positive C—reactive protein
	Prolonged P-R interval

- Etiology/Incidence

  1. RF is thought to be an autoimmune response to infection with group A beta-hemolytic streptococcus

  2. Incidence generally declining; focal outbreaks reported in specific geographic areas in the 1980s; a common cause of heart disease in underdeveloped countries;

  Predisposing factors:

  3. First attack usually occurs 5 to 15 years; peak 6 to 8 years; rare under 4 years of age

  4. Family history—RF may occur in more than one member of same family

  5. More common in winter and spring (similar to streptococcal pharyngitis)

  6. Recurrent streptococcal infections; approximately 3% of streptococcal

pharyngitis infections are followed by RF

■ Clinical Findings: Usually begin 1 to 5 weeks following upper respiratory infection

1. Polyarthritis—affects large joints primarily and migrates from one to another over a period of several days; swelling, tenderness and redness and limitation of movement apparent; most common manifestation occuring in 60 to 85% of patients

2. Signs of carditis occur in 40 to 50% of patients—tachycardia out of proportion to fever, significant cardiac murmurs

3. Subcutaneous nodules—occur in only 2 to 10% of patients; found on exterior surfaces and bony prominence of arms and legs, and scapula, and mastoid processes; usually indicates severe carditis

4. Chorea—found in 15% of cases; late manifestation are involuntary uncoordinated jerky movements, hypotonia, and emotional instability

5. Erythema marginatum—occurs in less than 10% of cases; area of erythema over the trunk and proximal parts of limbs

6. Fever—usually mild

7. Epistaxis (5 to 10%)

8. Loss of weight

9. Pleurisy and signs and symptoms of pneumonia

10. Arthralgia

11. Anemia, pallor

12. Abdominal pain

13. Malaise, fatigue

■ Differential Diagnosis

1. Juvenile rheumatoid arthritis

2. Systemic lupus erythematosus

3. Septic arthritis

4. Osteomyelitis

5. Sickle cell anemia

6. Myocarditis, pericarditis, secondary to viral infection

7. Drug sensitivity reactions

8. Henoch-Schönlein purpura

9. Acute leukemia

- Diagnostic Tests/Findings

    1. ESR—elevated

    2. C-reactive protein test—positive

    3. WBC elevated, Hgb and Hct decreased

    4. May have positive throat culture from Group A-beta hemolytic streptococcal infection

    5. ASO titers elevated (80%)

    6. Other strep antibodies elevated

    7. Chest radiograph—may demonstrate cardiac enlargement

    8. ECG—may suggest carditis

- Management/Treatment

    1. Referral to pediatrician/cardiologist as soon as suspected for diagnosis and management. Treatment will include: bed rest, antibiotic therapy (penicillin, erythromycin for penicillin sensitivity), aspirin, corticosteroids and treatment of CHF, as indicated

    2. Prevention

        a. Prompt and accurate diagnosis and treatment of streptococcal pharyngitis

        b. Prevention of recurrence of RF with monthly injections of long-acting penicillin (gantrisin or erythromycin for penicillin sensitivity) until adulthood

        c. Those with rheumatic heart disease require antibiotics prior to dental work plus the usual preventive therapy

Hypertension

- Definition

    1. "Average systolic and/or diastolic blood pressure equal to or greater than the 95th percentile for age on at least 3 separate occasions" (Report of the second task force on Blood Pressure Control in Children, 1987)

    2. May be primary or essential hypertension (no underlying cause known)

or secondary hypertension (identifiable cause)

3. Blood pressure norms related to height and weight in addition to age and sex appear to be more valuable in detecting abnormal blood pressure measurements

4. Most children prior to adolescence suffer from secondary hypertension; most often caused by renal disease but, recent consideration is being given to presence of primary hypertension in this age group

- Etiology/Incidence

    1. *Primary Hypertension*—no clearly defined pathophysiologic component; may have a genetic component; family history of hypertension or cardiovascular disease suggestive (most common in adolescents)

    2. *Secondary Hypertension*—(most common in infants and children)

        a. Renal disease—most common reason for secondary hypertension in children

            (1) Glomerulonephritis; polycystic kidneys, nephrosis

            (2) Systemic lupus erythematosus

            (3) Trauma

            (4) Neurofibromatosis

        b. Endocrine Disorders

            (1) Hypertension—may be pregnancy induced in adolescent

            (2) Cushings syndrome; congenital adrenal hyperplasia

            (3) Hyperthyroidism

            (4) Pheochromocytoma

        c. Cardiac disorders—coarctation of aorta (5%)

        d. Drugs or toxins

            (1) Oral contraceptives

            (2) Corticosteroids

            (3) Sympathomimetic substances

            (4) Cocaine, amphetamines, PCP

            (5) Heavy metal or lead poison

        e. Increased intracranial pressure

- Clinical Findings

  1. May discover elevated BP on routine screening; need at least three consecutive readings at different visits

  2. Proper measurement of BP is essential (see Growth & Development chapter)

  3. With substantial elevation headaches, dizziness, visual disturbances, chest pain, epistaxis and seizures may occur

  4. Detailed history including past medical history, family history, history of trauma and drug/medication use should guide physical examination in order to detect underlying causes of secondary hypertension

- Differential Diagnosis

  1. Primary hypertension—rare in young child before adolescence

  2. Secondary hypertension (see Etiology)

- Diagnostic Tests/Findings—Extent of testing determined by history and physical examination and severity of hypertension

  1. Urinalysis—to identify presence of nephritis, nephrosis, UTI

  2. BUN/Creatinine—renal function

  3. Peripheral plasma renin levels—elevated values significant

  4. Renal imaging

  5. CBC—anemia

  6. Lipid profile

  7. Echocardiogram—cardiomegaly

  8. Additional tests based on suspected cause of secondary hypertension

- Management/Treatment

  1. Depends on cause and degree of elevation

  2. Acute symptomatic severe elevation requires immediate referral

  3. Other types of secondary hypertension require surgery or pharmacologic management, e.g., coarctation of aorta, chronic renal disease

  4. Management of high normal or elevation without cause requires

     a. Weight reduction, if indicated

     b. Moderate sodium restriction—limit use of salt in meal preparation and restrict consumption of foods with high amounts of sodium

c. Increased potassium and calcium intake may be beneficial

d. Exercise and behavior modification

e. Pharmacotherapy

(1) Diuretics, e.g., hydrochlorthiazide, furosemide

(2) Adrenergic inhibitors, e.g., metoprolol atenolol

(3) Vasodilators, e.g., hydralazine, minoxidil

(4) Angiotensin—converting enzyme inhibitors, e.g., captopril

f. Counseling to increase compliance

g. Long term follow-up necessary

5. Prevention

Syncope

■ Definition: A transient loss of consciousness produced by alterations in the supply of oxygen and/or glucose to the brain

■ Etiology/Incidence: May be due to circulatory, metabolic or neuropsychologic causes

1. Circulatory causes

a. Common faint (Vasopressor syncope)—most frequent form due to activation of the cholinergic vasodilator system; this causes a fall in blood pressure and an increased blood flow to muscles; both sympathetic and parasympathetic systems are affected; It is associated with emotional stress, pain, fasting, and hot, humid or crowded environments

b. Orthostatic hypotension—inadequate response of usual vasoconstriction of arterioles and veins in the upright position resulting in hypotension without the reflex increase in heart rate; there is no autonomic response

c. Decreased systemic venous return—may occur from increased intrathoracic pressure from repetitive coughing or breath holding or decreased intravascular volume from hemorrhage or dehydration

2. Cardiac causes

a. Obstructive Lesions—e.g., pulmonary hypertension; usually precipitated by exercise

        b. Arrhythmias—e.g., severe tachycardia or bradycardia; complete heart block

    3. Metabolic causes

        a. Hypoglycemia

        b. Hypoxia

        c. Hyperventilation syndrome

    4. Neurologic causes

        a. Epilepsy

        b. Brain tumor

        c. Migraine

        d. Hysteria

■ Clinical Findings

    1. Signs and symptoms

        a. Vasopressor Syncope

           (1)   Almost always occurs while patient is standing

           (2)   Prodrome of weakness, generalized numbness, pallor, tachycardia, lightheadedness, blurring of vision (pupillary dilatation) sweating, nausea, and stomach discomfort

           (3)   Followed by brief loss of consciousness or cessation of symptoms on lowering of head

           (4)   Clonic movements may occur if patient remains unconscious longer than 15 to 20 seconds

           (5)   Physical examination—completely normal following event

        b. Orthostatic hypotension—differs from vasopressor syncope in that there is no perspiration, pallor or hyperventilation (autonomic response); unusual in children; may occur in adolescents who have stood motionless for long periods of time

■ Differential Diagnosis

    1. Cardiac causes—usually occur during or after exercise

    2. Epilepsy—sometimes difficult to differentiate but usually last longer and often occur when patient is sitting or lying down

    3. Hypoglycemia—usually does not produce true syncope, more often a

feeling of faintness; pallor, weakness and sweating

4. Conversion reaction—often more dramatic reaction, may faint while sitting and standing; fluttering of eyes, moaning or other sounds may occur, sequence of events and positions not typical

5. Other causes as indicated by history and physical examination

- Diagnostic Tests/Findings
  1. Depends on suggested causes
  2. CBC, blood sugar, ECG or EEG if indicated

- Management/Treatment
  1. Place patient in supine position
  2. Counsel patient to avoid precipitating factors
  3. Refer to appropriate specialist if syncope caused from other than common vasopressor syncope, for further evaluation and management

Disturbances of Rate and Rhythm

- Definition: Heart rates above or below norms for age or any irregularity of heart beat
- Etiology/Incidence
  1. Results from disturbance in formation and/or conduction of the cardiac impulse
  2. May be transient
  3. Can be secondary to inflammation and other systemic diseases, e.g., myocarditis, rheumatic fever, collagen, vascular disease, endocrine disorders
  4. Due to toxins, e.g., theophylline, cocaine
  5. Secondary to surgical repair for congenital heart disease
  6. Other systemic causes
     a. Myocarditis
     b. Metabolic abnormalities (hypoglycemia)
     c. Electrolyte imbalance (hyper/hypokalemia)
     d. Acidosis/hypoxia
     e. Diseases of CNS (increased ICP)
     f. Collagen vascular disease (SLE, R.A.)

g. Endocrine disorders (hyper-/hypo thyroidism)

h. Drugs (Sympathomimetics, cardiac drugs, illicit drugs, many others.)

7. Second in frequency to CHD as a pediatric cardiac problem in the U.S. Increase in incidence reported. May be due to more long-term survivors of cardiac surgery and better diagnostic capabilities

■ Clinical Findings

1. Children usually asymptomatic—often discovered on routine physical examination

2. Pallor and fatigue during feeding (infant)

3. Syncope/dizziness, palpitations (older infant)

4. Signs/symptoms of CHF (especially in infant)

5. Seizures

6. Physical findings, e.g., tachycardia, bradycardia, irregular pulses

■ Diagnostic Tests/Findings

1. ECG taken at rest and after exercise—will usually document an arrhythmia; children with intermittent episodes may have normal ECG between attacks

2. Continuous ECG monitor (Holter monitoring)—can document infrequent arrhythmias

■ Differential Diagnosis

1. Normal sinus arrhythmia—most common cause of irregular heart beat; represents the acceleration and deceleration of the heart rate that occurs with respiration; asymptomatic always (normal ECG)

2. Sinus tachycardia—very common in children; normal with exercise and fever; may indicate cardiac failure; may be associated with hyperthyroidism, myocarditis, or ingestion of atropine-like substances; heart rate is regular and rapid > 190 infants; > 140 to 200 children; > 100 to 150 adolescents; ECG is normal

3. Supraventricular tachycardia—most common tachyrhythmia or clinically significant arrhythmia in children (approximately 1:25,000); more common in infants under 1 year; more common in boys, 50% present by 4 months of age; CHD presents in 25% of cases; most

children have normal hearts; heart rate is usually regular, but rapid (220 to 300), usually paroxysmal with abrupt onset and termination; normal ECG except for rapid rate, P-wave may be absent; treatment necessary in rapid, sustained or recurrent attacks (digitalization and or cardioversion)

4. Ventricular tachycardia—much less common; rare in children with normal hearts but can occur; heart rate varies but rapid; usually < 250 with average of 120 to 180; with infants may be higher; abnormal ECG; three or more PVCs in sequence with widened QRS

5. Sinus Bradycardia—normal in athlete; may be associated with increased intracranial pressure or hypothyroidism; also seen in premature infants with apnea and following cardiac surgery; heart rate is regular but slow < 90 infants; < 60 children; < 50 adolescents; ECG is normal

6. Complete A-V block—less common; congenital or acquired following cardiac surgery; no conduction of atrial impulses to ventricle, i.e., ventricular rate regular but slow and below normal for age; abnormal ECG

■ Diagnostic Tests/Findings

1. ECG

2. Other tests based on history and clinical findings

■ Management/Treatment
Treatment depends on cause and presence of signs/symptoms; any sustained or recurrent arrhythmia requires referral and evaluation even if child is asymptomatic and has normal examination; infant requires immediate referral

Kawasaki Syndrome (Mucocutaneous Lymph Node Syndrome)

■ Definition: A febrile, exanthematous, multisystem illness affecting infants and young children involving a unique and distinctive clinical spectrum with acute vasculitis and associated with severe cardiac involvement including coronary (arteritis), aneurysm and thrombocytic occlusion

■ Etiology/Incidence

1. Etiology unknown—thought to be infectious; hypersensitivity reaction or environmental toxin exposure; first described in Japan in 1967

2. In the U.S. it is the leading cause of acquired heart disease in children

3. Occurs predominantly in children less than 5 years of age; peak age in U.S. between 6 months and 5 years

4. Increased incidence in Asians; male-female 1.6:1

5. Occurs in epidemic 2 to 3 year cycles, winter and spring, temperate climate

6. Coronary artery aneurysms or ectasia develop in 15 to 25% of children and may lead to myocardial infarction (MI), sudden death or chronic heart disease

■ Clinical Findings

1. Acute phase

a. Abrupt onset of fever (high, to 40 °C) lasting for 5 or more days (nonresponsive to antibiotics)

b. Conjunctival congestion—bilateral without exudate

c. Erythematous mouth and pharynx, strawberry tongue, red, cracked lips

d. Induration of hands and feet with erythematous palms and soles

e. Erythematous rash over trunk, accentuated in creases and joints

f. Cervical adenopathy—usually unilateral, enlarged to more than 1.5 cm

g. Drying, cracking, fissuring of lips usually by 6th day of illness

2. Periungal desquamation and peeling of the palms and soles occur during the 2nd to 3rd week

3. For the diagnosis to be made fever and at least 4 of the other 5 features (1. b, c, d, e, f) must be present (AAP, 1994)

4. Those with fever and fewer than 4 features may be diagnosed with atypical disease when coronary artery disease is present (AAP, 1994)

5. Subacute phase

a. Marked irritability

b. Anterior uveitis (80%)

c. Sterile pyuria (70%)

d. Diarrhea (watery)

e. Arthralgia, arthritis (can develop during acute and subacute phases)

f. Cardiac findings (can develop during acute and subacute phases)

   (1) Tachycardia and gallup rhythms out of proportion to degree of fever and anemia (myocarditis)

   (2) Heart murmurs (aortic or mitral regurgitation)

   (3) S/S of CHF

- Differential Diagnosis

   1. Polyarteritis

   2. Scarlet fever

   3. Erythema multiforme/Stevens-Johnson syndrome

   4. Measles and other viral exanthems

   5. Toxic shock syndrome

   6. JRA

   7. Infectious mononucleosis

   8. Rocky mountain spotted fever

   9. Leptospirosis

   10. Mercury poisoning

   11. Drug reaction

- Diagnostic Tests/Findings

   1. WBC—leukocytosis > 15,000 with left shift seen in acute phase and may remain elevated for 1 to 3 weeks

   2. CBC—mild normochromic, normocytic anemia

   3. Blood culture—usually negative

   4. Erythrocyte sedimentation rate—elevated (acute phase)

   5. C-reactive protein—increased (acute phase)

   6. Thrombocytosis— > 700,000/mm^3 after 10th day of illness (subacute phase)

   7. Urine—sterile pyuria

   8. ECG—nonspecific ST segment and T wave changes, prolonged P-R interval

   9. Two-dimensional echocardiogram—shows coronary vascular disease, coronary vascular dilatation, aneurysm formation

■ Management/Treatment

1. Immediate referral to pediatrician and/or subspecialist if suspected; goal of management to detect and prevent coronary aneurysm and myocardial infarction

2. Hospitalization

   a. Immune Globulin Intravenous (IGIV)—initiated within 10 days of onset of fever; concurrent aspirin therapy decreases prevalence of coronary artery dilation and aneurysms

   b. Cardiac care

   c. Corticosteroid use contraindicated except in unusual circumstances; may result in increased coronary aneurysms

3. Long term follow-up necessary

4. Parents, teachers and child care providers of children with cardiac complications of Kawasaki Syndrome should be instructed in CPR

5. Children should be monitored closely for other high-risk factors for CHD, such as hyperlipidemia or hypertension

6. Immunizations

   a. Measles vaccination deferred for 11 months for those who have received IGIV unless risk of exposure is high

   b. Other childhood immunizations not interrupted

   c. Yearly influenza vaccination indicated in patients undergoing long-term aspirin therapy (possible increased risk for Reye syndrome)

Hyperlipidemia/Hypercholesterolemia

■ Definition: Hyperlipidemia is a total cholesterol, LDL cholesterol or triglyceride levels that are above the 95th percentile for age and sex. Hypercholesterolemia is considered Type II hyperlipidemia when total cholesterol is at or above 200 mg/dl and/or the LDL is above 130 mg/dl. Children with total cholesterol levels above the 75th percentile and a family history of early coronary artery disease are considered at risk for developing atherosclerotic heart disease.

■ Etiology/Incidence

1. It is believed that atherosclerotic lesions begin to develop in childhood and may progress to irreversible lesions by the fourth decade of life

2. The degree of atherosclerotic changes correlates with blood cholesterol

levels, smoking and hypertension.

3. Risk factors in addition to an elevated serum cholesterol, include genetics, hypertension, obesity, diabetes mellitus, cigarette smoking and lack of physical activity

■ Clinical Findings

1. Family history—parents or grandparents with history of coronary or peripheral vascular disease before the age of 55; parents with hypercholesterolemia at or greater than 240 mg/dl

2. Diet history—look for high intake of total fats, saturated fats and cholesterol

3. Physical examination—look for signs of obesity, hypertension or diabetes

4. Habits—look for tobacco and alcohol use especially in adolescents; look for lack of physical activity

■ Differential Diagnosis: Rule out secondary causes of hyperlipidemia

1. Diabetes mellitus

2. Hypothyroidism

3. Nephrotic syndrome

4. Lupus erythematosus

5. Steroids

6. Congenital biliary atresia

■ Diagnostic Tests/Findings

1. Lipid Profile—total cholesterol, HDL, triglycerides after 12 hour fast

2. Estimate LDL cholesterol = total cholesterol − HDL cholesterol + triglycerides/5

3. Repeat tests if borderline or elevated

4. Additional studies to evaluate secondary causes as indicated

■ Management/Treatment

1. Weight reduction to ideal weight for height

2. Screen all family members

3. Dietary Restrictions—a nutritionist should be consulted if possible

    a. Step I diet—decrease fat intake to 30% of total calories with less than 10% as saturated fat and less than 300 mg of cholesterol per day. Increase fiber to 10-20 g/1000 calories

b. Step II diet—if desired decrease in lipid levels is not achieved after repeated testing, decrease level of saturated fat to less than 7% of total calories and decrease cholesterol to less than 200 mg/day

4. Increase exercise

5. Counsel to abstain from smoking and alcohol

6. Pharmacologic therapy—referral to appropriate specialist considered for children over 10 years of age who have not responded to an adequate trial of diet therapy. Bile acid sequestrants such as Cholestyramine or Colestipol are the drugs recommended for children. These children should be monitored carefully for growth and other side effects

7. Prevention—anticipatory guidance during all well child maintenance visits to maintain a well balanced diet according to the recommended dietary goals; encourage daily exercise, avoid known risk factors for heart disease; and encourage proper screening for those children considered at risk.

Questions

Select the best answer

1. During a well child examination, a 5 year old girl is found to have a grade II/VI vibratory—low pitched systolic ejection murmur at the LLSB radiating over the precordial area. The murmur disappears in the standing and sitting position. S_I and S_2 are otherwise normal. The rest of the examination is completely normal and there is no family history of heart disease. The most likely diagnosis is

   a. A venous hum murmur
   b. Pulmonary ejection flow murmur
   c. ASD murmur
   d. Still Murmur

2. In considering the management of this child the nurse practitioner should

   a. Document the findings in the chart and refer the child for a cardiac evaluation
   b. Document the findings in the chart and reassure the parent that this is an innocent heart murmur that requires no further evaluation or treatment
   c. Order an ECG and chest x-ray and ask the child to return in 2 weeks for re-evaluation of the murmur
   d. Revaluate in 3 months

3. The characteristics of an innocent heart murmur include all of the following except

   a. Always systolic
   b. No louder than III/VI
   c. Normal S_2
   d. Occasional thrill present

4. Of the following perinatal risk factors which of the following is least likely to lead to CHD?

   a. Rubella exposure during the first trimester
   b. Maternal alcohol use during pregnancy
   c. Maternal drug therapy with dilantin during pregnancy
   d. Family history of CHD in a distant relative

5. A 13 month old girl has a history of slow growth. She has been falling off the curve for both height and weight and is now below the 5th percentile. On examination you note a grade II/VI blowing systolic ejection murmur at the 2nd LIS that radiates around the axilla to the back. The S_2 appears widely split and does not change with respiration. The rest of the examination is normal. The nurse

practitioner suspects the presence of CHD. Which of the following lesions would most likely produce these findings:

   a. Patent Ductus Arteriosus
   b. Ventricular Septal Defect
   c. Atrial Septal Defect
   d. Coarctation of the aorta

6. The following statements are true about acute rheumatic fever except

   a. ARF is thought to be an autoimmune response to infection with Group A, beta hemolytic streptococcus
   b. Signs/symptoms usually appear 1 to 5 weeks following a URI
   c. Incidence declining, generally
   d. Most common under 5 years of age

7. The following laboratory test might be suggestive of acute rheumatic fever except

   a. Elevated ESR
   b. Positive C-reactive protein
   c. Elevated WBC
   d. Elevated Hgb/Hct

8. A 7 year old boy is found to have a BP of 130/85 on a routine well check up. The initial management of this child would include the following

   a. Have mother purchase electronic BP device to measure BP at select intervals and return at usual scheduled visit
   b. Repeat measurement
   c. Have child return for two consecutive repeat measurements
   d. Order a UA, BUN and IVP

9. The most likely cause of hypertension in this child would be

   a. Primary hypertension with unknown etiology
   b. Coarctation of the aorta
   c. Pheochromocytoma
   d. Renal disease

10. During an admission physical examination on a 16 hour old newborn you note a heart murmur. It is a grade II/VI soft, vibratory systolic murmur at the 2nd LIS. It does not radiate and the infant is otherwise completely normal. The infant is due to be discharged at 24 hours. The best course of action would be

   a. Order a stat chest x-ray and ECG
   b. Refer to the cardiologist before discharge
   c. Explain your findings to the parents, document your findings on the chart and advise parents to make a follow up appointment with the physician or nurse

practitioner within 48 hours

d. Consider this a normal finding and do nothing

11. The following statements are true about congenital heart disease except

a. The etiology probably involves a multifactorial inheritance pattern
b. The incidence is approximately 8 out of 1000 live births
c. Signs and symptoms of the abnormal heart are usually evident in the prenatal period before birth
d. Signs and symptoms during infancy might include poor weight gain and a history of feeding problems

12. The most common murmur of early childhood is

a. A carotid bruit
b. Pulmonary ejection flow murmur
c. ASD murmur
d. Still murmur

13. A Venous Hum can be identified as

a. Always disappearing when child is put in a supine position or when the jugular vein is compressed
b. A very rare murmur
c. Usually heard only in newborns
d. Heard best at the LLSB

14. A cyanotic congenital heart lesion that consists of an absent pulmonary valve and represents about 1% of congenital heart disease is

a. Tetralogy of Fallot
b. Tricuspid atresia
c. Pulmonary atresia with intact ventricular septum
d. Transposition of the Great Vessels

15. The following lesions are usually consistent with Tetralogy of Fallot except

a. Pulmonary stenosis
b. ASD
c. Dextroposition of the aorta
d. Right ventricular hypertrophy

16. A congenital heart lesion that is fatal within the first year of life without surgical intervention is

a Dextrocardia
b. Truncus Arteriosus
c. Ventricular Septal Defect
d. Hypoplastic Left Heart Syndrome

17. The most common cardiac abnormality in children that accounts for 25% of congenital heart disease is

    a. Patent Ductus Arteriosus
    b. Coarctation of the Aorta
    c. Ventricular Septal Defect
    d. Atrial Septal Defect

18. A cardiac lesion that is the most common cause of congestive heart failure in the first month of life is

    a. A large Ventricular Septal Defect
    b. Coarctation of the Aorta
    c. Atrial Septal Defect
    d. Aortic Stenosis

19. The following statements are true about mitral valve prolapse except

    a. It is more common in males
    b. It is often not recognized until adolescence
    c. The murmur is a mid-late SEM at the apex which is usually preceded by a click
    d. The syndrome results from an abnormal mitral valve mechanism that causes billowing of one or both mitral leaflets into the L atrium at the end of systole

20. A vascular anomaly that may compress the trachea and cause stridor, recurrent respiratory infections and dysphagia is

    a. Coarctation of the Aorta
    b. Tetralogy of Fallot
    c. Transposition of the Great Vessels
    d. Vascular Ring

21. The nurse practitioner who is participating in the care of a child with congenital heart disease would do all of the following except

    a. Assist in the coordination of care
    b. Monitor growth and development and nutritional status
    c. Provide preventive care through active and passive immunizations and recommendations for prophylactic antibiotics
    d. Order cardiac catheterization to diagnose specific lesion

22. An acquired heart disease that includes polyarthritis, carditis, subcutaneous nodules, chorea and erythema marginatum is

    a. Juvenile rheumatoid arthritis
    b. Acute leukemia
    c. Rheumatic Fever
    d. Systemic lupus erythematosus

23. The most common type of hypertension that might be found in the adolescent period would be

    a. Primary hypertension with no known cause
    b. Hypertension secondary to renal disease
    c. Hypertension secondary to oral contraceptive use
    d Hypertension secondary to illicit drug use

24. A 6-month-old infant is noted to have a tachyrhythmia with a heart rate of 220. The rate is regular and remains rapid for several hours then terminates without intervention. There is no history or evidence of congenital heart disease. The ECG is normal. The most likely diagnosis would be

    a. Normal sinus arrythmia
    b. Ventricular tachycardia
    c. Sinus tachycardia
    d. Supraventricular tachycardia

25. A 3-year-old boy presents with high fever of 5 days duration, an enlarged cervical node, acute erythema and congestion of both conjunctivae, severe erythema of the pharynx and tongue and cracking of the lips. There is a fine erythematous papular rash over the trunk, and the hands and feet appear red and edematous. Your differential would include all of the following except

    a. Scarlet fever
    b. Erythema Multiforme
    c. Kawasaki Syndrome
    d. Varicella

26. Diagnostic studies at this time that would help to determine if this child could have Kawasaki Syndrome would include

    a. Complete CBC with differential, blood culture, C-reactive protein and ECG
    b. Complete CBC with differential, platelets, blood culture, C-reactive protein and ESR
    c. CBC, blood culture, urinalysis
    d. CBC, platelets, 2D Echocardiogram

27. Laboratory findings that would be consistent with a diagnosis of Kawasaki Syndrome would be

    a. An elevated WBC (> 15,000), an elevated sedimentation rate and elevated C-reactive protein and a thrombocytosis after the first week of illness
    b. An elevated WBC, an elevated ESR, an elevated C-reactive protein and a thrombocytopenia after the first week of illness
    c. Decreased Hct, increased platelets and normal WBC

  d. An elevated WBC, positive blood culture, thrombocytopenia after the first week of illness

28. A clinical finding that is often seen in patients with the diagnosis of Kawasaki Syndrome but does not occur until after the first week of illness is

   a. Strawberry tongue
   b. Edema and erythema of the hands and feet
   c. Cervical adenopathy
   d. Desquamation of the skin on hands and feet

29. In addition to immediate referral to a pediatrician and/or cardiologist, the management of a child with Kawasaki would most likely include

   a. Hospitalization and IV antibiotics
   b. Hospitalization and IV immunoglobulins and salicylate therapy
   c. Outpatient follow up with salicylate therapy
   d. Hospitalization and IV corticosteroids

30. Hypercholesterolemia is defined as total cholesterol at or above

   a. 100 mg/dl
   b. 150 mg/dl
   c. 200 mg/dl
   d. 300 mg/dl

31. A child is found to have an elevated total cholesterol on screening. The child has a positive family history for early coronary artery disease. The best course of action would be

   a. Refer immediately to a cardiologist for evaluation
   b. Initiate Step I diet
   c. Order a complete lipid profile after 12 hour fast and initiate Step I diet
   d. Repeat test

32. Risk factors for coronary vascular disease include all of the following except

   a. Obesity
   b. Smoking
   c. Elevated serum cholesterol
   d. Vigorous physical exercise

Answer Key

1.	d	17.	c
2.	b	18.	b
3.	d	19.	a
4.	d	20.	d
5.	c	21.	d
6.	d	22.	c
7.	d	23.	a
8.	c	24.	d
9.	d	25.	d
10.	c	26.	b
11.	c	27.	a
12.	d	28.	d
13.	a	29.	b
14.	c	30.	c
15.	b	31.	d
16.	d	32.	d

Bibliography

American Academy of Pediatrics, Committee on Nutrition. (1992). Statement on cholesterol. *Pediatrics, 90*(3), 469-472.

American Academy of Pediatrics (1994). *Report of the committee on infectious diseases* (23rd ed.). Elk Grove Village, IL: American Academy of Pediatrics.

American Heart Association, Special Writing Group. (1992). Guidelines for the diagnosis of rheumatic fever. *Journal of the American Medical Association, 268*, 2069-73.

Carter, C., & Goldring, D. (Eds.). (1992). Prevention of heart disease. *Pediatric Annals, 21*, (4).

Cohen, D. (1992). Surgical management of congenital heart disease in the 1990s. *American Journal of Diseases of Children, 146*, 1447-1451.

Cowell, J. (1992). Cardiovascular risk stability: From grade school to high school. *Journal of Pediatric Health Care, 6*(6), 349-354.

Dajani, A. S., Ayoub, E., & Bierman, F. Z. (1992). Guidelines for the diagnosis of rheumatic fever (Jones Criteria updated 1992). *Journal of the American Medical Association, 268*, 2069-2073.

Flynn, P., Engle, A., & Ehlers, K. (1992). Cardiac issues in the pediatric emergency room. *Pediatric Clinics of North America, 39*(5), 955-986.

Gersong, W. (1991). Diagnosis and management of Kawasaki disease. *Journal of the American Medical Association, 265*, 20.

Gillette, P. C. (1990). Congenital heart disease. *Pediatric Clinics of North America, 37* (1).

Kaug, R. E. (1992). Preventive cardiology for the pediatrician. *Current Problems in Pediatrics, 22* (6), 258-279.

Monett, Z., & Moynihan, P. (1991). Cardiovascular assessment of the neonatal heart. *Journal of Perinatology/Neonatal Nursing, 5*(2), 50-59.

Oski, F. A., DeAngelis, C. D., Feign, R., & Warshaw, T. (1990). *Principles and practice of pediatrics.* Philadelphia: J. B. Lippincott.

Park, N. (1988). *Pediatric cardiology for practitioners.* (2nd ed.). Chicago: Yearbook Medical Publishers.

Roberts, K. (1991). Kawasaki syndrome: In the eye of the beholder. *Contemporary Pediatrics, 8,* 126-142.

Task Force on Blood Pressure Control in Children. (1987). Report of the Second Task Force on Blood Pressure Control in Children. *Pediatrics, 79,* 1-25.

Neurological Disorders

Elizabeth Hawkins-Walsh

Microcephaly

- Definition
    1. A head circumference that is 3 SD or more below the mean for sex and age or one that is not increasing with age
    2. A head circumference of 2 SD below the mean and falling off in repeated evaluations is also significant
- Etiology/Incidence
    1. Chromosomal/genetic disorders producing a variety of dysmporphic syndromes
    2. Intrauterine infections including Rubella, Cytomegalovirus, Toxoplasmosis, Syphilis, Neonatal Herpes Virus
    3. Fetal exposure to alcohol producing Fetal Alcohol Syndrome or exposure to other chemical toxins such as anticonvulsants
    4. Fetal exposure to ionizing radiation in the first 2 trimesters
    5. Severe malnutrition in early infancy
    6. Other metabolic disorders, head trauma, or degenerative central nervous system disorders
- Clinical Findings
    1. Chest circumference exceeds head circumference in the full term newborn or infant up to 6 months of age
    2. There may be marked backward slope of the forehead with narrowing of the temporal diameter and occipital flattening. This is indicative of hereditary or familial microcephaly. Disproportionately large ears may be present
    3. Skull asymmetries may be seen with many dysmorphic and chromosomal disorders. The palate may be high-arched and the teeth may be dysplastic
- Differential Diagnosis
    1. Craniosynostosis
    2. Hypopituitarism
    3. Severe malnutrition
- Diagnostic Tests/Findings

1. Karyotyping may be diagnostic of a variety of chromosomal and hereditary disorders

2. TORCHS screening—T = Toxoplasmosis; O = Other infections, R = Rubella; C = Cytomegalovirus; H = Herpes; S = Syphilis

3. Screening for amino acid abnormalities

4. Skull radiographs are indicated in dysmorphic syndromes and intrauterine infections. CT brain scanning may discover calcification, malformations or atrophy

-   Management/Treatment

    1. Most forms are not treatable, but correct diagnosis is important for genetic counseling and prognosis

    2. Management is supportive and directed at the various effects of the microcephaly and underlying disorder

Hydrocephalus

-   Definition: Condition which arises when production of cerebral spinal fluid (CSF) is greater than absorption of CSF or when absorption of CSF is compromised

-   Etiology/Incidence

    1. Multiple causes and conditions can lead to hydrocephalus

    2. Both congenital and acquired etiologies

    3. Obstructive hydrocephalus (99%)

        a. Impaired absorption of CSF within subarachnoid space (communicating hydrocephalus) or

        b. Obstruction to flow of CSF within ventricles (noncommunicating) caused by

            (1) Aqueductal stenosis

            (2) Obstruction of the foramina of Luschka and magendie

            (3) Postinfectious ventriculitis

            (4) Posthemorrhagic intraventricular hemorrhage

    4. Communicating and noncommunicating obstructive hydrocephalus occur with equal frequency in infants

    5. In children and adolescents, tumors are the most common cause

- Clinical Findings
    1. Time of onset and presence of pre-existing structural lesions affect clinical picture
    2. Infancy
        a. Head enlargement
        b. Anterior fontanel-wide open and bulging
        c. Dilated scalp veins
        d. Positive Macewen sign ("cracked-pot")
        e. Bossing (frontal enlargement)
        f. Eyes—"setting sun sign"
        g. Separated suture lines
        h. Sluggish pupils
        i. Irritability
        j. Lethargy
        k. Poor feeding
        l. High pitched cry
    3. Childhood
        a. Signs and symptoms caused by increased intracranial pressure and related to focal lesion
        b. Headache on awakening
        c. Vomiting
        d. Strabismus
        e. Papilledema; decreased visual activity
        f. Extrapyramidal tract signs (ataxia)
        g. Irritability
        h. Lethargy
        i. Confusion
        j. Personality changes
        k. Decline in academic performance
- Differential Diagnosis

1. Meningitis

2. Sepsis

3. Macrocephaly

4. Megalencephaly

5. Benign large head

6. Tumor

■ Diagnostic Tests/Findings

   1. Head circumferences (daily)

   2. Skull x-ray—will show widened cranial sutures

   3. CT scan/ultrasound—will show ventricular enlargement

   4. Ventriculography—identification of obstruction

■ Management/Treatment

   1. Treatment—surgical

   2. Relief of hydrocephalus with ventriculoperitoneal shunt

   3. Treatment of complications

   4. Management of problems with psychomotor development

   5. Teach caregiver signs and symptoms of increasing intracranial pressure

   6. Anticipatory guidance for families regarding potential problems encountered as the child grows and develops

   7. Referral to appropriate support group

Erb Palsy

■ Definition: Damage to the upper (C 5-6) roots of the brachial plexus

■ Etiology/Incidence

   1. Occurs following traction injury of plexus, secondary to breech delivery or cephalopelvic disproportion

   2. Most common brachial plexus injury

■ Clinical Findings

   1. Internal rotation of arm with pronation of forearm

   2. Biceps reflex absent or diminished

3. Moro reflex absent on affected side

4. Possible sensory defect over lateral aspect of arm

5. Normal grasp and normal forearm strength

- Differential Diagnosis

 1. Klumpke-Dejerine paralysis

 2. Fractured clavicle

 3. Phrenic nerve injury (accompanies 5 to 10% upper plexus injuries)

- Diagnostic Tests/Findings—none

- Management/Treatment

 1. Referral

 2. Treatment—fixation of affected limb in abduction with external rotation of shoulder and supination of forearm

 3. Accomplished by splinting or fixation to bed with towels or pins

 4. Passive range of motion exercises to prevent contractures 7 to 10 days after injury

 5. 75% regain complete function within 2 to 3 months

Cerebral Palsy

- Definition: A nonprogressive disorder of the developing brain characterized by disorders of posture and movement

 2. Most common movement disorder of childhood

 a. Classification

 (1) Spastic

 (2) Athetosis

 (3) Rigid

 (4) Ataxia

 (5) Tremor

 (6) Mixed

- Etiology/Incidence

 1. Definite cause not established in most cases; multiple factors probably involved

2. Low birth weight is major risk factor

3. Perinatal asphyxia, cardiorespiratory arrest and intraventricular hemorrhage may be involved in 1/3 of cases

4. Incidence is approximately 2 per 1000 live births

- Clinical Findings

    1. Early presentations are very subtle

        a. Feeding difficulties

        b. Behavioral disturbances

        c. Difficulty diapering

        d. Asymmetries in movement

        e. Persisting primitive reflexes (ATN)

        f. Scissoring

        g. Hypo, hypertonia

    2. Later

        a. Motor delay

            (1) Excessive, prolonged primitive reflexes

            (2) Absent postural responses

            (3) Asymmetries

        b. Hyperreflexia

        c. Ankle clonus

        d. Contractures

        e. Persistent toe walking

        f. Pathologic reflexes

    3. Associated deficits

        a. Processing impairments

            (1) Communicative disorders

            (2) Learning disabilities

        b. Mental retardation

        c. Strabismus

        d. Deafness

       e. Oral motor dysfunction

- Differential Diagnosis

    1. Normal variants of hypo, hypertonia

    2. Normal development premature infant

    3. Global nonspecific mental retardation

    4. Spinal cord abnormality secondary to injury, tumor or congenital defect

    5. Hypotonia and muscle weakness secondary to myopathy or neuropathy

    6. Neurodegenerative disease

- Diagnostic Tests/Findings

    1. No single diagnostic test exists

    2. Diagnosis depends heavily upon birth and developmental histories and multiple physical and neurologic examinations over time

    3. Laboratory tests may rule out other etiologies

        a. Urine screening for amino and organic acidurias

        b. Serum uric acid for Lesch-Nyhan syndrome

        c. Chromosomal studies if significant dysmorphia

        d. Thyroid function for hypothyroid

        e. Serum muscle enzymes, muscle biopsy for congenital myopathies

    4. CT or MRI may suggest underlying events which resulted in CP, (e.g., central atrophy; infarction; intracranial hemorrhage)

    5. Severe periventricular echodensities with large cyst formation is highly sensitive and specific predictor for development of CP in premature infants

    6. Other tests may be indicated dependent upon clinical findings, e.g., EEG

- Management/Treatment

    1. Treatment directed toward maximizing function and preventing secondary handicaps

        a. Maximize motor function

        b. Enhance communicative abilities

        c. Master activities of daily living

2. Refer to multidisciplinary team

3. Treat associated deficits

4. Family support

Brain Tumors

- Definition: Expanding intracranial lesion; most common primary childhood tumors are astrocytoma and medulloblastoma

- Etiology/Incidence

  1. Unknown

  2. Certain genetic predisposition (neurocutaneous disorders)

  3. Congenital? Environmental? Secondary malignancies?

  4. Most common solid tumor of childhood; 2.2 to 2.4 per 100,000 population at risk per year (Hoekelman, 1992)

  5. Second only to Leukemia as most prevalent malignancy

- Clinical Findings

  1. Depend primarily on tumor location

  2. Headache; usually intermittent and most commonly appears in the morning

  3. Vomiting; occurs more frequently in the morning; usually occurs without nausea and may be projectile

  4. Neuromuscular changes

  5. Behavioral changes or alterations in personality are often the first symptoms, irrespective of location (Behrman, Kliegman, Nelson & Vaughn, 1992)

  6. Fatigue, anorexia

  7. Bulging fontanel and increasing head size in an infant

  8. Changes in dexterity, weakness in lower extremities, spasticity, paralysis

  9. Vital signs disturbance with decreased respirations pulse rate or increased blood pressure with wide pulse pressure

  10. Visual problems (diplopia, strabismus, papilledema, or nystagmus)

  11. Seizures

- Differential Diagnosis
    1. Hydrocephalus
    2. Intracranial hemorrhage
    3. Arteriovenous malformation
    4. Subdural hematoma, effusion or empyema
    5. Infarction
    6. Brain abscess
    7. Migraine
- Diagnostic Tests/Findings
    1. MRI—considered to be more reliable than CT scan
    2. CT SCAN—will show tumor density, presence of hydrocephalus and calcifications or hemorrhage
    3. Angiography—determine tumor's blood supply
    4. Lumbar puncture NOT done if ICP suspected
- Management/Treatment
    1. Surgery (therapy of choice, if possible)
    2. Radiation therapy
    3. Chemotherapy—controversial; has not been as effective as in other malignancies because of difficulty in crossing blood-brain barrier
    4. Multidisciplinary support
    5. Coordination of primary care and specialties

Neuroblastoma

- Definition: Tumor arising from cells in the sympathetic ganglia and adrenal medulla
- Etiology/Incidence
    1. Familial occurrence has been reported
    2. Most common malignancy of infants
    3. Slightly more common in white children than in black and in males than in females
    4. About 75% of these tumors are diagnosed in children < 5 years of age

- Clinical Findings

    1. Depend on location and stage of disease

    2. Many presenting signs are caused by compression of adjacent structures

    3. Firm, nontender, irregular mass in abdomen may be the first sign

    4. Metastatic disease presentation is not uncommon with associated symptomatology, such as

        a. Bluish skin nodules which may be noted in infants

        b. Hepatic neoplasm manifested as marked abdominal distension

        c. Skeletal system involvement which usually causes pain that may be elicited as irritability and restlessness in the young child or infant

    5. General symptoms include failure to thrive, anorexia, fever of unknown origin, diarrhea, pallor and irritability

    6. Symptoms associated with excess catecholamine production are sweating, flushing, pallor, headaches

- Differential Diagnosis

    1. Wilms Tumor

    2. Renal masses

    3. Medulloblastoma

    4. Glioma

- Diagnostic Tests/Findings

    1. CBC

    2. Urinalysis

    3. Bone marrow biopsy—for staging purposes and evaluation of tumor cells

    4. Urinary catecholalmines—elevated levels indicative diagnostic feature

    5. Tumor examination—definitive diagnosis based on histologic characteristics

    6. Ultrasonography

    7. CT scan; MRI—tissue density, metastases

    8. Bone scans—may show multiple destructive lesions of bone with "moth eaten" appearance

9. X-rays—determined by presenting findings

■ Management/Treatment

1. Surgery

2. Radiation

3. Chemotherapy

4. Survival inversely related to age of child at diagnosis—the younger the child at time of diagnosis (< 2 years of age) the better the prognosis for cure

5. Multidisciplinary support

6. Coordination of primary care and specialties

von Recklinghausen Disease (Neurofibromatosis-1)

■ Definition: Neurocutaneous syndrome characterized by tumor formation of peripheral nervous system (spinal and cranial)

■ Etiology/Incidence

1. Autosomal dominant disorder

2. Negative family history not unusual

3. Highly variable expression—within family

4. Incidence 1/4000

5. A parent with neurofibromatosis has a 50% chance of transmitting the disease with each pregnancy

■ Clinical Findings: Diagnostic criteria are met if two or more of following are found (NIH Consensus Development Conference on Neurofibromatosis, 1987)

1. Six or more (CLS) over 5mm in greatest diameter in prepubertal individuals and over 15mm in post-pubertal

2. Two or more neurofibromas of any type, or one plexiform neurofibroma

3. Freckling in axillary or inguinal regions

4. Optic pathway glioma

5. Two or more Lisch nodules (iris hamartomas)

6. A distinctive osseous lesion, such as sphenoid dysplasia or thinning of

long bone cortex with or without pseudoarthrosis

7. A first degree relative with Neurofibromatosis-1 by the above criteria

■ Differential Diagnosis

1. Albright's Syndrome

2. Benign café-au-lait spots

■ Diagnostic Tests/Findings—clinical findings; CT scan and MRI confirmatory for optic glioma or hamartoma; slit lamp confirmatory for Lisch nodules

■ Management/Treatment

1. Treatment is symptomatic

2. Commonly associated problems which may require assessment and management

    a. Seizures

    b. Headaches

    c. Hyperactivity

    d. Learning disabilities

    e. Renovascular hypertension

3. Surgery is mainstay of treatment

4. Multidisciplined support for a chronic, progressive disease

5. Genetic counseling

Head Injury

■ Definition: Craniocerebral trauma; includes any injury sustained to the scalp, skull, meninges, or any portion of the brain caused by an external force; degree of severity may range from a slight bump to a severe brain-damaging injury

■ Etiology/Incidence

1. Results from physical force impacting on the skull and its contents

2. One of the most common causes of disability and death in children

3. Greatest incidence occurs in children < 1 year and > 15 years

4. Etiology related to age

    a. Infant—falls, child abuse

  b. Less than 2 years of age—falls

  c. Pre-school/school—auto accidents

  d. Older child/adolescent—accidents involving motor vehicles, cycles, sports injury

 5. Males outnumber girls by a ratio of 2:1

■ Clinical Findings—level of consciousness most important observation in a child with head injury

 1. Scalp injuries

  a. Hemorrhage is most prominent feature

  b. Significant blood loss can occur with minor lacerations because of the scalp's increased vascularity

 2. Concussion

  a. Temporary, brief loss of consciousness with transient impairment of neurological function

  b. May have amnesia for events preceding and events immediately following the injury; reflects extent and severity of injury

  c. Acute phase—loss of tone, flaccidity, dilatation of pupils; brief apnea, transient loss of vision

  d. Recovery phase—tachycardia, vomiting, pallor, lethargy and confusion lasting less than 24 to 48 hours

  e. Recovery is usually without sequelae

  f. Occasionally a post-concussion syndrome may occur with personality and behavior changes, shortened attention span and continued headaches for 6 months or longer

 3. Contusion

  a. Focal bruising or tearing of cerebral tissues with bleeding and edema

  b. Neurological signs depend upon precise site of injury; frontal and temporal lobes most common sites; may vary from transient weakness to paralysis and prolonged unconsciousness

  c. May be disturbances of strength and sensation

  d. Changes in behavior

  e. Symptoms of increased intracranial pressure (ICP)

4. Hematomas

    a. Epidural hematoma (bleeding between skull and dura mater)

        (1) Can be life-threatening

        (2) Initially, brief period of unconsciousness followed by lucid period for a variable time of minutes to hours

        (3) Increase in hematoma leads to progressive loss of consciousness with severe headache, vomiting, seizures and coma

        (4) Prognosis can be good to excellent if treatment is initiated early and if underlying brain injury does not exist

    b. Subdural hematoma (bleeding between the dura mater and cerebrum)

        (1) May be found in physically abused infant who is repeatedly shaken

        (2) Infantile subdural presents with history of poor feeding, failure to thrive, irritability, lethargy, vomiting and fever; examination reveals tense bulging anterior fontanel and enlarged head circumference; eyes may show "setting sun" sign secondary to increased intracranial pressure

        (3) Acute subdural hematomas—within 48 hours of head injury, usually have increased symptoms starting with headache and progressing to agitation, confusion to decreased levels of consciousness with ICP

        (4) Chronic subdural hematomas—may occur days to several months following injury

            (a) Presenting symptoms may include irritability, drowsiness, vomiting, seizures, increased head circumference

            (b) Older children may complain of headache; academic performance may decline

5. Skull fracture

    a. Does not always indicate damage to the underlying brain

    b. Conversely, severe brain injury is not always associated with skull fractures

    c. Type, extent, symptomatology depend on area involved, age of child, velocity and force

    d. Linear nondepressed

        (1) Most common

        (2) Outcome usually excellent

        (3) Serious, if blood vessels involved or impinges on brainstem or cranial nerves

    e. Depressed

        (1) Skull is indented at point of impact

        (2) May cause significant damage to intracranial contents

    f. Basilar

        (1) Occurs frequently in children; temporal, frontal, ethmoid, sphenoid, occipital bones may be involved

        (2) Bloody discharge from middle ear

        (3) Cranial nerve palsies

        (4) Edema and ecchymosis of periorbital areas ("raccoon eyes")

        (5) Bruising behind ear ("battle sign")

■ Differential Diagnosis

    1. Child abuse

    2. Primary seizure disorder

■ Diagnostic Tests/Findings

    1. Skull radiographs

        a. Often overused

        b. Fractures infrequent in subdural hematomas

        c. Basilar skull fracture may not be evident on x-ray—80% missed

    2. Criteria for radiographs

        a. History

            (1) Age—younger than 1 year

            (2) Prolonged unconsciousness (usually more than 5 minutes)

            (3) Penetrating scalp wound

        b. Physical Findings

      (1)   Cephalohematoma

      (2)   Skull depression

      (3)   Discharge from nose or ear

      (4)   Hemotympanum (discolored tympanic membrane)

      (5)   Battle/Raccoon sign

      (6)   Focal neurologic signs including irregular pupils

      (7)   Persistent alteration in level of consciousness

      (8)   Hemiparesis

  3.   CT scan: Increasing use for diagnosis of intracranial bleeding

  4.   MRI—especially for detection of intracranial injury caused by shaking

■ Management/Treatment

  1.   Decision to admit less severely injured child for observation difficult one which must be individualized. Indicators include

     a. Deterioration in level of consciousness

     b. Continuous confusion and lethargy

     c. Focal neurologic signs

     d. Excessive and copious vomiting

     e. Seizure activity

     f. Uncertain history or circumstances of trauma

  2.   Referral and hospitalization for injuries associated with

     a. Severe impact secondary to motor vehicles or motorcycles; blows sustained by golfballs, baseballs, rocks, miscellaneous dense objects

     b. Fall from a significant distance, e.g., second story of building, roof, tree, full flight of stairs

     c. Suspicious events related to injury

  3.   Home observation dependent upon

     a. History of head injury, child cries for a few moments and resumes normal activities

     b. No loss of consciousness, vomiting or change of color

     c. Complaints of a mild headache

    d. Parental ability (instructions to parents to return to health facility)

        (1) Excessive drowsiness (initially test by awakening child at 15 minute intervals)

        (2) Changes in vital signs—slow pulse, irregular respirations, increased temperature

        (3) Persistent vomiting

        (4) Weakness on one side, limping

        (5) Double vision

        (6) Dilation or constriction of pupils or unequal

        (7) Convulsion

        (8) Swelling of scalp

Febrile Seizures

- Definition: Generalized tonic-clonic seizure usually lasting less than 15 minutes associated with an acute, benign febrile illness
- Etiology/Incidence
  1. Cause is uncertain
  2. Many episodes occur at upward phase of temperature
  3. Occurs in children between 9 months and 6 years; most frequently between 18 months and 3 years
  4. Boy: girl—2:1
  5. Most common seizure disorder of childhood; incidence 3 to 4%
- Clinical Findings
  1. Fever usually 102 °F or above
  2. Tonic-clonic seizure of less than 15 minutes duration
  3. May be first manifestation of illness
  4. No evidence of disease of CNS
- Differential Diagnosis
  1. Epilepsy
  2. Meningitis
  3. Lead poisoning

- Diagnostic Tests/Findings
  1. Focuses on finding cause for fever
  2. Examination of CSF if meningitis suspected
  3. EEG not warranted for simple febrile seizure—recordings are usually normal
- Management/Treatment
  1. Usually seizure activity has ceased by the time child is examined; if not, then anticonvulsant therapy, e.g., diazepam should be given
  2. Measures to reduce body temperature
     a. Sponging
     b. Anti-pyretics
  3. Treat underlying infection
  4. 20-30% children have recurrent febrile seizure
  5. Both short-term and prolonged anticonvulsant prophylaxis for the prevention of recurrent febrile convulsions is controversial
  6. Cognitive function may be decreased in those children treated with prophylactic phenobarbital (Behrman et al., 1992; Avery & First, 1994)

Seizure Disorders

- Definition: "Seizure (convulsion) is defined as a paroxysmal involuntary disturbance of brain function that may be manifested as an impairment of loss of consciousness, abnormal motor activity, behavioral abnormalities, sensory disturbances, or autonomic dysfunction" (Behrman, 1992, p. 1491)
- Etiology/Incidence
  1. Cause usually unknown
  2. Potential causes include
     a. Trauma
     b. Infection
     c. Asphyxia
     d. Biochemical factors
     e. Genetic factors/disorders

  f. Metabolic disorders

  g. Hemorrhage (intracranial)

  h. Tumors (intracranial)

 3. Occurrence rate is 4 to 6 cases for every 1000 children

■ Clinical Findings

 1. Partial seizures—caused by abnormal electric discharges, no interruption in consciousness with *simple* seizures; usually impaired with *complex* seizures

  a. Simple partial

   (1) Consciousness usually maintained

   (2) Abnormal movements of an arm or leg (Jacksonian march); orderly sequence of movements

   (3) Olfactory or auditory sensations

   (4) Tachycardia, diaphoresis, flushing, pallor, nausea

   (5) Anger, fear or hallucinations

   (6) Length of seizure approximately 10 to 20 seconds

  b. Complex partial—originates in a circumscribed portion of one cerebral hemisphere with impaired level of consciousness

   (1) May begin with a simple partial seizure and progress to brief unconscious period

   (2) In another presentation child may demonstrate altered state of consciousness; may have no other symptoms

   (3) An *aura* consisting of visual or auditory sensations (unpleasant feelings), nausea, vomiting, weakness is present in 1/3 of children with *simple* and *complex* seizures

   (4) Amnesic *automatisms* are common feature (picking at bed linens, clothing, rubbing objects repetitively, nondirective walking, running

   (5) Length of seizure 1 to 2 minutes

 2. Generalized seizures—bilateral cerebral cortical involvement always accompanied by some degree of unconsciousness

  a. Absence (petit mal)

   (1) Brief period of unconsciousness (lasting seconds) with

cessation of any motor activity; transient staring episode may be only manifestation

(2) Automatisms such as "lip smacking" or eye blinking

(3) May occur several times a day

(4) Often mistaken as learning disability, inattention, or behavioral problem

(5) Uncommon prior to age 5 years and are more common in girls

b. Generalized tonic-clonic (grand mal)

(1) Most common seizure; may be preceded by an aura

(2) Tonic phase characterized by rigidity, extension of extremities and fixed jaw; cessation of respirations; nonreactive dilated pupils; usually lasts less than 1 minute

(3) Clonic phase follows tonic phase and is characterized by rhythmic jerking of all extremities; expiratory grunts may be evident in addition to bowel and bladder incontinence; usually lasts several minutes, but can vary

(4) Postictal phase—semiconscious initially and may sleep for a few minutes to several hours

(a) May be associated with visual and speech difficulties

(b) May awaken with severe headache, fatigue and generalized muscle soreness

(5) May be precipitated by infections, fatigue, fever, stress, drugs

c. Myoclonic—generalized brief abrupt muscle contractions with duation of a few seconds; seizures may be clustered with several in one day or can be siezure-free for weeks

d. Atonic—sudden loss of muscle tone with possible loss of consciousness; may cause child to drop to the floor ("drop attacks")

e. Infantile spasms—rare disorder with onset during first year of life

(1) Brief flexion of neck, trunk and/or legs lasting for a few seconds

(2) Peak age of onset between ages 4 and 12 months

(3) May experience hundreds each day

(4) Prognosis for normal development is poor; 75 to 90% are

abnormal (Burg, Ingelfinger & Wald, 1993)

    (5)   May mimic "colic"

■ Differential Diagnosis

1. "Day dreaming"

2. Apnea

3. Breath holding

4. Temper tantrums

5. Sleep disorders

6. Syncope

7. Benign paroxysm

8. Migraine

9. Intoxication

10. Psychosis

11. "Acting out"

■ Diagnostic Tests/Findings—seizure workup

1. Detailed history of event

2. Complete neurological examination and physical examination

3. Blood studies/urine studies

4. EEG to document changes in brain's electrical activity; useful for classification purposes

5. Brain Imaging (CT, MRI, SPECT, PET)

6. Neuropsychological testing

■ Management/Treatment

1. Management guidelines for all seizures: Eliminate seizures without compromising child's normal growth and development

2. Principles

    a. Proper treatment requires clear diagnosis and identification of seizure type

    b. Anti-epileptic drugs are often seizure specific

    c. Use fewest drugs possible with least side effects

    d. Ideal drug level highly individual

    e. Surgery may offer relief to intractable

    f. Ketogenic diet for recalcitrant seizures

3. Factors influencing choice of drug

    a. Seizure type

    b. Potential side effects

    c. Half-life

    d. Patient age

    e. Drug cost

    f. Acceptance/compliance

    g. Types of drugs

        (1) Carbamazepine—generalized tonic-clonic, partial seizures

        (2) Phenobarbital—partial, febrile, generalized tonic-clonic seizures

        (3) Phenytoin—generalized tonic-clonic, partial seizures

        (4) Sodium valproate—generalized tonic-clonic, absence, myoclonic seizures

        (5) Adrenocorticotropic hormone (ACTH)—infantile spasms

        (6) Ethosuximide—absence, myoclonic seizures

        (7) Primidone—partial, generalized seizures

        (8) Clonazepam—absence, myoclonic, infantile spasms, partial seizures

        (9) Nitrazepam—absence, myoclonic, infantile spasms

4. Anticipatory Guidance

    a. Recognition of seizures

    b. Exacerbation

    c. Instruction in first aid for all significant others

    d. Potential drug interactions

    e. Problems with generics

    f. Participation in activities

    g. Issues of discipline

      h. School issues

Tic Disorders

- Definition

    1. Tic—abrupt, brief, involuntary, repetitious, stereotyped movements or vocalization

    2. Range from mild, transitory condition to complex, persistent, disabling set of behaviors

    3. Categories

        a. Transient tic disorder (retrospective diagnosis)—duration of tics for less than 1 year occurs in 5 to 24% of school children

        b. Chronic tic disorder—tics present for more than 1 year

            (1) Chronic motor tic

            (2) Tourette's Syndrome—both motor and vocal tics; fluctuating disorder of variable severity

- Etiology/Incidence

    1. Cause unknown; often positive family history

    2. Transient tics are commonly related to stress

    3. Chronic tics are believed to be related to an inherited neurochemical imbalance

    4. Occasionally either transient tics or Tourete's syndrome can be seen with the use of stimulant medications

    5. Incidence of transient tics—commonly present between 4 to 7 years; between 5 to 24% of school children have transient tics

    6. Incidence of Tourette's—between 1 to 10 per 10,000 persons; 3 times more common in males; mean age of onset is 6 to 7 years

- Clinical Findings

    1. Signs/symptoms

        a. Facial tics—eye blinking, nose twitching, lip licking, grimacing, etc

        b. Complex tics—finger snapping, jumping, hitting, skipping

        c. Vocal tics—throat clearing, barking, grunting, coughing, humming, echolalia, coprolalia

  d. Tics

    (1) Wax and wane

    (2) Worsen during stress

    (3) Change over time

    (4) Occur while awake and asleep

 2. Physical findings

  a. Normal physical exam

  b. Some voluntary control/suppression

 3. Comorbid problems

  a. Obsessive compulsive disorder (50%)

  b. Attention-deficit—hyperactivity disorder (50 to 60%)

  c. Behavioral-emotional problems

  d. Learning disabilities

■ Differential Diagnosis: In addition to diagnosing comorbid problems, tics must be differentiated from

 1. Chorea

 2. Paroxysmal choreoathetosis

 3. Stuttering

 4. Focal motor seizures

■ Diagnostic Tests/Findings: None

■ Management/Treatment

 1. Transient—patient and family education and guidance

 2. Chronic

  a. Comprehensive multimodal individualized treatment

  b. Behavioral management

  c. Psychotherapy, if indicated

  d. Pharmacological treatment—indicated when tics are psychosocially or functionally disabling; treatment is symptomatic, not curative

    (1) Clonidine—sedation is major side effect

    (2) Pimozide—apparently fewer side effects

(3)   Haloperidol—frequent side effects, acute dystonic reactions and tardive dyskinesia

Meningitis

- Definition: Inflammation of the meninges
- Etiology/Incidence—age related
  1. Most commonly through hematogenous spread of organisms
  2. Other less common routes—following head trauma; sinus fracture; dermoid sinus tracts; complication of neurosurgery
  3. Bacterial pathogens—age related
     a. Newborn
        (1)   Group B streptococci
        (2)   *Eschericia coli*
        (3)   *Listeria monocytogenes* (less frequently encountered, but important)
     b. Infants and children
        (1)   *Haemophilus influenzae* type b—usually most common cause but is on the decline since the advent of the *Haemophilus influenzae* type b vaccines (McCracken, 1993)
        (2)   *Neisseria meningitidis*
        (3)   *Streptococcus pneumoniae*
  4. Viral (aseptic)—primarily enteroviruses
  5. Other—fungal, tuberculosis, spirochetes
  6. Ninety percent of cases occur between 1 month and 5 years; infants 3 to 8 months at greatest risk
- Clinical Findings
  1. Early-onset neonatal—typically presents as fulminant, overwhelming disease in "high risk" infant
  2. Newborns—signs and symptoms are generally non-specific and nonlocalizing, e.g., fever or temperature instability; poor feeding, hypotonia, lethargy, irritability, unusual cry, seizure
  3. Older infants and children—prodromal febrile illness with progression to high fever, vomiting, headache (older child), photophobia, nuchal

rigidity, listlessness or irritability and seizures; skin eruptions ranging from maculopapules to petechiae and purpura; cranial nerve involvement

- Differential Diagnosis

  1. "Flu"

  2. Bacteremia

  3. Aseptic vs bacterial meningitis

  4. Reye syndrome

  5. Kawasaki disease

  6. Rocky Mountain spotted fever

  7. Brain abscess

  8. Leptospiral infection

- Diagnostic Tests/Findings

  1. Fundoscopic examination prior to lumbar puncture to rule out papilledema

  2. CSF analysis—See Table 1

     a. Usually provides a definite diagnosis although findings are often variable; however, unlikely to have normal protein, glucose, and cell count in presence of meningitis

     b. CSF is characterized by absence of organisms on Gram stain and culture in aeseptic (viral) meningitis

     c. CSF culture and Gram stain—identify organisms; Gram stain will confirm diagnosis of bacterial meningitis in majority of cases

  3. Countercurrent immunoelectrophoesis (CIE) and Latex Particle Agglutination (LPA—rapid means of antigen detection)

  4. CT—if focal neurologic signs or papilledema present

Table 1—Common CSF Findings in Meningitis

CSF	Bacterial	Viral
Leukocytes	> 500	< 500
% PMNs	> 80%	< 50%
Glucose	< 40 mg/dl	> 40 mg/dL
% CSF: Blood	< 30%	> 50%
Protein	> 100 mg/dl	< 100 mg/dL
Stains	Gram stain	—

■ Management/Treatment—immediate referral to physician/acute care facility

1. Bacterial

   a. Hospitalization

   b. Appropriate antibiotic therapy initiated as soon as diagnosis of bacterial meningitis suspected based on clinical findings and CSF findings while awaiting CSF culture

   c. Therapy guided by age, clinical findings, gram stain and antigen detection results based on expected pathogen, e.g., cefotaxime, ceftriaxone, or ampillin with chloramphenicol (AAP, 1994)

2. Viral (aseptic) meningitis

   a. Children over 1 year may be managed expectantly

   b. Infants under 12 months, or if unclear etiology, antibiotic begun until culture data available

3. Prophylaxis—meningococcal and *H. influenzae* meningitis have significant risk of secondary spread within households (see Respiratory Disorders chapter)

   a. Rifampin prophylaxis to household contacts at time of diagnosis

   b. Index patient should receive prophylaxis at completion of parenteral therapy

4. Follow-up

   a. Significant risk of sequelae (25-50%)—significant hearing loss (10-11%); visual defects (2-4%); motor deficits (3-7%); seizures (2-8%); mental retardation (10-11%)

   b. Hearing evaluation at discharge and 3 to 6 months later

     c. Careful developmental evaluations

Headache

- Definition: Pain in the head
- Etiology/Incidence
  1. Majority are benign (functional) but may indicate severe underlying disorder (pathological)
  2. Pathophysiology of benigh is poorly understood; probable association with distention of extracranial vessels and contracture of scalp and neck musculature
  3. Threshold for expression of headache affected by genetic, hormonal, and exogenous factors (diet, stress, medications, alcohol)
  4. Minority are pathological—pain probably related to increased intracranial pressure and related distention, stretching, and compression of intracranial structures
  5. Common presenting complaint of childhood and adolescence; 5 to 20%
  6. Incidence increases with age
- Clinical Findings

  The goal of this section is to assist the practitioner in distinguishing headaches which are organic (pathologic) from those which are benign (functional). Headaches which are a symptom of other systemic febrile and non-febrile illnesses will not be dealt with here

  Crucial distinction between organic and benign is made on basis of

  1. Thorough history with particular emphasis on
     a. History of present illness—characteristics more suggestive of organic causes
        (1) Very young child
        (2) Initial; acute episode
        (3) Intense pain, precisely described and localized
        (4) Patient awakened by pain
        (5) Pain occuring in a.m.
        (6) Pain precipitated by strain, cough, sneeze
        (7) Vomiting without nausea

        b. Family history

        c. Social and habit history

    2. Physical examination

        a. Careful neurologic examination

        b. Ophthalmoscopy

        c. Visual field check

        d. Evaluation of ocular muscle balance and convergence

        e. Palpation and transillumination of sinuses

        f. Palpation and auscultation of skull, mastoid, optic globes

        g. Careful check of teeth, ears, throat, temporomandibular joint

        h. Blood pressure

■ Differential Diagnosis—see Table 2 for common functional headaches in children

    1. Sinusitis

    2. Meningitis

    3. Encephalitis

    4. Post head injury

    5. Hypertension

    6. Allergy

    7. Intracranial mass

    8. Anemia

    9. Lead encephalopathy

    10. Dental problem

■ Diagnostic Tests/Findings: Usually unnecessary, except with indications of infection or increased intracranial pressure

■ Management/Treatment

    1. Specific cause dictates specific management

    2. Headaches of organic nature require immediate referral to physician/neurologist

    3. Benign headaches

a. Process of meticulous evaluation and empathic response may affect symptom

b. Identification, elimination/reduction of exacerbating conditions

c. Reassurance

d. Cautious use of medication (Ergot, Fiorinal, Propranolol)

   (1) Acetaminophen 5 to 10 mg/kg/every 4 to 6 hours (response is not dose related)

e. Referrals may be necessary if pain is severe and unresponsive to above

   (1) Neurology

   (2) Biofeedback

   (3) Psychiatry

   (4) Allergy

Table 2—Differential Features of Functional Headaches in Children

	Migraine	Tension	Occipital	Neuralgia Cluster
Usual Age of onset	5-8	9-12	Adolescence	Older teen
Sex	Males 2:1	Females 2:1	Both	Male
Prodrome	Scotomas (less common in children)	Stress	No	No
Family History	Positive	No	No	?
Associated Findings	GI, transient paresthesia	Sleep disruption processes	Tenderness cervical spinous C-2	Ipsilateral eye tearing, nasal congestion
Pain	unilateral both sides	generalized, occiput	occiput, neck unilateral brief, frequent nocturnal	severe "suicidal"
Treatment	Ergotamine Propranolol Acetaminophen	stress reduction, sleep	physical therapy muscle relaxants aspirin	Ergotamine

Learning Disabilities

- Definition: Central processing disorders which create difficulties in learning. Includes perceptual handicaps, minimal brain dysfunction, and dyslexia. Learning disabilities might be categorized according to the step in learning apparently affected

1. Input disabilities—related to the central brain process of perceiving one's environment
   a. Visual perception disability
   b. Auditory perception disability
   c. Sensory integrative disorders
2. Integration disabilities—related to understanding information
   a. Sequencing disabilities
   b. Abstraction disabilities
   c. Organization disabilities
3. Memory disabilities—related to storage and retrieval
   a. Short-term memory disability
   b. Long-term memory disability (children with this are more likely to be considered mentally retarded)
4. Output disabilities—related to expressing information
   a. Language disability
   b. Motor disability

■ Etiology/Incidence
1. No clear pattern of etiology in majority of cases
2. Familial pattern in 40% of cases
3. Result of neurological dysfunction
4. Underdiagnosed—estimated 3 to 7% of general population
5. Between 35 to 50% of children seen in mental health clinics have learning disabilities
6. Frequent association with other neurologically based disorders, e.g., attention-deficit hyperactivity disorders; obsessive compulsive disorder; and tourette syndrome

■ Clinical Findings
1. Thorough history to include
   a. Precise family history

      b. Developmental history which may reveal motor, language, or other delays

      c. Current patterns of behavior, peer relations, school strengths and weaknesses, home activities, and sports participation

      d. School difficulties are most often cause of concern

  2. Physical examination

      a. Essential hearing and vision screening

      b. Particular attention to visual, auditory, and sensory examinations to rule out sensory deficits

      c. Thorough developmental and neurological examination may reveal subtle motor signs—clumsiness, choreoathetoid movements, overflow, difficulty with fine motor coordination and errors in cortical sensory tests

      d. Mild dysmorphic features may be evident

      e. Otherwise, an essentially normal physical examination expected

- Differential Diagnosis
  1. Visual deficits
  2. Hearing loss
  3. Motor handicaps
  4. Global mental retardation
  5. Environmental disadvantages
  6. Attention deficit disorders

- Diagnostic Tests/Findings: Beyond audiological testing, children will require comprehensive psychological and education testing

- Management/Treatment
  1. Medical evaluation is only one piece of a multifaceted approach to the child with learning disabilities
  2. Evaluation and management is an interdisciplinary process
  3. The extent of the involvement of the nurse practitioner will depend upon several factors. These include availability of community referral sources; individual practitioner's expertise; and a commitment and willingness to serve as an advocate for the child and family throughout a lengthy process of evaluation, management and follow-up
  4. Referrals are based on nature and degree of learning disability, but

may involve consultation with teachers, psychologist, pediatric practitioner, neurologist, audiologist, speech and language pathologist, occupational therapist and occasionally, child psychiatrist or social worker

5. Many unproven remedies and fad treatment are being advertised. Parents need education, support, and guidance in analyzing these "therapies"

6. A learning disability is a permanent, life-long processing disorder which may have tremendous or relatively little effect on child's success in school and beyond.

7. Opportunities for success will be enhanced for the child who can be assisted to utilize his strengths and to recognize alternative methods of mastering difficulties

8. The child who meets repeated frustrations and disappointment may begin a chronic pattern of failure with resulting behavioral and emotional problems

Questions

Select the best answer

1. In evaluating a child with a history of head trauma it is important to realize that basilar skull fractures

   a. May be signified by hemotympanum
   b. May not be evident on x-ray
   c. May be associated with positive Battle Sign
   d. All of the above

2. The most helpful indicator of degree of head trauma sustained by a child is

   a. Persistent vomiting
   b. Seizure immediately following trauma
   c. Level of consciousness
   d. Hypotension

3. All of the following facts about migraine headaches are true except

   a. Positive family history common
   b. Seldom appear before 10 years of age
   c. Description of unilateral pain
   d. Scotomas are less common in children

4. Which of the following is not usually associated with febrile seizures?

   a. Recurrent febrile seizures in 1/3 of cases
   b. Slightly increased risk for nonfebrile seizures
   c. Febrile illness lasting more than three (3) days
   d. Children between six (6) months and three (3) years of age

5. The following statements are true regarding von Recklinghausen Disease except

   a. Although it is an autosomal dominant disorder, a negative family history is not unusual
   b. The disease is highly variable in expression within a family
   c. A hallmark feature is six (6) or more cafe-au-lait spots, measuring 1.5 cm or more
   d. There is no evidence of predisposition to malignancy

6. Erb Palsy is characterized by all except

   a. Follows traction injury of brachial plexus
   b. Biceps reflex absent or diminished
   c. Moro reflex unaffected

    d. Normal grasp and forearm strength

7. A 16-month-old girl is admitted to the hospital with *Haemophilus influenzae* meningitis. Social history reveals that she lives at home with her parents and a 3-year-old brother; she attends a day care center two mornings a week. You are asked to advise about appropriate prophylaxis for contacts. Each of the following should receive rifampin prophylaxis, except

    a. The patient
    b. The sibling
    c. The parents
    d. A distant cousin

8. Of the following, the *most* common cause of cerebral palsy is

    a. An inborn error of metabolism
    b. A chromosomal abnormality
    c. Intrauterine infection
    d. Unknown

9. The highest age-specific attack rate for bacterial meningitis beyond the newborn period occurs in the following age group
    a. 3 to 8 months
    b. 1 to 2 years
    c. 5 to 9 years
    d. 10 to 14 years

10. A newborn who is microcephalic at birth most likely

    a. Has a head circumference that is 1 cm above the chest circumference
    b. Suffered from mild malnutrition during the last trimester
    c. Is a likely candidate for surgery
    d. Contracted an intrauterine viral infection

11. The least likely sign of increased intracanial pressure in a newborn is

    a. Separated suture line
    b. High pitched cry
    c. Sluggish pupillary reactions
    d. Papilledema

12. A tumor which arises from neural crest cells that normally give rise to adrenal medulla and sympathetic ganglia is

    a. Cerebellar asteocytoma
    b. Neuroblastoma
    c. Brain stem glioma
    d. Ependymoma

13. A firm nontender irregular mass in the abdomen is likely to raise concern about

    a. Dessicated stool
    b. Hepatosplenomegaly
    c. Osteosarcoma
    d. Neuroblastoma

14. Which of the following is least likely to be included in the diagnostic criteria for neurofibromatosis?

    a. Optic pathway glioma
    b. Iris hamartoma
    c. Café-au-lait spots
    d. Heterochromia

15. Which statement regarding Tic disorders is true?

    a. Transient tics commonly present between 10 to 13 years of age
    b. Transient tics occur in 1 to 2% of school children
    c. Tourette's syndrome more common in boys
    d. Transient tics are not associated with the use of stimulant medications

16. Children with Tourette's syndrome frequently have

    a. A positive family history
    b. No ability to suppress tics temporarily
    c. No increased incidence of attention deficit, hyperactivity disorder (ADHD)
    d. Extremely stressful family environments

17. Which of the following comorbid problems are not seen with Tourette Syndrome?
    a. Obsessive compulsive disorder
    b. Schizophrenia
    c. Learning disabilities
    d. Sleep disorders

18. A mother and her 3-month-old male infant just moved in from out of state and you are seeing the infant for the first time. The mother is concerned because she thinks the baby's head has been getting larger and he seems sleepy and "cranky" a lot of the time. In your judgment the best method of treatment at this time would be to

    a. Observe the mother's head size to determine if there is a familial tendency
    b. Examine the infant, record the findings, do a CBC and have the mother return the following day for further evaluation
    c. Examine the infant and make the appropriate medical referral immediately
    d. Measure the head circumference and start plotting the growth on a standardized graph and have the mother return with the infant in 2 weeks

19. The three most common causes of bacterial meningitis in the newborn are

    a. Group B Strep, *E. coli, Listeria Monocytogenes*
    b. *Haemophilus Influenzae*, Strep Pneumoniae, *Neisseria Meningites*
    c. Group A Strep, Mycoplasma pneumoniae and *Listeria monocytogenes*
    d. *Staph aureus,* Group B Strep, *E. coli*

20. Which of the following analyses of cerebral spinal fluid is likely to indicate bacterial meningitis?

    a. Protein of 80 mg/dl
    b. Glucose of 22 with serum glucose 88
    c. Leukocytes of 325
    d. 45% PMNs

21. Which of the following general statements regarding headaches is true?

    a. The younger the child, the more serious the complaint
    b. Pain in the evening is probably more serious than headache pain in the morning
    c. Headaches and nausea are usually more ominous than headaches with vomiting
    d. They are an uncommon complaint in school children

22. Often migraine headaches occur in a child who

    a. Is female
    b. Is between 12 to 15 years
    c. Has positive family history
    d. Is premenstrual

23. Which of the following seizure types carries the worst prognosis for future development?

    a. Petit Mal
    b. Jacksonian
    c. Grand Mal
    d. Infantile spasms

Answer Key

1. d
2. c
3. b
4. c
5. d
6. c
7. d
8. d
9. a
10. d
11. d
12. b
13. d
14. d
15. c
16. a
17. b
18. c
19. a
20. b
21. a
22. c
23. d

Bibliography

American Academy of Pediatrics. Committee on Infectious Disease (1994). *1994 Red Book: Report of the Committee on Infectious Disease* (23rd ed.). Elk Grove Village, IL: The American Academy of Pediatrics.

Avery, M. E., & First, L. R. (Eds). (1994). *Pediatric medicine* (2nd ed.). Baltimore, MD: William & Wilkins.

Behrman, R. E., Kliegman, R. M., Nelson, W. E., & Vaughn, V. C. (Eds.). (1992). *Nelson textbook of pediatrics (14th ed.).* Philadelphia: W. B. Saunders.

Burg, F.D., Ingelfinger, J. R., & Wald, E. R. (Eds.). (1993). *Gellis & Kagan's current pediatric therapy* (14th ed.). Philadelphia: W. B. Saunders.

Carter-Snead, P. (1990). Treatment of infantile spasms. *Pediatric Neurology, 6* (3), 147-149.

Castiglia, P. T., & Harbin, R. E. (Eds.). (1992). *Child Health Care.* Philadelphia: J. B. Lippincott.

Dooling, E. C. (1993). Neurologic problems. In R. Dershewitz, (Ed.). *Ambulatory pediatrics* (2nd ed.), (pp. 547-598).

Elser, J. M. (1991). Easing the pain of childhood headaches. *Contemporary Pediatrics, 8*(11), 108-123.

Fenichel, G. (1988). Clinical pediatric neurology. *A signs and symptoms approach.* Philadelphia: W. B. Saunders.

Fishman, M. A. (1990). Febrile seizures. In F. Oski & C. DeAngelis (Eds.). *Principles and practices of pediatrics*, (pp. 1876-1878).

Gardner, S., & Hagedorn, M. (1992). Physiologic sequelae of prematurity: Part VIII: Neurological conditions. *Journal of Pediatric Health Care, 6*, 263-270.

Hirtz, D. G. (1993). Treatment of seizure disorders in children. In F. D. Burg, J. R. Ingelfinger, & E. R. Wald (Eds.), *Gellis & Kagan's current pediatric therapy* (14th ed.). (pp. 80-90). Philadelphia: W. B. Saunders

Hoekelman, R. A., Friedman, S. B., Nelson, N. M., & Seidel, H. M. (Eds.). (1992). *Primary pediatric care* (2nd ed.). St. Louis: Mosby Year Book.

Jackson, P. L. (1990). Primary care needs of children with hydrocephalus. *Journal of Pediatric Health Care, 2*, 59-71.

McCracken, G. H., Jr. (1993). Bacterial meningitis. In S. L. Kaplan (Ed.), *Current therapy in pediatric infectious disease* (3rd ed.). (pp. 144-149). St. Louis: Mosby

Year Book.

Murphy, M., & Hagerman, R. (1992). Attention deficit hyperactivity disorder in children. *Journal of Pediatric Health Care, 6*, 2-11.

Pranzatelli, M. R. (1993). An approach to movement disorders of childhood. *Pediatric Annals*, 22(1), 13-17.

Riccardi, V. (1992). Type I neurofibromatosis and the pediatric patient. *Current Problems in Pediatrics, 22*, 66-99.

Rylance, G. W. (1990). Treatment of epilepsy and febrile convulsions in children. *The Lancet, 336*, 488-491.

Silver, L. B. (Ed.). (1993). Learning disabilities. *Child and Adolescent Psychiatric Clinics of North America*. 3, 2. Philadelphia: W. B. Saunders.

Singer, H. S. (1993). Tic disorders. *Pediatric Annals*, 22(1), 22-29.

Symposium on Tic Disorders in Childhood. (1988). *Pediatric Annals, 17*(6).

Trimble, M. R. (1990). Antileptic drugs, cognitive function, and behavior in children. *Epilepsia, 31* (Supple 4), 530-533.

Musculoskeletal Disorders

Elizabeth Hawkins-Walsh

Congenital Talipes Equinovarus ("Clubfoot")

- Definition: Complex congenital deformity of the foot: adduction of forefoot; foot is plantar flexed at the ankle (equinus) and the forefoot curves in (in varus)

- Etiology/Incidence
  1. Precise cause is not known
  2. Vascular, cartilaginous, neurologic and myopathic growth disturbances; possible etiologic factors
  3. Underlying genetic factor
  4. Mild cases may be due to utero postural-induced compression
  5. Present in 1 in 1000 births; male-to-female ratio is aproximately 2:1; risk in sibling is 1:50

- Clinical Findings
  1. Usually obvious at birth
  2. See definition (above)

- Differential Diagnosis
  1. Myelomeningocele
  2. Arthrogryposis
  3. Metatarsus adductus

- Diagnostic Tests/Findings: Radiographs show aberrant, bony, anatomic relationships

- Management/Treatment
  1. Complex problem requiring prompt diagnosis and early referral
  2. Refer to orthopedics for treatment
  3. Non-operative treatment most successful if begun in nursery (serial manipulation, casting)
  4. Surgical correction for severe cases and residual deformity

Metatarsus Adductus/Metatarsus Varus

- Definition: Bones of forefoot deviated medially on the bones of the hindfoot at the tarsometatarsal joint

- Etiology/Incidence

1. Unclear

2. Multifactorial

3. Genetic

4. Intrauterine mechanical factors

5. Incidence—1/1000

    a. 1/20 in siblings

    b. Increased in twins and breech births

- Clinical Findings

    1. Distinguish between supple vs. fixed supple

        a. Supple—foot straightens when lateral border of foot stroked or gentle pressure applied over base of 5th metatarsal and behind 1st metatarsal head

        b. Fixed

            (1) Rigidity of forefoot

            (2) Intoeing

            (3) Medial crease

            (4) Convex lateral curvature

            (5) Great toe widely separated from rest

            (6) Heel valgus in standing position

- Differential Diagnosis

    1. Fixed vs supple

    2. Clubfoot

- Diagnostic Tests/Findings—none

- Management/Treatment

    1. Early differentiation of supple vs fixed

        a. Supple

            (1) Spontaneous correction in 90% of cases

            (2) Gentle stretching exercises with each diaper change, probably not necessary

        b. Fixed

(1) Serial cast correction

(2) Straight-or reverse-last shoes after desired correction obtained may be indicated

Developmental Dysplasia of the Hip (DDH) "Congenital Hip Dysplasia"

- Definition

  1. A broad term that describes imperfect development of the hip that can affect the femoral head, the acetabulum or both

  2. Categories

     a. Complete congenital dislocation—femoral head is totally outside acetabulum

     b. Subluxation—femoral head is partially dislocated

     c. Unstable—femoral head can be pushed out from the acetabulum (dislocatable)

     d. Other dysplasia of hip joint—acetabular dysplasia, a condition in which the acetabulum is flattened

- Etiology/Incidence

  1. Precise etiology unknown

  2. Multifactorial

     a. Heredity

     b. Intrauterine position—breech birth at term; 14 times increased likelihood

     c. Simple capsular laxity

  3. Incidence

     a. Dislocated—1 to 11/1000

     b. Unstable—8 to 12/1000

     c. Four times more common in females

     d. Left hip affected 10 times more often than right hip

- Clinical Findings

  1. Vary with age and degree of dysplasia

  2. Newborn (birth to 3 months)

    a. Hip instability—primary manifestation

        (1) Ortolani maneuver—examiner feels femoral head slide into acetabulum with a "clunk"; "clicks can be found in approximately 10% of normal infants

        (2) Barlow maneuver—causes an abnormal hip to dislocate

  3. Older infant

    a. Signs of hip instability tend to disappear by 3 months

    b. Limited abduction of dislocated hip

    c. Thigh fold asymmetry (may be seen in normal infants)

    d. Leg length inequality

    e. Telescoping maneuver—femoral head and shaft can be pushed to and fro with hip held in 90° flexion

    f. Galleazzi/Allis sign—unequal knee heights when supine with knees flexed

    g. Lax hamstrings

  4. Older walking

    a. Lateral spine deviation to affected hip

    b. Limp—Trendelenburg gait; leg length discrepancy

- Differential Diagnosis

  1. Benign clicks of hip or knee

  2. Septic arthritis of hip

  3. Arthrogryposis

- Diagnostic Tests/Findings

  1. Radiograph (anterior/posterior view of pelvis)—most definitive diagnostic test after 3 months of age

  2. Sonogram/MRI—newer techniques; can be used from birth throughout infancy for identification and monitoring

- Management/Treatment

  1. Ideally, identification in nursery

  2. Importance of continued screening throughout first year of life

  3. Triple diapering not effective

4. Pavlik harness is treatment of choice under 6 months age

    a. Simple, effective, comfortable treatment that is usually successful

    b. The earlier the treatment, the better the prognosis

    c. Infants older than 6 months will probably require traction, reduction with cast immobilization

Legg-Calvé-Perthes Disease (LCPD)

■ Definition: Juvenile idiopathic avascular necrosis of femoral head (Behrman, 1992; Dyment, 1993)

■ Etiology/Incidence

1. Unknown

2. Trauma, transient synovitis, venous congestion, hyperviscosity, coagulation abnormalities, and other mechanisms have been suggested (Behrman, 1992)

3. Boys are affected approximately four times more often than girls; familial predisposition

4. Disease is associated with low birth weight; retarded bone age; poor socioeconomic status; white race

5. Age range—between ages of four and eight

■ Clinical Findings

1. Insidious onset of limp

2. History of pain usually, but sometimes knee pain is only presenting symptom

3. Pain worse with activity and relieved by rest

4. Thigh, knee pain

5. Restriction of voluntary motion

6. Limited, painful passive motion

7. Tenderness over anterior groin and adductor muscle

8. Limited abduction and rotation

9. May be atrophy of thigh or calf muscles and eventually shortened leg length

■ Differential Diagnosis

1. Septic or tuberculous arthritis
2. Acute transient toxic synovitis
3. Proximal femoral fracture
4. Slipped capital femoral epiphysis
5. JRA
6. Sickle cell anemia

- Diagnostic Tests/Findings
    1. Hip roentgenogram—definitive diagnosis
    2. Bone scan—decreased uptake in early stages; increased uptake in later stages
    3. MRI—shows necrosis

- Management/Treatment
    1. Refer to orthopedics—basic premise of treatment is containment by means of a "broomstick" abduction long leg cast or an abduction brace, both of which allow for ambulation
    2. Surgical containment may be required if compliance with bracing program is a problem

Transient Synovitis of the Hip (Toxic Synovitis)

- Definition: Transient, nonspecific, common, unilateral, inflammatory arthritis involving hip joint (Behrman, 1992)

- Etiology/Incidence
    1. Unknown
    2. Possible etiologic factors have been related to infectious causes; occult hip trauma
    3. Increased incidence in young boys, 2 to 12 years of age; peak 3 to 6 years of age
    4. Incidence 3 in 100; most common cause of limp with hip pain in this age group

- Clinical Findings
    1. Hip pain of acute onset without any history of trauma
    2. Child does not appear ill, although an upper respiratory infection may

be present or preceded onset of hip pain

3. Markedly restricted active and passive hip motion and limp (decreased hip extension and internal rotation)

4. Thigh, knee, hip pain

- Differential Diagnosis

    1. Legg-Calvé Perthes Disease

    2. Septic arthritis

    3. Slipped capital femoral epiphysis

    4. Osteomyelitis

    5. Tumors

- Diagnostic Tests/Findings

    1. Hip roentgenogram—usually normal hips

    2. CBC—slight leukocytosis or normal

    3. ESR—may be slightly elevated or normal

- Management/Treatment

    1. Usually self-limiting disease

    2. Bed rest; no weight bearing on involved joint, if possible

    3. Recovery expected in 3 to 5 days

    4. Gradual resumption of full activity

    5. Anti-inflammatory agents, e.g., ibuprofen, 40 to 50 mg/kg/day, two to three times daily

    6. Follow-up

Slipped Capital Femoral Epiphysis (SCFE) (Coxa Vara)

- Definition: A displacement of the femoral head from the femoral neck in a downward and backward position relative to the neck of the femur

- Etiology/Incidence

    1. May result from severe trauma

    2. Usually are more often due to a more gradual slip from chronic, abnormal, shear forces

    3. Occurs before epiphyseal plate closes

4. Incidence is approximately two per 100,000; twice as often in boys than girls and in blacks more than whites

5. Seen between ages of 11 and 15 years, in boys later than girls

6. Almost 90% of affected children are obese

7. Associated with a variety of endocrine and systemic disorders

■ Clinical Findings

1. In an acute slip, pain may be preceded initially by injury or strain; patient cannot walk, and affected femur is held in external rotation; passive movements of the hip are painful

2. In the chronic form, pain is more varied and often located in anterior thigh or knee; hip kept in external rotation; abduction and flexion of the hip are limited

3. Limb shortening common with chronic SCFE

■ Differential Diagnosis

1. Legg-Calvé-Perthes

2. Transient toxic synovitis

3. Osteochondritis dissecans

4. Rheumatological disorders

■ Diagnostic Tests/Findings

1. Bilateral Roentgenograms

2. AP (and "froglateral" radiography—mild slip more obvious)

3. Earliest radiologic change—irregularity and widening of growth plate of proximal femur

4. Later—displacement of femoral head; diffuse osteopenia of metaphysis and widening of the physis

■ Management/Treatment

1. Refer to orthopedics

2. Patient is usually hospitalized immediately

3. Operative fixation of the epiphysis

Osteomyelitis (Acute)

- Definition: Infection of bone
- Etiology/Incidence
    1. *Staphylococcus aureus* most common organism
    2. Is usually spread from another primary site, such as skin trauma, skin, ear or throat infection
    3. Relationship between age and organism; occurs more often in children less than one year and between three and 10 years of age
    4. Two to four times more common in boys than girls
    5. Occurs most commonly in the long bones, but can affect any bone
- Clinical Findings
    1. Vary with age
    2. May range from acute febrile illness and/or loss of active movement in an extremity in infants to local and systemic symptoms in the older child
    3. Initial symptoms present with redness, tenderness, swelling at the site
    4. Systemic symptoms follow with fever, lethargy, chills
    5. Unwillingness to use affected extremity
    6. Guarding of area
    7. If extremity involved warmth, edema and erythema directly related to periosteal and deep tissue involvement
    8. Vertebral or pelvis involvement may present with gate disturbances, back or thigh pain, abdominal pain
- Differential Diagnosis
    1. Septic arthritis
    2. Acute rheumatic fever
    3. Rheumatoid arthritis
    4. Leukemia
    5. Cellulitis
    6. Bone infarction

7. Bone tumors

- Diagnostic Tests/Findings
  1. CBC—leukocytosis with shift to the left
  2. ESR—elevated in most patients
  3. C-reactive protein—elevated in most patients
  4. Blood cultures—positive 50% of the time
  5. Needle aspiration for long bone osteomyelitis to identify organism and drain periosteal abscess if present
  6. Radiographs—usually negative first 10 to 14 days; evidence of bone destruction and lysis follow

- Management/Treatment
  1. Immediate referral
  2. Initial hospitalization
  3. Intravenous antibiotic therapy for four to six weeks
  4. Failure to respond—surgical decompression

Juvenile Rheumatoid Arthritis (JRA)

- Definition
  1. Any child under 17 years of age with persistent arthritis of more than six weeks duration, involving one or more joints; subgroups include polyarticular-onset disease, pauciarticular-onset, and systemic-onset disease
  2. JRA is further classified into subtypes based on clinical course over first six (6) months of illness
     a. Polyarticular—30-35% involving five (5) or more joints. Often chronic and symmetric
     b. Pauciarticular—50%—Four (4) or fewer joints
        (1) Large joints
        (2) Asymmetric distribution
     c. Systemic onset—15% extra-articular manifestations are hallmark

- Etiology/Incidence
  1. Etiology unknown

        a. May be due to infection from microorganisms in an immunologically predisposed host

        b. May be due to a hypersensitivity or autoimmune response

    2. Approximately 250,000 children affected in the U.S. (Behrman, 1992)

    3. About 50% of cases begin in childhood

- Clinical Findings

    1. Polyarticular-onset

        a. Multiple joints including small joints of hands involved

        b. Subgroups

            (1) Rheumatoid factor—negative

                (a) May begin at any time in childhood

                (b) Usually mild or minimal symptoms and rarely associated with rheumatoid nodules

            (2) Rheumatoid factor—positive

                (a) Onset in late childhood

                (b) Arthritis is more severe

                (c) Rheumatoid nodules are frequent with occasional rheumatoid vasculitis

        c. Arthritis onset may be subtle with gradual joint stiffness, swelling, and loss of motion; joints are swollen and warm, not red

        d. Systemic manifestations include slow growth, low-grade fever, malaise, anorexia, irritability

    2. Pauciarticular-onset

        a. Limited to four or fewer large joints for first six months; distribution of arthritis often asymmetric

        b. Types

            (1) Type I (early onset)

                (a) Includes girls primarily who are young at onset, 2 to 4 year-olds

                (b) Most common manifestation of JRA

                (c) Most patients are positive for antinuclear antibodies (ANA)

        (d)   Knees, ankles, elbows most often affected

        (e)   At high risk for eye complications (iridocyclitis)

   (2)   Type II (late onset)

        (a)   Affects 15% of JRA patients, mostly boys over eight years of age

        (b)   Tests for rheumatoid factor and ANA are negative; 75% have HLA-B 27

        (c)   Large joints affected, especially those of lower extremity

        (d)   Hip girdle involvement early in disease process

        (e)   Some patients may develop ankylosing spondylitis of lumbodorsal spine and Reiter syndrome

3.   Systemic-onset

   a.   Characterized by extra-articular symptomatology, especially high fevers and rheumatoid rash

   b.   Affects about 20% of JRA patients

   c.   Boys and girls equally affected

   d.   Hepatosplenomegaly present in most cases

   e.   Most children have joint manifestations at onset or within a few months

■ Differential Diagnosis

1.   Septic arthritis

2.   Other rheumatic diseases to include systemic lupus erythematosus

3.   Acute rheumatic fever

4.   Tuberculous joint infection

5.   Lyme disease

6.   Legg-Calvé-Perthes disease

7.   Osgood-Schlatter disease

8.   Osteomyelitis

9.   Acute leukemia

10. Slipped capital femoral epiphysis

11. Inflammatory bowel disease

12. Benign limb pain

12. Benign hypermobile joint syndrome

- Diagnostic Tests/Findings

  1. Diagnosis of JRA is based on persistence of arthritis or typical systemic symptomatology for three or more consecutive months and exclusion of other known causes of arthritis, arthropathy

  2. No specific laboratory tests exist

     a. WBC—often elevated

     b. CBC—anemia is common

     c. Erythrocyte sedimentation rate (ESR)—may be elevated

     d. ANA—may be found in polyarticular-onset and pauciarticular (type I), but rarely in pauciarticular (type II) or systemic

     e. Rheumatoid factor—usually found in children with older age of onset

     f. C-reactive protein (CRP)—usually, but not always, elevated

     g. Roentgenography—soft tissue swelling, osteoporosis and periostitis in affected joints

- Management/Treatment

  1. Overall prognosis is good, although pauciarticular JRA shows a more favorable prognosis regarding long-term joint function than children with multiple joint involvement

  2. Pharmacologic therapy

     a. Control of inflammation is goal of drug therapy

     b. Nonsteroidal anti-inflammatory drugs

        (1) Salicylates remain the standard treatment

           (a) For children less than 25 kg, 70 to 100 mg/kg/day

           (b) For older children total daily doses of 2400 to 3600 mg/day

           (c) Considerable variation in dose requirement and toxic symptoms

        (2) NSAID

(a) Tolmetin sodium (Tolectin), 20 to 30 mg/kg/day; can be initial agent or substituted for aspirin; well tolerated, but not as effective as aspirin or naproxen

(b) Naproxen—10 to 20 mg/kg/day; well tolerated

c. Slow acting antirheumatic drugs (SAARD)

(1) Reserved for those children with aggressive, multi-joint disease at risk for crippling and disability; at high risk for side-effects; require close surveillance

(2) Gold preparations

(3) Penicillamine

(4) Hydroxychloroquine

(5) Sulfasalazine

d. Corticosteroid—only reserved for otherwise unresponsive cases

(1) Significant adverse reactions

(2) Use as small a dose as possible

(3) Wean as soon as possible

e. Cytoxic drugs—reserved for those children whose disease is crippling and unresponsive to conventional therapies

3. Physical/occupational therapy

a. Forms cornerstone of management; imperative to preserve joint integrity

b. Physical therapy—passive, active and resistive exercises to preserve full range of motion and muscle strength

c. Occupational therapy—goal is to preserve independence in activities of daily living and age-appropriate function

4. Support family and child in achieving an optimal psychosocial adjustment

Scoliosis (Idiopathic Adolescent)

■ Definition: Lateral curvature of the spine

■ Etiology/Incidence

1. Idiopathic (80%)

2. Familial and some genetic influence

3. Incidence is same in boys and girls for small curves, but increases in girls as curves progress

4. Most frequent onset is during pubertal growth spurt; 2 to 3% incidence of curves less than 10 degrees in those under 16 years of age. 3% of adults have curves of 10 degrees or more

- Clinical Findings
  1. Usually painless
  2. Asymmetric shoulder levels
  3. Forward bend test shows rib hump and can be measured with "scoliometer"
  4. Right thoracic curve most common
  5. Asymmetry of waistline or flank contour
  6. Unequal leg length

- Differential Diagnosis
  1. Distinguish between structural scoliosis and functional scoliosis
  2. Paralysis and neuromuscular disease

- Diagnostic Tests/Findings
  1. Radiography reserved for patients with more significant deformities; those with milder manifestations can be observed clinically and monitored with scoliometer

- Management/Treatment
  1. Early detection through screening
  2. Preadolescent and adolescent with idiopathic curves less than 25 degrees require regular observation at 4 to 6 mo intervals
  3. Curves that progress to 25 to 40 degrees require bracing (Milwaukee brace, Boston brace, Charleston Bending Brace)
  4. Bracing is not curative but will slow progression until spine reaches more adult size
  5. Curves greater than 45 degrees require surgical management (Cotrel-Dubousset system has largely replaced Harrington rod)

Torticollis ("Wry Neck")

- Definition: Congenital or acquired condition in which neck is flexed and deviates toward affected side as a result of shortening of sternocleidomastoid muscle

- Etiology/Incidence
    1. Wide spectrum of underlying causes
    2. May be a manifestation of self-limiting muscular or inflammatory process
    3. May be a sign of a serious disease
    4. Congenital
        a. Fibrous shortening of sternocleidomastoid muscle (most common cause)
        b. Possible factors are birth trauma, intrauterine positioning, hemorrhage
    5. Acquired
        a. Minor, soft tissue trauma
        b. Viral myocitis
        c. Inflammatory problems affecting the neck, e.g., adenitis, pharyngitis, retropharyngeal abscess
        d. Less common causes include medications (especially phenothiazines), ocular strabismus, and tumors
    6. Incidence unknown
- Clinical Findings
    1. Head tilted toward affected side
    2. Palpable mass over muscle during first month of life
    3. Abnormal head position may cause deformities of face and skull
- Differential Diagnosis
    1. Congenital cervical vertebral anomalies
    2. Acute bacterial/viral infection with cervical lymphadenopathy
    3. Vertebral, spinal cord tumors
    4. Cervical fracture
- Diagnostic Tests/Findings
    1. Roentgenogram—to identify disorders of the spine and disk spaces
    2. Computed tomography—may be necessary to exclude suspicious

vertebral anomalies since abnormality may not be demonstrated on radiograph

- Management/Treatment
    1. Failure to diagnose cause of torticollis accurately may result in neurologic catastrophe if physical therapy is attempted (Mier, 1993)
    2. Treatment directed toward underlying pathology
    3. Early therapy indicated for congenital muscular torticollis
        a. Gentle, stretching exercises and positioning
        b. Conservative therapy should result in resolution of head tilt within 3 to 4 months
        c. If not, surgical correction/brace
    4. Acquired torticollis directed at correction of underlying disorder; surgery may be indicated if conservative approaches not effective

Muscular Dystrophy

- Definition: Group of chronic diseases characterized by progressive degeneration of skeletal musculature leading to atrophy, weakness and increasing disability
- Etiology/Incidence
    1. Basic defect uncertain
    2. Duchenne muscular dystrophy (DMD) most common hereditary neuromuscular disease
    3. Affects all races and ethnic groups
    4. Occurs 1 in 3600 live male births
- Clinical Findings (DMD)
    1. Symptoms usually not present at birth
    2. Onset—early childhood, 1 to 3 years of age, before 6; developmental milestones may be achieved at appropriate age or slightly delayed
    3. Walking usually within normal age range
    4. Hip girdle weakness may be apparent as early as two years of age
    5. Gower's sign (climbs up legs with hands) at three years of age and clearly evident by five to six years
    6. Trendelenburg gait or hip waddle appears at about five or six years

7. Pseudohypertrophy (enlargement) of calves and wasting of thigh muscles is a classic feature

8. Cardiac muscle involvement is universal

9. Delayed or impaired cognitive development

10. Death usually occurs at about 18 years of age

- Differential Diagnosis

  1. Becker muscular dystrophy

  2. Scapulohumeral muscular dystrophy

  3. Myotonic dystrophy

  4. Periodic paralyses

  5. Hyper- and hypothyroidism

  6. Myasthenic syndromes

  7. Botulism

- Diagnostic Tests/Findings

  1. Diagnosis based upon clinical findings and positive tests

  2. Creatinine phosphokinase (CPK)—consistently greatly elevated (15,000 to 35,000 Iu/L)

  3. Mucle biopsy shows characteristic changes (absent or abnormal dystrophia)

  4. Electromyography shows classic myopathic characteristics

- Management/Treatment

  1. No effective drug treatment; corticosteroids will increase strength temporarily

  2. Goal—maintenance of function as long as possible

  3. Supportive

     a. Physical therapy; various techniques and equipment used to minimize deformity, prolong ambulation, and assist with activities of daily living

     b. Nutrition—according to ambulatory level

     c. Weight control

     d. Aggressive response to cardiopulmonary problem

   e. Surgery (contracture deformities)

   f. Knee-ankle-foot orthoses may prolong ambulation

   g. Ongoing assistance of caregivers in coping with disease outcome; referral to child and family support groups

4. Genetic counseling

Malignant Bone Tumors

- Definition

  1. Osteosarcoma—rapidly growing malignant tumor of bone

  2. Ewing Sarcoma—round-cell tumor of bone

- Etiology/Incidence

  1. Osteosarcoma

      a. Arises from osteoblasts; found in areas of active skeletal growth, distal femur, proximal tibia and humerus

      b. Most common malignant bone tumor

      c. Found mostly in adolescents and young adults 10 to 25 years of age with equal incidence in males and females

  2. Ewing sarcoma

      a. Originates in myelogenic cells of bone marrow

      b. Affects individuals between 10 and 30 years of age, with highest incidence in 2nd decade

      c. Males affected twice as often as females

      d. Common sites are pelvis, humerus, femur, clavicle and fibula

- Clinical Findings

  1. History

      a. Localized pain at night (knee)

      b. Awakens child

      c. Unilateral

      d. Unrelated to activity

      e. Trauma—incidental (not causative) finding in 25%

  2. Physical Findings

a. Bony tenderness

b. Rarely extends into adjacent joint

c. Mild joint stiffness may exist

d. Rarely demonstrates instability

e. Normal neurovascular examination

f. Absence of effusion

g. Systemic manifestations may be present with Ewings sarcoma—low grade fever, anorexia, fatigue, weight loss

■ Differential Diagnosis

1. "Growing" pains

2. Trauma

3. Osteochondroses

4. Orthopedic or postural defects

5. Osteomyelitis

6. Tendonitis

7. JRA

8. Septic arthritis

9. Soft tissue sarcomas

10. Leukemia

11. Eosinophilic granuloma

■ Diagnostic Tests/Findings

1. Osteosarcoma

a. Radiography—often diagnostic

b. Bone biopsy—confirms diagnosis

c. Total body technetium bone scans and computed tomography (CT)—to identify metastatic lesions

d. Alkaline phosphatase—may be increased; may be used as marker in tracking therapy

2. Ewing Sarcoma

a. WBC—leukocytosis with left shift

      b. Erythrocyte sedimentation rate (ESR)—increased

      c. Radiography—diagnostic features

      d. Surgical biopsy—confirmatory

      e. Bone marrow aspiration—confirmatory

- Management/Treatment/Referral
  1. Osteosarcoma
     a. Surgery—amputation/limb salvage procedures
     b. Chemotherapy
  2. Ewing sarcoma
     a. Chemotherapy and radiation have been recommended in lieu of surgery; now radiation is avoided because of risk, decreased bone growth and development of osteosarcomas (Behrman, 1992; Carroll, 1993)

Fractured Clavicle (Collarbone)

- Definition: Break in bone structure
- Etiology/Incidence
  1. Most frequent birth injury, especially in difficult vertex and breech presentations
  2. Most common fracture in pediatric age group
  3. May follow a fall onto a shoulder
- Clinical Findings
  1. Newborn
     a. Arm not moved freely on affected side
     b. Occasionally discoloration over fracture site
     c. Moro absent on affected side
  2. Child/adolescent
     a. Pain; limited motion
     b. May have lowered shoulder on affected side
     c. Arm is held against body supported by opposite hand
- Differential Diagnosis

1. In newborns — brachial plexus injury; epiphyseal separation of humerus in brachial plexus traction injuries

2. Fracture of humerus in older child and adolescent

- Diagnostic Tests/Findings: Usually none required unless problems encountered

- Management/Treatment

1. In newborn, prognosis is excellent; comfort measures employed or immobilization of arm and shoulder on affected side

2. For older child and adolescent, sling immobilizatin for comfort; figure-of-eight brace used to maintain length of clavicle in overlap fractures

3. Union occurs in 10 to 14 days in infants

4. Usually three weeks immobilization is sufficient for the older child and adolescent, although return to sports should be restricted for several additional weeks to lessen the risk of refracture (Avery & First, 1994)

Subluxation of Radial Head (Nursemaid's Elbow)

- Definition: Dislocation injury involving immature radial head and annular ligament

- Etiology/Incidence

1. Results from sudden longitudinal traction on the hand while the elbow is fully extended and forearm pronated

2. Common in children less than four years of age

- Clinical Findings

1. History of sudden onset of elbow pain following arm being pulled

2. Child usually refuses to move arm, which is held in slight flexion with forearm pronated

3. Flexion and extension normal

4. Supination is limited

5. No swelling or other evidence of injury

- Differential Diagnosis

1. Fracture of proximal radius

2. Dislocation of elbow

3. Fracture of clavicle

- Diagnostic Tests/Findings—none (radiographs normal)
- Management/Treatment
    1. Application of pressure to head of radius with supination with arm in 90-degree flexion; no further treatment usually necessary
    2. If treated shortly after injury, relief of pain is dramatic
    3. With longer standing symptoms, relief not as immediate

Stress Fractures

- Definition: An overuse injury; common sites of fracture are the metatarsals, distal fibula, calcaneus, proximal medial tibial metaphysis in runners, and the pars interarticularis in the vertebral bodies of gymnasts, divers, and football linemen (Gregg & Ergin, 1993)
- Etiology/Incidence
    1. Muscle envelope becomes fatigued, its stress attenuating capability becomes progressively more limited and more force is taken by the underlying bone, leading to subsequent stress fracture (Stanitski, DeLee, & Drez, 1994)
    2. A significant source of sports disability
    3. Direct relationship to age, e.g., children have fewer fractures than adolescents, who have fewer than adults
    4. Occur most commonly in the fibula and the second metatarsal
- Clinical Findings
    1. Gradual onset of pain which increases with activity
    2. May be pain over fracture site
    3. Usually no history of direct trauma to affected site
- Differential Diagnosis
    1. Osteoid osteoma
    2. Osteomyelitis
    3. Bone tumors
    4. Leukemia
    5. Rickets
- Diagnostic Tests/Findings: CBC, ESR and roentgenography usually normal;

bone scan may be needed for follow-up

- Management/Treatment
  1. Identification of the offending factor or factors prior to treatment; possible referral
  2. Rest
  3. Ice
  4. Possibly anti-inflammatory drugs
  5. Education of the athlete, parents, and coaches must be a major part of treatment program
  6. Further specific management choices may include, e.g., orthotics, training modification, surgery

Osgood-Schlatter Disease (Tibial Tubercle Apophysitis)

- Definition: Painful self-limited swelling of tibial tubercle
- Etiology/Incidence
  1. Athletic activity associated with a recent growth spurt causes detachment of cartilage fragments from tibial tuberosity
  2. An overuse syndrome that occurs commonly in physically active males and females during adolescence
- Clinical Findings
  1. Symptoms usually begin during rapid growth at the time of tibial tubercle maturation
  2. Knee pain; aggravated by extension of knee against resistance or by application of pressure over tibial tubercle
  3. Swelling and point tenderness over tibial tubercle
  4. Examination of knee and lower extremity may be normal
  5. Pain worsened by activity; relieved by rest
  6. Self limiting
- Differential Diagnosis
  1. Osteosarcoma
  2. Patellar tendonitis
  3. Osteomyelitis

■ Diagnostic Tests/Findings

    1. Roentgenogram (may or may not be necessary)

        a. To rule out other disorders

        b. More severe involvement will show bony particles

■ Management/Treatment

    1. Disease is usually self-limited

    2. Activity modification

    3. Ice; nonsteroidal anti-inflammatory drugs

    4. Quadriceps stretching and strengthening program

    5. Restriction of activity may be suggested

    6. Knee pads are sometimes recommended to control symptoms

Little League Elbow

■ Definition: Overuse injury of the elbow; injury includes pathologic entities in and about the elbow joint

■ Etiology/Incidence

    1. Physical stresses of throwing produce exceptional forces in and about the elbow

    2. Condition may be less frequent since recent rule changes regarding the number of games pitchers can play per week

■ Clinical Findings

    1. Pain in elbow is usually presenting complaint

    2. Related, but less frequent problems may include

        a. Decreased elbow motion

        b. Mild flexion contracture

        c. Swelling, point tenderness

        d. Decreased performance

        e. Duration of pain related to severity of the problem

■ Differential Diagnosis

    1. Osteoid osteoma

    2. Osteomyelitis

3. Bone tumors

4. Leukemia

■ Diagnostic Tests/Findings: Radiography essential in elbow pathology (Stanitski et al., 1994)

■ Management/Treatment

1. Rest

2. Progressive rehabilitation program once healing has taken place (3 to 4 weeks)

3. Best treatment is prevention

   a. Pitchers should pitch no more than six innings per week with 3 days off between games

   b. Managers should observe technics and fatigue levels of pitchers

Questions

Select the best answer

1. The most common malignant bone tumor in pediatrics is

   a. Osteosarcoma
   b. Ewing's sarcoma
   c. Osteochondroma
   d. Rhabdomyosarcoma

2. Which of the following is associated with forefoot adduction?

   a. Talipes equinovarus (clubfoot)
   b. Talipes calcaneovalgus
   c. Lateral tibial torsion
   d. Pes planovalgus

3. Which of the following disorders is least likely to present with a limp?

   a. Legg-Calvé-Perthes disease
   b. Osgood-Schlatter disease
   c. Slipped capital epiphysis
   d. Toxic synovitis

4. Signs and symptoms consistent with transient synovitis of the hip may include all, except

   a. Mild URI
   b. Pain
   c. Decreased ROM
   d. Swelling

5. During a newborn admission examination, a "clunk" is felt while performing the Ortolani procedure on the hips. The following statements regarding dislocation of the hip are true, except

   a. Dislocation occurs more frequently in females
   b. A palpable "clunk" is highly suggestive of a dislocated hip
   c. X-ray is not very helpful in diagnosis in newborns
   d. The Barlow procedure reduces a hip that is dislocated while the Ortolani procedure evaluates a dislocatable hip by dislocating a hip that is unstable.

6. Club Foot (Talipes Equinovarus) commonly does not include which deformity?

   a. Plantar flexion at ankle
   b. Varus of heel

    c. Adduction of forefoot
    d. Internal tibial torsion

7. Immediate orthopedic referrals include which of the following?

    a. A 3-year-old with minimal knock knees
    b. A 2-year-old with flexible flat feet
    c. A 3-month-old with internal tibial torsion
    d. A four-week-old with fixed metatarsus adductus

8. Which statement concerning subluxation of radial head is *not* true?

    a. It is one of the most common injuries in children less than four years of age
    b. Radiographs are diagnostic
    c. It results from longitudinal pull on the hand
    d. Pain relieved almost immediately following treatment

9. Fractured clavicles may present at or immediately after birth with all except

    a. Discoloration over fracture site
    b. Limited use of affected arm
    c. Mora absent on affected side
    d. Palpable callus mass

10. The most common fracture in children of all ages is a

    a. Femur
    b. Supracondylar
    c. Clavicle
    d. Humerus

11. Diagnostic criteria for Juvenile Rheumatoid Arthritis (JRA) includes

    a. Arthritis lasting for at least 6 weeks
    b. Positive family history for JRA
    c. Arthritis of at least three joints
    d. Positive rheumatoid factor

12. The most common type of JRA is

    a. Systemic onset
    b. Polyarticular onset
    c. Acute onset
    d. Pauciarticular onset

13. Early onset pauciarticular JRA most typically presents in

    a. 2- to 4-year-old females
    b. 3- to 6-year-old males
    c. 10- to 12-year-old males and females

    d. 14- to 18-year-old males and females

14. Dysplasia of the hip in an older infant may typically be evidenced by

    a. Limited adduction of dislocated hip
    b. Positive Ortolani and Barlow
    c. Positive Galleazzi sign
    d. Negative telescoping maneuver

15. Correct management of a dislocated hip in a newborn is most likely to include

    a. Triple diapering for first six months
    b. Traction and surgical reduction
    c. Following carefully for two to three months; then referring to orthopedist if no improvement
    d. Use of Pavlik harness to insure flexion

16. The most common hereditary neuromuscular disease in pediatrics is

    a. Cystic fibrosis
    b. Myasthenia gravis
    c. Multiple Sclerosis
    d. Duchenne muscular dystrophy

17. A classic feature of Duchenne muscular dystrophy is

    a. Delay in rolling over from front to back
    b. Delayed speech
    c. Pseudohypertrophy of calf muscles
    d. Positive Allis sign

18. The following statements regarding Osgood Schlatter disease are true, except

    a. Quadriceps stretching contraindicated
    b. A contributing factor is rapid growth
    c. Pain worse with activity
    d. Involves a painful prominence of tibial tubercle

19. Which of the following statements regarding scoliosis is true?

    a. The majority of cases are idiopathic
    b. Most cases have their onset in preschool years
    c. The frequency in males is three times that in females
    d. Inspection of the spine in a standing position is required to detect minor curvatures

20. The most common elbow injury in childhood is

    a. Fracure of head of radius
    b. Subluxation of radial head

   c. Acute tendinitis

   d. Fracture of proximal ulna

21. A young adolescent comes in with a complaint of pain in the hip. The PNP notices his hip is held in external rotation; the rest of the physical examination is normal. A most likely diagnosis is

   a. Legg-Calvé-Perthes

   b. Osgood-Schlatter

   c. Blount's disease

   d. Slipped capital femoral epiphysis

22. The most common organism causing acute osteomyelitis is

   a. *Mycoplasma pneumoniae*

   b. *Haemophilus influenza*

   c. *Pseudomona aeruginosa*

   d. *Staphylococcus aureus*

23. In Ewings sarcoma the following systemic findings may be present

   a. Localized pain at night

   b. Pain in lower extremity following recent trauma

   c. Low-grade fever, fatigue and weight loss

   d. Limitation in movement and visible swelling

24. Which of the following statements regarding acute osteomyelitis is not true?

   a. Prevalent during adolescence

   b. It occurs more frequently in boys

   c. It occurs most frequently in long bones

   d. There is a relationship between age of child and likely organism

Answer Key

1. a
2. a
3. b
4. d
5. d
6. d
7. d
8. b
9. d
10. c
11. a
12. d
13. a
14. c
15. d
16. d
17. c
18. a
19. a
20. b
21. d
22. d
23. c
24. a

Bibliography

Avery, M. E., & First, L. R. (Eds.). (1994). *Pediatric medicine* (2nd. ed.). Baltimore, MD: Williams & Wilkins.

Behrman, R. E., Kliegman, R. M., Nelson, W. E., & Vaughan, V. C. (Eds.). (1992). *Nelson textbook of pediatrics* (14th ed.). Philadelphia: W. B. Saunders

Brown, L. M. (1993). Development dysplasia of the hip. In R. A. Dershewitz (Ed.). (1993). *Ambulatory pediatric care*, (pp. 494-497). Philadelphia: J. B. Lippincott

Burg, F. D., Ingelfinger, J. R., & Wald, E. R. (Eds.). *Gellis & Kagan's current pediatric therapy*. Philadelphia: W. B. Saunders

Carroll, N. C. (1993). Treatment of bone tumors and limb salvage. In F. D. Burg, J. R. Ingelfinger & E. R. Wald (Eds.), *Gellis & Kagan's current pediatric therapy* (14th ed.). (pp. 447-449). Philadelphia: W. B. Saunders

Castiglia, P. T., & Harbin, R. E. (Eds.). (1992). *Child health care*. Philadelphia: J. B. Lippincott.

Chauvenet, A., & Wofford, M. (1990). Cures in childhood cancer. *Pediatrics in Review, 11* (10), 311-317.

Dyment, P. G. (1993). The hip. In F. D. Burg, J. R. Ingelfinger & E. R. Wald (Eds). *Gellis & Kagan's current pediatric therapy* (14th ed.). (pp. 442-444). Philadelphia: W. B. Saunders

Gregg, J. R., & Ergin, T. M. (1993). Orthopedic trauma. In F. D. Burg, J. R. Ingelfinger, & E. R. Wald. *Gellis & Kagan's current pediatric therapy* (14th ed.). (pp. 459-469). Philadelphia: W. B. Saunders.

Hoekelman, R. A., Friedman, S. B., Nelson, N. M. & Seidel, H. M. (Eds.). (1992). *Pediatric primary care* (2nd ed.). St. Louis: Mosby Year Book.

Killam, P. E. (1989). Orthopedic assessment of young children: Developmental variations. *Nurse Practitioner, 14*, 27-36.

Landry, G. (1992). Sports injuries in childhood. *Pediatric Annals, 21*(3), 165-170.

MacEwen, G., & Millet, C. (1990). Congenital dislocation of the hip. *Pediatrics in Review, 11*(8), 249-252.

Mier, R. S. (1993). Torticollis. In F. D. Burg, J. R. Ingelfinger & E. R. Wald (Eds), *Current pediatric therapy* (pp. 470-471). Philadelphia: W. B. Saunders.

Moe, P., & Seay, A. (1993.). Musculoskeletal disorders. In Hathaway, H., Groothius,

& Parsley (Eds.). *Current pediatric diagnosis and treatment* (pp. 674-747). Norwalk, CT: Appleton & Lange.

Skinner, S. R. (1991). Orthopedic problems in pediatrics. In R. Ary (Ed.). *Pediatrics* (pp. 1937-1938). Norwalk, CT: Appleton & Lange.

Staneli, L. T. (1987). Rotational problems of the lower extremities. *Orthopedic Clinics of North America, 18*, 503-512.

Stanitski, C. L., DeLee, J. C., & Drez, D. Jr. (Eds.). (1994). *Pediatric and adolescent sports medicine*. Vol. 3. Philadelphia: W. B. Saunders.

Genitourinary and Gynecologic Disorders

Elizabeth Hawkins-Walsh

Cryptorchidism

■ Definition: Unilateral or bilateral undescended testicles

1. "Ectopic"—has completed descent through inguinal canal through external ring; has become lodged in perineum, thigh, or proximal scrotum

2. "True"—has never been in scrotal sac; lies somewhere along normal path of descent (usually unilateral)

■ Etiology/Incidence

1. Congenital interference in descent of testicles into scrotum which normally occurs between 7th and 9th month of gestation

2. Theoretical

   a. Hormonal deficiency

   b. Intrinsic abnormality of testis

   c. Mechanical causes

3. Higher incidence in prematures; 3 to 4% of full-term infants

4. Usually spontaneous descent before end of first year

■ Clinical Findings

1. Scrotum smaller and softer than normal

2. Absence of testis in scrotal sac upon physical examination

3. Higher incidence of inguinal hernias and hydroceles

■ Differential Diagnosis

1. Anorchia

2. Retractile testes

3. Chromosomal abnormality

4. Bilateral—ambiguous genitalia

■ Diagnostic Tests/Findings

1. Ultrasonography—to determine location of non-palpable testes

2. Serum testosterone levels prior to and after administration of human chorionic gonadotropin (hCG)—increase in testosterone levels indicates presence of testicular tissue

■ Management/Treatment

1. Bilateral and nonpalpable anywhere in canal—refer to urologist

2. Unilateral—refer to urologist for evaluation by 1 year

3. Hormonal therapy

   a. Has not replaced surgical treatment

   b. Treating with hCG over long periods can hasten onset of puberty and cause sterility

4. Surgery

   a. Orchiopexy—at 1 to 3 years; usually not before 1 year

   b. Earlier timing

      (1) Higher fertility

      (2) Fewer psychological effects

5. Rationale for surgery

   a. Prevent damage to undescended testis from exposure to higher degree of body heat; decrease incidence of infertility

   b. Decrease incidence of tumors

   c. Avoid trauma/torsion

   d. Close processus vaginalis

   e. Cosmetic/psychological effects

Hypospadias

■ Definition

1. Condition in which the urinary meatus is located on the ventral surface of penis (most often on the glans) or anywhere along the penile shaft

2. Types range from mild (meatus just off center from tip of penis) to severe (meatus located on perineum with bifid scrotum)

■ Etiology/Incidence

1. Incomplete fusion of urethral folds along the midline

2. Incidence—occurs in less than 1% of newborn males but is the most common penile abnormality

■ Clinical Findings

1. Abnormal urinary stream indicating location of urethral meatus

2. Dystonic meatus—occurring anywhere along penile shaft

3. Chordee—a ventral band of fibrous tissue which causes ventral curvature

- Differential Diagnosis

    1. Associated G.U. abnormalities

    2. Meatal stenosis?

    3. Vestigial vagina?

- Diagnostic Tests/Findings

    1. Severe

        a. Radiography; sonography or excretory urography—to determine presence of an associated anomaly

        b. Chromosomal analysis

    2. Mild—none

- Management/Treatment

    1. Refer to urology

    2. Surgery for cosmetic, functional, psychological reasons

    3. Mild cases without chordee may not require treatment

    4. Preparation of parents for type of procedure (if surgical) to be done and expected cosmetic results

    5. If children are old enough to understand, they, too, require preparation

Hydrocele

- Definition: Presence of fluid between layers of tunica vaginalis

- Etiology/Incidence

    1. Noncommunicating

        a. Upper segment of processus vaginalis has been obliterated, but tunica vaginalis still contains peritoneal fluid

        b. Common in newborns

        c. Often subsides spontaneously as fluid is gradually absorbed

    2. Communicating

    a. Caused by fluid from peritoneal cavity passing through patent processus vaginalis into scrotum

    b. May be present at birth or appear later

  3. Acquired

    a. Secondary to epididymitis with orchitis

    b. Secondary to testicular tumors

- Clinical Findings

  1. Translucent upon transillumination

  2. Scrotum becomes swollen as day progresses, usually smaller in a.m. (communicating)

  3. Nonfluctuating volume of fluid (noncommunicating)

  4. Nonpainful

- Differential Diagnosis

  1. Inguinal hernia

  2. Hematoma

  3. Hematocele

- Diagnostic Tests/Findings—Ultrasound

- Management/Treatment

  1. Refer communicating to M.D.

  2. Observe for concomitant hernia

  3. Generally surgical repair indicated if spontaneous resolution doesn't occur by 1 year (communicating)

Testicular Torsion

- Definition: Torsion or twisting of testicle on its spermatic cord; can lead to decreased blood supply with ischemic necrosis

- Etiology/Incidence

  1. May result from irregular development of tunica vaginalis and spermatic cord

  2. Most commonly seen between 10 to 14 years of age; not specific to this age group

  3. Also seen in infancy

- Clinical Findings
  1. Sudden onset of acute unilateral scrotal pain (may follow physical activity or awaken child from sleep)
  2. Nausea, vomiting may occur
  3. Younger child may present doubled over, limping
  4. Acutely tender scrotum makes adequate examination difficult
  5. Edematous, red, taut scrotal skin
  6. Firm, fixed, swollen testicle
- Differential Diagnosis
  1. Epididymitis
  2. Orchitis
  3. Trauma
  4. Incarcerated hernia
- Diagnostic Tests/Findings: Usually not recommended because of delay in executing surgical procedure
- Management/Treatment: Prompt sugical exploration

Inguinal Hernia

- Definition: Protrusion of abdominal contents into inguinal or scrotal areas
- Etiology/Incidence
  1. Congenital
  2. Derived from persistence of processus vaginalis
  3. Eight times more common in boys
  4. Right-sided hernias are more frequent
  5. May be bilateral
  6. Increased incidence in prematures; 13 to 30% of male prematures
  7. More common in children with increased intra-abdominal pressure; VP shunts, ascites, bronchopulmonary dysplasia (BPD)
- Clinical Findings
  1. An intermittent or constant bulge lateral to the pubis
  2. Bulge may appear when child is crying, straining or standing; usually reduces when child is relaxed or supine

3. Often detected at 2 to 3 months when intra-abdominal pressure increases

4. Reducible, usually

5. "Silk glove" sign elicited by rubbing sides of hernial sac together

6. Thickening of cord in groin can be palpated

7. Symptoms of irreducible or incarcerated hernias
   a. Irritability
   b. Anorexia, nausea, vomiting (if bowel is involved)
   c. Groin or abdominal discomfort
   d. Constipation

8. Incarceration usually leads to strangulation
   a. Groin becomes tender and swollen
   b. As process progresses area may become red

- Differential Diagnosis
  1. Hydrocele
  2. Undescended testis
  3. Femoral hernia
  4. Lymphadenopathy
  5. Abscess

- Diagnostic Tests/Findings: Ultrasound of inguinal region and scrotum to differentiate hydrocele from true hernia if diagnosis is unclear

- Management/Treatment
  1. Managed by surgical correction
  2. Timing of surgery may be semi-elective for an asymptomatic inguinal hernia
  3. Emergency is indicated in the case of a strangulated hernia
  4. Education of patient and parent regarding surgical procedure and discussion of concerns or fears

Phimosis

- Definition: Tightening or narrowing of the foreskin that prevents its retraction over glans penis*

- Etiology/Incidence

  1. Unknown

  2. Theoretical

    a. Trauma from forcible retraction

    b. Congenital abnormalities

    c. Recurrent infections of foreskin

    d. Improperly performed circumcisions

    e. Poor hygiene

  *The majority of newborns have foreskins which are not retractable due to adhesions between the glans and foreskin; this is a normal situation, and the foreskin should not be forcibly retracted. By three years of age, most adhesions have disappeared

- Clinical Findings

  1. Dysuria

  2. Hematuria

  3. Decreased urinary stream

  4. Foreskin tenderness

  5. Ballooning of foreskin during urination (severe)

  6. Foreskin that cannot be retracted over glans

  7. Whitish, scarred stenotic foreskin

- Differential Diagnosis

  1. Developmentally normal unretractable foreskin

  2. Balanoposthitis

  3. Paraphimosis

- Diagnostic Tests/Findings: None indicated

- Management/Treatment

  Prevention

  1. Teach caregivers not to forcibly retract foreskin; may cause inflammation and scarring

  2. Hygiene

  3. Treatment

    a. Mild

(1) Gentle, manual retraction; cleanse during bath

(2) Replace foreskin over glans

b. Severe

(1) Surgery (circumcision)

Urinary Tract Infection

- Definition: Bacterial invasion of urinary tract structures by microorganisms

  1. May involve upper urinary tract (ureters, renal pelvis, calyces, renal parenchyma)

  2. May involve lower urinary tract (urethra and bladder)

- Etiology

  1. Predisposing factors

      a. Urinary Stasis—anatomic and functional factors which produce incomplete drainage and stasis in urinary system

          (1) Contribute to infection of urinary tract

          (2) Promote renal parenchymal damage by allowing infected urine to reach renal parenchyma

      b. Anatomic factors

          (1) Reflux—retrograde flow of urine into ureters

          (2) Anatomic abnormalities (especially ureters)

          (3) Neurogenic bladder

      c. Functional obstruction

          (1) Constipation

          (2) Pregnancy

          (3) Infrequent voiding

      d. Hygienic factors

      e. Uncircumcised

      f. Miscellaneous disorders

          (1) Malnutrition

          (2) Diabetes

          (3) Nephrocalcinosis

     g. Trauma

       (1)   Irritation

       (2)   Instrumentation

  2. Bacterial Pathogens

     a. *Escherichia coli* (75 to 90% of all female infections followed by *Klebsiella* and *Proteus*)

     b. *Staphylococcus saprophyticus* is most common pathogen following *E. coli* in sexually active adolescent

  3. Viral Pathogens

     a. Decreased; relatively unimportant

     b. Adenovirus (cystitis)

■ Incidence—varies with sex and age

  1. Newborn

     a. Symptomatic UTIs in approximately 1.4/1000 infants with slightly more males than females

     b. Prematurity—increased incidence

  2. Post neonatal:

     a. Incidence unknown

     b. Female incidence 10 times greater than males

     c. Peak incidence—2 to 6 years of age (excluding structural abnormalities and sexually active females)

  3. Recurrent:

     a. Most common in females

     b. Eighty percent recurrence within 2 years in white females; 60% in black

     c. Recurrences infrequent after 2 years

■ Clinical Findings

  1. Asymptomatic bacteriuria

     a. All age groups may present with no symptoms

     b. Careful history may elicit symptoms in previously believed "asymptomatic"

2. Symptomatic

   a. Newborns (descending route—hematogenous spread)

      (1) Nonspecific manifestations—malaise, anorexia, feeding difficulties, failure to thrive, jaundice, fever of unknown origin, malnutrition, "colic," diarrhea, vomiting, irritability

      (2) Urinary tract symptoms—changes in caliber and force of stream; diapers continuously wet

   b. Young children

      (1) Nonspecific still common— fever

      (2) Gastrointestinal symptoms—abdominal pain, vomiting, diarrhea

      (3) Urinary—dysuria, frequency, enuresis, urgency, foul-smelling urine

      (4) Bedwetting in a previously dry child

   c. Older child

      (1) Upper tract—fever, chills, flank pain, CVA tenderness, abdominal pain

      (2) Lower tract—frequency, urgency, dribbling, hesitancy, dysuria, daytime incontinence

3. Physical Findings—may be of limited value

   a. Vital signs/temperature/blood pressure

   b. Rule out other foci of infection

   c. Abdominal examination

      (1) Abdominal mass (obstructed and distended urinary structures)

      (2) Abdominal tenderness—suprapubic pain

      (3) Kidneys (may be enlarged in acute pyelonephritis)

   d. Costovertebral angle percussion tenderness—upper tract involvement

   e. Genitalia

   a. External irritation/discharge

   b. Erythema of urinary meatus

- Differential Diagnosis

  1. Inflammation of external genitalia secondary to miscellaneous irritants, poor hygiene, masturbation, etc.

  2. Pinworms

  3. Foreign bodies

  4. Trauma

  5. Sepsis (newborns)

  6. Gastroenteritis

- Diagnostic Tests/Findings

  1. Urinalysis—may raise or lower index of suspicion; not diagnostic

     a. Specific gravity—preferred specimen above 1.005 (less dilute); ability to concentrate urine may be compromised with upper tract involvement

     b. Hematuria—may indicate blood in urinary tract or any organ; increased exercise

     c. Proteinuria—may be transient and intermittent (fever, exercise); may be significant of upper tract involvement, especially in presence of blood

     d. pH—highly alkaline, suspect bacteria

  2. Urine Culture

     a. Urine specimens

        (1) Fresh specimen—properly handled

        (2) First a.m. urine

        (3) Methods

            (a) Clean catch (midstream)

            (b) Suprapubic

            (c) Catheterization

     b. Method of collection

        (1) Clean catch, midstream

            (a) Colony count greater than 100,000/ml of single organism—indicative (90% accuracy) of infection

            (b) Less than 10,000 colonies—likely negative

       (c) Between 50,000 and 100,000 — highly suggestive, but not diagnostic

       (d) Mixed organisms more commonly seen in contaminated specimens and recurrent infections

    (2) Catheterization

       (a) Used for infants who cannot voluntarily void

       (b) When urine specimen required due to illness

       (c) To confirm questionable cultured specimens

       (d) Almost any number of colonies significant

    (3) Suprapubic

       (a) Same indications as above under catheterization

       (b) Presence of any bacteria on culture significant

3. Screening tests for detection of bacteriuria

4. Radiologic evaluation — indicated in children with UTI to identify those patients with vesicoureteral reflux (VUR), obstruction or other urinary tract abnormalities (Elerian & Adelman, 1993; Avery & First, 1994)

- Management/Treatment

1. Goals

  a. Elimination of acute infection

  b. Prevent recurrence

    (1) Education

    (2) Identification and correction of organic abnormalities

  c. Early detection of correctable abnormalities

2. Indications for possible hospitalization and IV antibiotics

  a. Newborns

  b. Infants under 3 to 6 months

  c. Children with severe systemic manifestations, dehydration, or inability to tolerate oral fluids

  d. Pyelonephritis

  e. Urinary obstruction

3. Outpatient management

   a. Uncomplicated infections

      (1) Antibiotics selected on basis of sensitivity

      (2) Sulfisoxazole 120-150 mg/kg orally q.i.d.; amoxicillin 25-50 mg/kg t.i.d. or q.i.d.; TMP/SMX (TMP 10 mg/kg/day + SSMX 50 mg/kg/day) b.i.d.

      (3) Usually treated 7 to 14 days

      (4) Increase in fluid intake

      (5) Frequent and complete emptying of bladder

      (6) Proper hygiene

4. Duration of therapy debatable

   a. Factors

      (1) Age of patient

      (2) Severity of symptoms

      (3) Previous history

   b. Uncomplicated primary infections in child over 6 months in absence of high fever, etc.; 10-day course

5. Follow up

   a. Urine culture at 48 hours and again, approximately one week following completion of therapy

   b. Urine culture at 3-month intervals for 1 to 2 years (time frames may vary)

6. Recurrent infections—treat acute infection

7. Prophylactic therapy

   a. Usually 3 documented infections in 1 year

   b. Nitrofurantoin given nightly

   c. TMX/SMX given nightly or on alternate nights

   d. Therapy should be continued for 6 months to 2 years, or longer if indicated (Elerian & Adelman, 1993)

Acute Poststreptococcal Glomerulonephritis (APSGN)

- Definition: An immune mediated disease characterized by diffuse changes in the glomeruli of the kidneys

- Etiology/Incidence
    1. Group A ß—hemolytic streptococcal antigens provoke antibody response
    2. Generally occurs in children over 2 years of age; more common in males
    3. May follow streptococcal pharyngitis or streptoccal infections by 8 to 14 days
    4. The most common form of nephritis in children
- Clinical Findings
    1. Signs and symptoms
        a. Dark colored urine
        b. Lethargy, anorexia, abdominal pain, vomiting
        e. Headache (with severe hypertension)
        f. Oliguria
    2. Physical Findings
        a. Facial puffiness, worse in a.m.; may involve extremities and abdomen as day progresses
        b. Elevated blood pressure
        c. CVA tenderness
- Differential Diagnosis
    1. Henoch-Schönlein purpura
    2. Nonstreptococcal glomerulonephritis
    3. Benign hematuria
    4. Membranoproliferative glomerulonephritis
    5. Chronic glomerulonephritis
    6. Systemic lupus erythematosus
- Diagnostic Tests/Findings
    1. Urinalysis shows
        a. High specific gravity
        b. Low pH

      c. Hematuria

      d. Leukocyturia

      e. RBC casts; epithelial casts

      f. Proteinuria (dependent on hematuria)

  2. Titers

      a. Serum ASO—elevated in up to 80% of cases

      b. Anti-DNase B (antideoxyribonuclease B) titers—elevated

      c. Streptozyme test—detects antibodies to streptolysin O, DNase B, hyaluronidase, streptokinase, NADase

  3. Cultures (often negative by time nephritis develops)

      a. Throat

      b. Skin lesions

  4. Serum C3—usually reduced

- Management/Treatment

  1. No specific treatment

  2. Supportive therapy related to clinical manifestations

  3. Outpatient or hospitalization dependent upon severity of illness

  4. Antibiotics usually do not alter course of illness

  5. Usually complete recovery in greater than 95% of children

Enuresis

- Definition: Involuntary voiding after control should be established

  1. Primary (persistent)—no history of consistent dryness

  2. Secondary (regressive)—occurs in children who have previously been bladder-trained at least 6 months or more

  3. Types

      a. Primary nocturnal—wetting during nighttime sleep (85%)

      b. Diurnal—wetting during daytime

- Etiology/Incidence

  1. In both types of enuresis organic pathology can be found in only a small number of cases

2. Possible organic factors

   a. Obstruction

   b. Urinary tract infections

   c. Diabetes mellitus

   d. Diabetes insipidus

   e. Sickle cell anemia

3. Developmental delay

4. Deep sleep (controversial)

5. Psychological-emotional factors

   a. Recent move

   b. New sibling

   c. Divorce

   d. Death in family

   e. Parental attitudes

6. Persistent nocturnal enuresis is often due to inappropriate toilet training

7. Prevalence at age 5 is 7% for males and 3% for females

8. Prevalence at age 10 is 3% for males and 2% for females

■ Clinical Findings

1. Demonstration by history of nocturnal, diurnal enuresis or both

2. Complete physical examination to rule out organic disorders

3. Psychosocial evaluation to rule out psychosocial disturbances/disorders

■ Differential Diagnosis

1. Urinary tract infection or anatomic abnormalities

2. Diabetes mellitus; diabetes insipidus

3. Increased fluid intake

4. Seizure disorder; neurological disorder

5. Renal insufficiency

■ Diagnostic Tests/Findings

1. Urinalysis and urine culture to rule out organic or infectious disorders

2. Further evaluation usually not warranted unless physical examination

findings are abnormal

■ Management/Treatment

1. Principles

   a. Primary nocturnal enuresis is usually a benign, self-limiting disorder

   b. Avoid excessive laboratory investigation and overly aggressive treatment

   c. Child should be involved in the treatment plan and decision to treat

   d. In some cases the decision not to treat may be most therapeutic

   e. Treatment is justified when help is sought since it appears that children can have improved self concept following successful treatment

2. Treatment

   a. Pretreatment Phase

      (1) Education—reassurance and support to avoid adverse secondary effects on self esteem and interpersonal relationships

      (2) Observation

         (a) Open discussion

         (b) Track symptoms with chart

         (c) Positive reinforcement for dryness

      (3) Simple steps

         (a) Fluid restriction at night

         (b) Voiding prior to sleep

         (c) Voiding once during night

      (4) The pretreatment phase alone may yield remission of symptoms

   b. Treatment phase—multiple treatment plans exist

      (1) "Enuresis Alarm"—most effective; a conditioning alarm device worn at night which is triggered by voiding

         (a) Children over 8 years
            • Use until 21 consecutive dry nights are achieved

- Typical course—4 months
- Address compliance
- Good success rate—60 to 80% initial response
- Some relapse
- May require second course

(2) Other treatments—much less effective unless used in conjunction with alarm

(3) Bladder-training program—daytime increase in fluid intake with concomitant delay in voiding; requires motivation and compliance

(4) Medication—most useful in situation where rapid, short term relief is important (camp, etc.)

    (a) Imipramine (25-75 mg/day)
- Decrease in frequency of wetting usual
- Drug tolerance is common
- Significant relapses
- Side-effects (cardiac)
- Risk of fatal overdose

    (b) Desmopressin acetate (DDAVP)—may be effective with those children who have abnormal circadian variation of antidiuretic hormone secretion
- Provides physiological control of nighttime production of urine in children over 6 years of age
- May be used adjunctive to behavioral conditioning or other nonpharmacological interventions
- Effectiveness still controversial
- Available as a nasal spray 20 to 40 mg in each nostril until response obtained
- Expensive, does not cure problem and has high relapse rate

Vulvovaginitis in Prepubertal Child

- Definition: Inflammation of the vulva and vagina

- Etiology/Incidence

    1. Predisposing factors

      a. Anatomy—lack of labial fat pads and pubic hair in younger child; proximity of anal orifice to vagina

      b. Poor perineal hygiene practice

   2. Common causes

   a. Irritation from bubble bath, improper wiping after defecation, tight clothing, panty hose, plastic coated paper diapers

   b. Masturbation

   c. Foreign bodies

   d. Sexual abuse

   e. Associated systemic illness

   f. Secondary to antibiotics (candidiasis)

   g. Infections

   (1) Nonspecific vulvovaginitis—coliform bacteria; ß-hemolytic streptoccoccus; staphylococcus

   (2) Nonsexually transmitted pathogens—*Yersinia enterocolitica*, *Enterobius vermicularis*, *Candida albicans*, *shigella*

   (3) Sexually transmitted disease—Trichomonas vaginalis, Neisseria gonorrhoeae, Herpes progenitalis, Human papillomavirus, *chlamydia trachomatis*

- Clinical Findings

   1. Dependent upon cause

   2. Patient may complain of

   a. Itching, burning, discharge, bleeding

   b. Dysuria

   3. Physical findings may include

   a. Erythema, excoriation, bruising, rashes

   b. Vaginal discharge

   c. Lacerations

   d. Blood

   e. Labial adhesions—may result from chronic vulvar irritation

- Differential Diagnosis: See causes above, including normal physiologic leukorrhea

- Diagnostic Tests/Findings

   1. Vaginal discharge

      a. Gram stain

      b. Wet mount

      c. KOH

      d. Cultures

■ Management/Treatment

    1. Treat for specific etiology

    2. Symptomatic

      a. Sitz baths

      b. Antibiotics as indicated

      c. Education regarding perineal hygiene

      d. Avoidance of potential irritant

    3. Labial adhesions

      a. Mild—require no treatment

      b. Significant

        (1) Forceful separation should be avoided

        (2) Estrogen containing cream applied to adhesions twice a day for 2 weeks; then nightly 1 to 2 weeks

        (3) Application of A&D ointment at bedtime may prevent reformation

Toxic Shock Syndrome

■ Definition: An acute, multisystem disease which primarily affects menstruating females

■ Etiology/Incidence

    1. Association with staphyloccal enterotoxin F which is produced by 10% of strains of *Staphylococcus aureus*

    2. 9% of females are culture positive for *Staphylococcus aureus* from vagina or labia

    3. Menstrual blood and microabrasions may contribute to release of toxins

    4. Incidence peaked in 1980

    5. Peak age of incidence is 16 to 17 years

      6.   95% of cases in females occur at or near menstruation

      7.   Risk factors—superabsorbent tampon use; skin and wound infections

      8.   10% of cases occur in males

- Clinical Findings

      1.   Prodrome

          a. May or may not occur

          b. Includes headache, vomiting, diarrhea, fatigue

      2.   High fever (> 38.9 °C)

      3.   Diffuse macular rash

          a. Prominent around perineum and thighs

          b. Desquamation 1 to 2 weeks after onset, especially palms and soles

      4.   Hypotension

      5.   Additional findings may include hyperemia of conjunctival, vaginal or oropharyngeal mucous membranes; disorientation or alterations in consciousness unrelated to fever; and severe myalgia

- Differential Diagnosis

      1.   Kawasaki's disease

      2.   Meningococcemia

      3.   Septicimia/septic shock

      4.   Rocky Mountain spotted fever

      5.   Streptococcus toxic shock-like syndrome

      6.   Acute pyelonephritis

- Diagnostic Tests/Findings

      1.   Cultures of blood, vagina, oropharynx—*Staphylococcus aureus*

      2.   CBC—platelets < 100,000 mm^3

      3.   Urinalysis—BUN, creatinine 2 times normal or > 5 WBC/HPF in absence of UTI

      4.   Total bilirubin, AST, ALT—two times normal levels

- Management/Treatment

      1.   Immediate referral for management of this potentially lethal disease

2. Prevention/education

   a. Because of recurrent infections in up to 30% of cases, these individuals should not continue to use tampons

   b. Superabsorbent tampons should not be used

   c. When tampons are used, they should be changed frequently, reserved for times of heavier flow and not used at night

   d. Careful hand washing when changing tampons

   e. Notification of health care provider should any febrile illness occur during menstruation

Genital Tract Infections

Bacterial Vaginosis (BV)

- Definition: A vulvovaginitis syndrome found in sexually active adolescents and adult women

- Etiology/Incidence

   1. Microbiologic cause not clearly delineated; *Gardnerella vaginalis, Mycoplasma hominis,* predominate flora

   2. Most prevalent vaginal infection in sexually active adolescents and adults

   3. Rarely reported in prepubescent females; unless found in children who have had sexual contact

   4. Role of sexual transmission unclear; sexually associated rather than a sexually transmitted syndrome

- Clinical Findings

   1. Vaginal discharge

      a. Homogenous gray-white, adheres to vaginal walls

      b. "Fishy" odor

      c. Amount varies widely

      d. Onset not related to menses

   2. Infrequent pruritus, dysuria, dyspareunia

   3. Perineum usually has normal appearance

   4. Up to 50% of patients are asymptomatic

- Differential Diagnosis
    1. Foreign body (tampon, IUD, toilet tissue, diaphragm)
    2. *Trichomonas vaginalis* (pruritus)
    3. Physiologic leukorrhea (nonodorous)
- Diagnostic Tests/Findings—should have 3 or more of the following
    1. Vaginal pH—> 4.5
    2. Wet mount—should see at least 20% clue cells (epithelial cells heavily coated with bacteria)
    3. Positive amine/whiff test—vaginal fluid mixed with 10% KOH produces fishy, amine odor
    4. Homogenous gray-white adherent vaginal discharge
- Management/Treatment
    1. Metronidazole 500 mg orally b.i.d. for 7 days
        a. For contraindications and side-effects, see Trichomoniasis
        b. Routine treatment of male sexual partners not recommended since relapse or recurrence rates not affected (AAP, 1994)
        c. Abstinence or use of condom during treatment
    2. Alternative—clindamycin 300 mg orally b.i.d. for 7 days
    3. HIV-infected female treated the same as above
    4. Stress no alcohol intake during treatment and for 72 hours following treatment (GI symptoms may occur)
    5. Other STDs may coexist
    6. Education regarding prevention, early symptoms, risk of other STDs (HIV) and follow-up

Vulvovaginal Candidiasis

- Definition: A fungal infection of the vulva and vagina
- Etiology/Incidence
    1. Most common—*Candida albicans* (85 to 90%)
        b. *Candida tropicalis*—< 5% cases
        c. *Torulopsis glabrata*—< 5% cases

2. Common and frequent recurrences

3. Incidence of symptomatic candidiasis increases with

   a. Broad-spectrum antibiotic use

   b. Diabetes mellitus

   c. Corticosteroid or oral contraceptive use

   d. Depressed cell-mediated immunity

   e. Pregnancy

   f. Increased local heat, irritation and moisture

   g. Chemical irritation (douches)

   h. Obesity

4. Sexual transmission may play a role in some cases

- Clinical Findings

   1. Usually severe vulvar or vaginal pruritus

   2. Marked mucosal erythema (cervical)

   3. Diffuse erythema and hyperemia of vulva

   4. Linear perineal fissures/excoriations

   5. Papulopustular perineal dermatitis

   6. Discharge—characteristically nonodorous thick, white, curd-like, resembling cottage cheese

- Differential Diagnosis

   1. Allergic/contact dermatitis

   2. Mucopurulent cervicitis

   3. Genital herpes

   4. Trichomonas, bacterial vaginosis, chlamydia or gonococcal infection

- Diagnostic Tests/Findings

   1. KOH wet-mount—presence of hyphae, pseudohyphae, spores or buds

   2. pH—between 3.5 and 5

   3. Gram stain—presence of hyphae, pseudohyphae

- Management/Treatment

   1. Topical imidazole therpay remains first choice for treatment of

infrequent cases; includes butoconazole (Femstat); clortrimazole (Gyne-Lotrimin, Mycelex); miconazole (Monistat); and terconazole (Terazole)

   a. Wide range of doses and forms available; both creams and suppositories

   b. Seems to be no difference in cure rates between the different imidazole agents or between suppository and creams

2. Sitz baths may provide relief; cotton undergarments; discontinuation of perfumed vaginal hygiene products

3. Frequent recurrences require thorough assessment and reevaluation of risk factors

4. In cases of recurrence, prophylactic postmenstrual therapy with intravaginal clotrimazole (500 mg each month) or suppressive therapy with low-dose oral ketoconazole (100 mg daily for 6 months) may be beneficial (Ray, Jones & Muram, 1994)

5. Treatment of sexual partner not routinely required

6. Use of abstinence/condom until symptoms subside

Trichomonas Vaginalis (Trichomoniasis)

- Definition: Sexually transmitted, anaerobic, flagellated protozoan infection
- Etiology/Incidence
   1. *Trichomonas Vaginalis*
   2. One of the most frequent STDs in the U.S. (2.5 to 3 million cases per year
   3. Almost always sexually transmitted
   4. Correlates with level of sexual activity and number of partners
   5. Peak rates 16 to 35 years
   6. Found in 30 to 40% of male partners of symptomatic females
   7. Found in 80 to 85% of female partners of symptomatic males
   8. Frequently occurs with chlamydia, gonorrhea and bacterial vaginosis
- Clinical Findings
   1. Incubation 4 to 30 days
   2. Copious, watery, yellow or green colored, frothy, odorous vaginal

discharge—present in 50%

3. Vulvovaginal pruritus

4. Dyspareunia, dysuria, frequency

5. Vaginal walls and cervix may have erythematous, granular ("strawberry spots") appearance from subepithelal hemorrhages

6. Lower abdominal pain with excoriation of vulva and thighs

7. May be asymptomatic—25% of females

9. Males

   a. Usually asymptomatic

   b. Urethral discharge, dysuria

   c. Usually self-limiting disease

■ Differential Diagnosis

1. Bacterial vaginosis

2. Chlamydia infection

3. Gonorrhea

4. Urinary tract infection

■ Diagnostic Tests/Findings

1. Saline wet mount—to demonstrate trichomonads; positive wet-mount will show many or few pear-shaped motile organisms with anterior flagellae and undulating membrane (**slide must be examined immediately after collection**)

2. Trichomonads may also be detected through urinary sediment, Pap smears, cultures, stained smears and direct monoclonal antibody tests

3. pH > 4.5

■ Management/Treatment

1. Metronidazole

   a. Adolescents and adults—2 g orally in a single dose

   b. Prepubertal girls—15 mg/kg/day in 3 divided doses (maximum dose 250 mg)

   c. Treatment failures should be retreated with metronidazole (1 g in two divided doses for adolescents and adults) for 7 days (AAP, 1994)

      d. Should not be used in first trimester of pregnancy or during lactation

  2. Side-effects of metronidazole

      a. GI disturbances, headache, dizziness, metallic taste

      b. Alcohol interaction similar to disulfiram (antabuse)

      c. Drug interactions (potentiates warfarin; phenobarbital decreases its half life; cimetidine prolongs its half life)

  3. Partner requires concurrent treatment

  4. Abstinence/condom use during treatment

  5. Education regarding prevention, treatment, additional risks of STDs (HIV), follow-up

Chlamydia Trachomatis

- Definition: Sexually transmitted pathogen which can cause urethritis in both sexes, vaginitis in prepubertal females, cervicitis in postpubertal females and epididymitis in males

- Etiology/Incidence

  1. *Chlamydia trachomatis*

  2. Most common bacterial sexually transmitted infection in the U.S.

  3. Sharp increase in past 20 years

  4. Risk factors

      a. Young age

      b. Multiple sexual partners

      c. Presence of other STDs

      d. Use of oral contraceptives

      e. Abnormal pap smear

  4. Occurs in about 50% of infants born vaginally of infected mothers; these infants are at risk for conjunctivitis and pneumonia

- Clinical Findings

  1. Female—often asymptomatic

      a. Lower abdominal pain

      b. Abnormal vaginal discharge

    c. Intermenstrual or post-coital bleeding

    d. Dysuria, frequency

    e. RUQ pain, fever, tenderness, and abdominal wall spasm

    f. Mucopurulent discharge

    g. Hypertrophic cervix

    h. Spontaneous or easily induced cervical bleeding

    i. Cervical tenderness

    j. Suprapubic tenderness

2. Males

    a. Whitish, clear or purulent urethral discharge

    b. Dysuria

    c. Epididymitis

3. Neonate

    a. Chlamydial conjunctivitis

    b. Develops a few days to several weeks after birth and lasts 1 to 2 weeks

    c. Asymptomatic infection of rectum/vagina of infant can persist for up to 2 years

- Differential Diagnosis
  1. Urethritis
  2. Salpingitis
  3. Endometritis
  4. Vaginitis
  5. Gonorrhea

- Diagnostic Tests/Findings
  1. Gold standard is cervical tissue culture—positive if inclusion bodies present
  2. Rapid antigen detection tests
     a. Direct fluorescent staining for elemtary bodies in clinical specimens using monoclonal antibody (DFA)
     b. Enzyme immunoassay (EIA)

       c. DNA probe—test has been evaluated primarily in adult females; utility in other populations not yet well documented

    3. Presumptive diagnosis made when the gram stain reveals > 30 polymorphonucleocytes (PMNs) hpf in cervical mucus, few bacteria and *no* gram-negative intracellular diplococci

■ Management/Treatment

    1. Drainage/secretion precautions for duration of illness in patients with conjunctivitis or genital tract disease

    2. Genital tract infections in adolescents

       a. Oral doxycycline 200 mg/day in 2 divided doses for 7 days *OR*

       b. Azithromycin in a single 1 g oral dose

       c. Alternatives are oral erythromycin base 2.0 g/day in 4 divided doses for 7 days *OR* erythromycin ethylsuccinate 3.2 g/day in 4 divided doses for 7 days; also recommended therapy for pregnant patients and young children; a second course of therapy may be needed because of decreased efficacy

    3. Conjunctivitis and pneumonia in young infants

       a. Oral erythromycin 50 mg/kg/day in 4 divided doses for 14 days

       b. Oral sulfonamides after immediate neonatal period for infants who do not tolerate erythromycin

       c. Topical treatment of conjunctivitis ineffective

       d. Second course of treatment may be required

    4. Treatment for gonorrhea should include treatment for chlamydia since infections frequently coexist

    5. Emphasize importance of complete treatment

    6. Avoid sexual intercourse until patient and partner(s) complete treatment

    7. Education regarding increased risk of PID and fertility problems with repeated infections; risk of HIV

    8. Preventive measures

       a. Pregnancy—treat infected women during pregnancy to prevent infant disease

       b. Screen those women less than 25 years of age and those with new or multiple sex partners

   c. Neonatal conjunctivitis—topical prophylaxis with silver nitrate, erythromycin, or tetracycline for prevention of gonococcal ophthalmia *will not* prevent neonatal chlamydia conjunctivitis

   d. Infants with conjunctivitis or pneumonia—mothers and sexual partners should be treated

   e. Sexually active adolescents—should be routinely tested for *Chlamydia* infection

   f. Sexual contacts of patients with *C. trachomatis* infection, nongonococcal urethritis, mucopurulent cervicitis, epididymitis, or PID should be evaluated for exposure to *C. trachomatis* (AAP, 1994)

Gonococcal Infections

- Definition: A major, sexually transmitted disease of concern for adolescents; one of the most common causes of lower genital tract infections in females involving the cervix

- Etiology/Incidence

  1. *Neisseria gonorrhoeae*

  2. Male-to-female transmission highter than female-to-male

  3. 1,000,000 reported cases to CDC yearly

  4. Young men 20 to 24 years of age have highest incidence followed by 15 to 19 year olds; in females highest rates in 15 to 19 year olds

  5. High infectivity, short incubation (2 to 5 days) and frequent asymptomology contribute to problem

  6. Concurrent infection with *Chlamydia trachomatis* is very common

- Clinical Findings

  1. Large percentage (80% of females) are asymptomatic in the early disease stage

  2. Infection usually localized to vagina in prepubertal girls

  3. Infection in newborn usually involves the eye

  4. Abnormal vaginal discharge

  5. Dysuria, frequency

  6. Labial tenderness, swelling (Bartholin's glands)

7. Abnormal vaginal bleeding, pelvic pain, lower abdominal pain (ascending infection)

8. Extragenital mucosal infections (pharyngitis)

9. In adolescent males, primary site of infection is usually urethra

- Differential Diagnosis

    1. *Chlamydia trachomatis* infection

    2. Urinary tract infection

    3. Extra-genital infections

    4. Pelvic inflammatory disease

    5. Fitz-Hugh-Curtis syndrome

    6. Disseminated gonorrhea

- Diagnostic Tests/Findings

    1. Culture—Thayer-Martin in 5 to 10% CO_2 to confirm diagnosis

    2. Gram stain—presence of gram negative intracellular diplococci

    3. Serologic test for syphilis—rapid plasma reagin (RPR); high coinfection rates

- Management/Treatment

    1. Goals

        a. Eliminate gonococcal infections

        b. Treat coexisting chlamydia infection (33 to 50%)

        c. Eradicate associated disease—incubating syphilis

        d. Treat sexual partner

    2. Neonatal disease—hospitalization for infants with ophthalmia, scalp abscess or disseminated infections

    3. Beyond neonatal period and in adolescents

        a. Prepubertal who weigh < 45 kg with uncomplicated vulvovaginitis, urethritis, proctitis and pharyngitis

            (1) Ceftriaxone 125 mg IM in a single dose *OR*

            (2) Spectinomycin 40 mg/kg (max 2 g) IM in a single dose *PLUS*

            (3) Erythromycin 40 mg/kg/day in divided doses for 7 days

        b. Patients who weigh ≥ 45 kg and are 9 years or older with

uncomplicated endocervicitis or urethritis

    (1)   Ceftriaxone, 125 mg IM in single dose *OR*

    (2)   Ciprofloxacin, 500 mg, orally in single dose *OR*

    (3)   Cefixime, 400 mg, orally in single dose *OR*

    (4)   Ofloxacin, 400 mg, orally, in single dose *OR*

    (5)   Spectinomycin, 2 g, IM, in a single dose *PLUS*

    (6)   Doxycycline, 100 mg, orally, twice daily for 7 days *OR*

    (7)   Azithromycin, 1 g, orally, in single dose

4. Patients with uncomplicated gonorrhea who are asymptomatic after treatment need not be cultured for a test of cure

5. Preventive measures

    a. Neonatal ophthalmia

        (1)   1% silver nitrate solution *OR*

        (2)   1% tetracycline *OR*

        (3)   0.5% erythromycin instillations to both eyes immediately after birth

    b. Infants born to infected mothers—Ceftriaxone, 125 mg, IV or IM; low birth weight, 25 to 50 mg/kg

    c. Children and adolescents with sexual exposure to infected patient— should be examined, cultured and treated

    d. Adolescents—abstain from intercourse or use condoms

    e. Identification and management of high risk groups, e.g., sexually active adolescents, street youths, drug and alcohol abusers (APA, 1994)

Herpes Genitalis 2 (HSV-2)

- Definition: One of the most common sexually transmitted diseases characterized by painful vesicular lesions of the genitals

- Etiology/Incidence

1. Herpes simplex virus (HSV) type 2 (85 to 90%); type 1 (5 to 10%)

2. Due to reactivation of latent herpes virus

3. Most common in adolescents and young adults

    4.   Incubation period 2 to 14 days

■ Clinical Findings

    1.   Primary infection

        a. Symptoms may vary from none to widespread erosions

        b. Usually more symptomatic than recurrent infections

        c. Lymphadenopathy

        d. Severe pain, dysuria, dyspareunia

        e. Ulcerative lesions with an erythematous base, often covered with a purulent exudate

        f. Systemic symptoms common, e.g., fever, headache, malaise, myalgia

    2.   Recurrent infections

        a. May present with a prodrome of burning, irritation or severe pain

        b. Grouped vesicles on erythematous base can be found in localized area of genitalia following prodrome; less in number and shorter mean duration of viral shedding

    3.   In females, lesions are characteristically found around the introitus, urethral meatus or labia

    4.   In males, lesions are found on the glans penis, penile shaft or perianal region

    5.   In both sexes, lesions may spread to thighs, buttocks and surrounding areas

■ Differential Diagnosis

    1.   Traumatic lesions

    2.   Granuloma inguinale

    3.   Chancroid

    4.   Syphilis

    5.   Granuloma venereum

■ Diagnostic Tests/Findings

    1.   Tissue culture—viral detection is gold standard

    2.   Newer diagnostic techniques—direct fluorescent antibody staining of vesicle scrapings or enzyme immunoassay detection of HSV antigens

yields a more rapid diagnosis; as specific but less senstive than culture (AAP, 1994)

- Management/Treatment
  1. Symptomatic treatment
     a. Good genital hygiene
     b. Topical anesthetics
     c. Cool compresses, sitz baths
     d. Analgesia
     e. Topical (5%) acyclovir (questionable benefit)
     f. Avoidance of tight, restrictive clothing
  2. Children—acyclovir and vidarabine have been used for potentially serious infections in neonates and immunocompromised children
  3. Use of these drugs in less serious conditions has been limited to adults
     a. Primary—diminishes duration of symptoms and viral shedding
     b. Recurrent—minimal effect
  4. Encourage consistent and proper use of condoms
  5. Avoid sexual activity until lesions have healed
  6. Advise regarding increased risk of HIV

Pelvic Inflammatory Disease (P.I.D)

- Definition: Syndrome of inflammatory disorders occurring as a result of migration of microorganisms from the vagina and cervix to uterus, fallopian tubes, and contiguous structures
- Etiology/Incidence
  1. Most frequent organisms are *Neisseria gonorrhoeae* and *Chlamydia trachomatis*
  2. Other etiologic agents can include Bacteroides species; Peptostreptococcus species; *Gardnerella vaginalis*; coliform bacteria; *Mycoplasma hominis*
  3. Major consequence of sexually transmitted diseases
  4. In prepubertal females, ascending infection is uncommon
  5. Additional etiological risk factors include multiple sex partners, use of

an IUD, douching and previous episode of P.I.D.

- ■ Clinical Findings
    1. Onset of symptoms usually follows menses
    2. Clinical presentation may vary depending upon causative organism, affected structures and severity of the disease; may be asymptomatic
    3. Lower abdominal pain
    4. Fever
    5. Increased vaginal discharge
    6. Irregular vaginal bleeding
    7. Pelvic examination reveals a purulent cervical discharge
    8. Tenderness on motion of the cervix (chandelier's sign)
    9. Adnexal tenderness
    10. Diagnostic criteria according to Centers for Disease Control and Prevention (1991)
        a. Oral temperature > 38.3 °C
        b. Abnormal cervical or vaginal discharge
        c. Elevated ESR and/or C-reactive protein
        d. Culture or gram stain antigen/detection assay evidence of cervical infection with *N. gonorrhoeae* or *C. trachomatis*
- ■ Differential Diagnosis
    1. Cervicitis/vaginitis
    2. Acute abdomen
    3. Urinary tract infections
    4. Ectopic pregnancy
- ■ Diagnostic Tests/Findings
    1. Pregnancy test—to rule out pregnancy
    2. ESR, WBC, C-reactive protein (CRP)
        a. Elevated values suggest inflammation
        b. Non of these tests are specific for P.I.D.
    3. Microbiologic work-up confirms diagnosis
        a. Cervical culture for *N. gonorrhoeae*

    b. Cervical culture or antigen detection test for *C. trachomatis*

- Management/Treatment
  1. Goals
     a. Treat infection
     b. Prevent infertility and other chronic residua
  2. Inpatient/outpatient controversy
     a. Aggressive inpatient treatment minimizes risk of noncompliance and inaccurate diagnosis
     b. Outpatient
        (1) Early intervention
        (2) Broad spectrum antibiotics to address polymicrobial nature
        (3) Reevaluation within 48 hours
        (4) Evaluate and treat partners
        (5) Pharmacotherapy (ambulatory)—cefoxitin 2 g, IM with concurrent probenecid 1 g, orally *OR* equivalent cephalosporin *PLUS* Doxycycline 100 mg, orally, 2 times a day for 14 days *OR* for patients older than 18 years, oxfloxacin 400 mg, orally, 2 times a day for 14 days *PLUS* Clindamycin 450 mg, orally 4 times a day, or metronidazole 500 mg, orally, 2 times a day for 14 days (AAP, 1994)
        (6) Test of cure 4 to 7 days following treatment for isolated pathogens
  3. Criteria for hospitalization
     a. Possibly all adolescents
     b. Presence of pelvic or tubo-ovarian abscess
     c. Pregnancy
     d. T > 38.3 °C
     e. Nausea and vomiting precluding oral medications
     f. I.U.D. in place
     g. Failure of outpatient treatment in 48 hours
  4. Sequelae
     a. Short term

              (1)   Perihepatitis (Fitz-Hugh-Curtis syndrome)

              (2)   Tubo-ovarian abscess and rupture

      b. Long term

              (1)   Involuntary infertility (21%)

              (2)   Ectopic pregnancy (5%)

              (3)   Chronic pelvic pain

              (4)   Dyspareunia

              (5)   Pelvic adhesions

  5. Education

      a. Prevention

      b. Early recognition

      c. Partner treatment

      d. Sequelae

      e. Follow-up

Urethritis

■ Definition: Inflammation of the urethra

■ Etiology/Incidence

  1. Almost always sexually acquired

  2. Most common cause is infection with *Chlamydia trachomatis, Neisseria gonorrhoeae, Mycoplasma, Trichomonas vaginalis*, herpes simplex virus or coliform bacteria

■ Clinical Findings

  1. Symptoms may be absent

  2. Urethral discharge (especially purulent, mucoid yellow-green)

  3. Urinary frequency

  4. Burning, itching at distal urethra

■ Differential Diagnosis

  1. Normal discharge

  2. Gonococcal or nongonococcal

■ Diagnostic Tests/Findings

1. Gram stain smear of urethral secretions > 5 leukocytes—urethritis; gram negative intracellular diplococci; probable gonococcal

2. Urine—> 10 to 15 WBC in sediment of first catch

3. Cultures for *C. trachomatis* and *N gonorrhea*—positive for offending organism

- Management/Treatment

    1. Antibiotics based on source of infection

    2. Treat sexual partners presumptively

    3. Education regarding prevention, detections, risks (HIV)

    4. Follow-up

Questions

Select the best answer

1. Which of the following statements regarding undescended testes is true?

   a. Decreased incidence of inguinal hernias
   b. Primarily due to increased testosterone levels
   c. Tendency toward later repair leads to increased chance for adult fertility
   d. Usually spontaneous descent before end of first year

2. Which of the following findings are typical of an inguinal hernia?

   a. A painless intermittent or constant inguinal swelling
   b. Irritability, groin or abdominal discomfort common symptoms
   c. Translucent upon transillumination
   d. Found more frequently in full-term females

3. Which of the following statements regarding acute poststreptococcal glomerulonephritis is true?

   a. It is the most common form of nephritis in children
   b. It typically occurs in the 18 months to 3-year age range
   c. It can be prevented by penicillin
   d. The interval between infection with nephritogenic group A ß-hemolytic strep and onset of glomerulonephritis is typically 4 to 6 months

4. Acute poststreptococcal glomerulonephritis recovery is

   a. Usually complete in greater than 95% of children
   b. Dependent upon a full course of antibiotic treatment for 14 to 28 days
   c. Usually poor if hypertension is present
   d. Associated with a decrease in heterophil titer levels

5. An unretractable foreskin found upon physical examination in a 9-month-old is most probably

   a. Related to poor hygiene
   b. Reason to refer to a urologist to rule out phimosis
   c. A congenital abnormality
   d. Developmentally normal

6. A 12-year-old boy awakens suddenly with onset of severe, unilateral scrotal pain, nausea and vomiting. He is afebrile. Inspection reveals an acutely tender scrotum and marked scrotal edema. The most likely cause is

   a. Scrotal trauma

b. Mumps orchitis
c. Acute epididymitis
d. Testicular torsion

7. An 8-year-old boy has primary nocturnal enuresis. The history is otherwise unremarkable, and findings on physical examination are normal. Urinalysis, including a measure of concentrating ability, is normal; culture of the urine is sterile. His parents ask what they can do to assist in the treatment of this problem. Your response might suggest

   a. Maturation of the urinary tract is the best they can hope for
   b. That conditioning devices are probably worthless
   c. That fluid restriction and voiding prior to and during the night may be effective measures
   d. That medications such as imipramine will provide the best long-term relief

8. Amy, an 8-year-old female, is seeing you today for acute onset of dysuria. Which of the following is least likely to occur with a cystitis?

   a. Enuresis
   b. Colony count less than 10,000 colonies/mL
   c. Colony count greater than 100,000 colonies/mL
   d. Urgency, frequency

9. Which of the following laboratory findings is probably most helpful in differentiating an upper from a lower urinary tract infection?

   a. More than 100,000 organisms/mL
   b. Hematuria and proteinuria
   c. Presence of occasional casts
   d. Presence of 1 or 2 WBCs

10. Significant labial adhesions are best treated

    a. With forceful separation
    b. With vitamin A and D ointment
    c. With estrogen containing cream applications
    d. Sitz baths t.i.d. followed by petroleum jelly applications

11. Which of the following facts regarding Toxic Shock Syndrome is true?

    a. It is associated with toxic strains of *Escherichia coli*
    b. Approximately 10% of cases occur in males
    c. The incidence peaked in 1985 and it is no longer seen in the U.S.
    d. Hypertension is a frequent finding

12. Orchiopexy for repair of undescended testicles is usually performed when?

    a. At birth

b. Before school age
c. Before onset of puberty
d. Between 1 to 3 years

13. The most common penile abnormality in the U.S. is

   a. Phimosis
   b. Paraphimosis
   c. Meatal atresia
   d. Hypospadias

14. Urinary tract infections are more common in females than males in all age groups except

   a. Newborns
   b. Toddlers
   c. School age children
   d. Adolescents

15. A child with a documented urinary tract infection has what kind of risk for further infections?

   a. No increased risk
   b. Increased risk greatest during two-year period following first infection
   c. Increased risk throughout life
   d. Increased risk only if first infection not treated effectively

16. Risk factors for development of UTI include

   a. Infrequent voiding
   b. Circumcision
   c. Hydrocoele
   d. Small for gestational age

17. The most common pathogens in UTIs in sexually active adolescents include

   a. *E. coli* and Staphylococcus saprophyticus
   b. Adenovirus and *E. coli*
   c. Group D streptococcus and enterobacter
   d. *Klebsiella* and *E. coli*

18. Almost any number of colonies growing in a urine culture are indicative of an infection, except for the following collection method

   a. Suprapublic tap
   b. Catheterization
   c. Urethral aspiration
   d. Clean catch midstream

19. Typical physical findings in a patient suspected to have acute poststreptococcal

glomerulonephritis include

a. Hypotension
b. Hepatosplenomegaly
c. Renal mass
d. Periorbital edema

20. The most common type of enuresis is

a. Primary diurnal
b. Secondary nocturnal
c. Primary nocturnal
d. Mixed

21. Which statement is true regarding nocturnal enuresis?

a. The male/female ratio is equal in all age groups
b. It occurs in 45% of 5-year-old boys
c. Treatment should begin by 4½ to 5 years
d. Prevalence at age 10 is 3% for males and 2% for females

22. Vulvovaginitis in a prepubertal child

a. Is most frequently an indication of child abuse
b. Is usually caused by *Neisseria gonorrhoeae*
c. May be a risk factor for development of labial adhesions
d. Is an infrequent finding

23. Which of the following is the most prevalent vaginal infection in sexually active females?

a. *Trichomonas vaginalis*
b. Physiologic leukorrhea
c. *Candida tropicalis*
d. Bacterial vaginosis

24. Characteristic clinical findings in bacterial vaginosis include

a. Vulvar edema
b. Cervical erosion
c. Cheesy, white vaginal discharge
d. Grey-white vaginal discharge

25. A positive amine test is expected with

a. Vulvovaginal candidiasis
b. Bacterial vaginosis
c. *Chlamydia trachomitis* cervicitis
d. Gonococcal cervicitis

26. Which of the following laboratory findings is not typical of vaginal candidiasis?

    a. Vaginal pH of 6.0 or greater
    b. Gram stain with pseudohyphae, hyphae
    c. KOH prep—presence of spores or buds
    d. Presence of *C. Albicans*

27. Treatment of bacterial vaginosis might include

    a. Topical miconazole (Monistat)
    b. Metronidazole orally
    c. Tetracycline orally
    d. Ceftriaxone IM

28. A gram stained smear of cervical mucous reveals 38 PMN/hpf; no gram-negative intracellular diplococci and a few bacteria. This is consistent with a diagnosis of of

    a. Gonococcal cervicitis
    b. Bacterial vaginosis
    c. *Trichomonas vaginalis*
    d. *Chlamydia trachomatis*

29. Which statement is true regarding gonococcal infections?

    a. Male to female transmission of *N. gonorrhoeae* is higher than female to male
    b. The majority of cases occur in the third decade of life
    c. Incubation period is long (14 to 28 days)
    d. Very few females are asymptomatic

30. The test that is regarded as the "gold standard" in detecting herpes simples virus is

    a. Tzanck smear
    b. Tissue culture/viral isolation
    c. RPR
    d. Gram stain

Answer key

1. d		16. a	
2. a		17. a	
3. a		18. d	
4. a		19. d	
5. d		20. c	
6. d		21. d	
7. c		22. c	
8. b		23. d	
9. b		24. d	
10. c		25. b	
11. b		26. a	
12. d		27. b	
13. d		28. d	
14. a		29. a	
15. b		30. b	

Bibliography

Abramowicz, M. (1990). Treatment of sexually transmitted diseases. *The Medical Letter on Drugs and Therapeutics*, Vol. 32, (pp. 5-10). New Rochelle, N.Y.

ACOG Technical Bulletin # 135 Nov, 1989 "Vulvovaginitis"

American Academy of Pediatris (1994). *Report of the committee on infectious disease* (23rd ed.). Elk Grove Village, IL: American Academy of Pediatrics.

Avery, M. E., & First, L. R. (1994). *Pediatric medicine* (2nd ed.). Baltimore: Williams & Wilkins

Berry, P., & Brewers, E. (1990). Glomerulonephritis and nephrotic syndrome. In Oski & DeAngelis (Eds.), *Principles and practices of pediatrics*, (pp. 1629-1637) Philadelphia: J. B. Lippincott.

Bullough, B., & Bullough V. (1991). Contraceptives for teenagers. *Journal of Pediatric Health Care, 5*, 237-244.

Centers for Disease Control and Prevention. *Pelvic inflammatory disease: Guidelines for prevention and management.* MMWR 1991; 40 (RR-5): 1-25.

Dashefsky, B. (1993). Sexually transmitted diseases. In R. Dershewitz (Ed.), *Ambulatory pediatric care* (pp. 730-742). Philadelphia: J. B. Lippincott.

Elerian, L. F., & Adelman, R. D. (1993). Urinary tract infections in children. In F. D. Burg, J. R. Ingelfinger, & E. R. Wald (Eds.). *Gellis & Kagan's current pediatric therapy* (pp. 379-381). Philadelphia: W. B. Saunders.

Emans, S. H., & Goldstein D. P. (1990). *Pediatric and adolescent gynecology (3rd ed.).* Boston: Little, Brown and Company.

Farmer, M., Hook, E., & Heald, F. (1986). Laboratory evaluation of sexually transmitted diseases. *Pediatric Annals, 5*(10), 715-724.

Forsythe, W. E., & Butler, R. J. (1989). Fifty years of enuretic alarms. *Archives Diseases of Children, 65*, 879-885.

Hawtrey, Charles. (1990). Undescended testes and orchiopexy: Recent observations. *Pediatrics in Review*, 10, 305-310.

Holmes, K. K. (1990). *Sexually transmitted diseases* (2nd ed.). New York: McGraw-Hill.

Johal, B., Ridgeway, G. L. & Siddle, N. C. (1990). Management of pelvic inflammatory disease. *International Journal of STD and AIDS* Vol. I, 401-403.

McCracken, G. H. (1987). Diagnosis and management of acute urinary tract infections in infants and children. *Pediatric Infectious Disease Journal, 6*(1), 107-112.

Neinstein, L. S. (1991). Toxic-shock syndrome. In *Adolescent health care* (2nd ed.). (pp. 529-534). Baltimore, MD: Urban & Schwarzenberg.

Oski, F. (1990). Urinalysis and culture to detect urinary tract infections. In *principles and practices of pediatrics*, (pp. 1968-1972): Philadelphia: J. B. Lippincott.

Oski, F., McMillan J., Arnold, W, & Harmon, E. (1992). UTI controversies: Circumcision, reflux, and more. *Contemporary Pediatrics, 9*(3), 75-101.

Rau, F. J., Jones, C. E., & Muram, D. (1994). Vulvovaginitis. In J. S. Sanfilippo, D. Muram, J. Dewhurst & P. A. Lee (Eds.). *Pediatric and adolescent gynecology* (pp. 187-201). Philadelphia: W. B. Saunders.

Smith, D., & Lohr, J. (1993). Vulvovaginitis. In R. Dershewitz (Ed.), *Ambulatory pediatric care* (pp. 462-467). Philadelphia: J. B. Lippincott.

Travis, L. B. (1991). Evaluating the kidney and renal function. Infections of the urinary tract. In A. M. Rudolph (Ed.), *Pediatrics* (19th ed.). (pp. 1236-1239, 1288-1293). Norwalk, CT: Appleton-Lange.

Gastrointestinal Disorders

Elizabeth Hawkins-Walsh

Hirschsprung Disease (congenital aganglionic megacolon)

- Definition
  1. Absence or deficiency of ganglion cells from the submucosal and intermuscular regions of the intestinal wall; not limited to the colon
  2. Peristalsis in involved segment absent or abnormal
  3. Results in continuous, smooth muscle spasm with partial or complete obstruction and massive dilation of proximal bowel
- Etiology/Incidence
  1. Caused by absence of ganglion cells from myenteric plexus
  2. More common in males
  3. Rare in low birth-weight infants; increased risk in siblings
  4. Incidence is 1 in 5000 live births
- Clinical Findings
  1. Neonatal
     a. Failure to pass meconium
     b. Abdominal distention (may be severe)
     c. Vomiting
     d. Poor feeding
  2. Later
     a. Chronic constipation
     b. Abdominal distention
     c. Poor feeding
     d. Diarrhea
     e. Loose, small infrequent stools
     f. Unexplained fever
     g. Failure to thrive
  3. Physical Findings
     a. Enlarged, distended abdomen; fecal masses palpable
     b. Empty rectal ampulla

   c. Respiratory distress (newborn)

   d. Growth failure

- Differential Diagnosis

   1. Meconium ileus

   2. Meconium plug syndrome

   3. Colonic inertia

   4. Ileal atresia

   5. Chronic idiopathic constipation

   6. Obstipation

- Diagnostic Tests/Findings

   1. Barium enema—can confirm localized constriction with proximal dilation; less useful with infants

   2. Rectal biopsy (absence of ganglion cells)

   3. Radiographic studies—gaseous distention and absence of gas in rectum with patient in prone position

   4. Anorectal manometry—rise in pressure with megacolon; newborns may not exhibit reflex

- Management/Treatment—surgical referral; resection of aganglionic segment followed by a pull through procedure of normal intestine to anal canal

Intussusception

- Definition: Intestinal obstruction caused by invagination of one segment of bowel, usually the terminal ileum, into the cecum

- Etiology/Incidence

   1. Cause is unknown

   2. Most common cause of intestinal obstruction in children 1 month to five years

   3. Highest incidence between 3 months and 2 years of age

   4. 2:1 male-to-female ratio

- Clinical Findings

   1. Previously healthy infant presents with intense pain which causes child

to draw knees to chest

2. Pain lasts for several minutes; child becomes quiet following pain

3. In early stages—nonbilious emesis

4. Bilious vomiting usually indicative of mechanical bowel obstruction

5. Diarrhea—"current jelly" stools usually occur several hours after the onset of pain

6. Physical findings—depend on duration of intussusception and degree of bowel involvement

   a. Sausage-shaped mass often palpable in right upper quadrant of abdomen

   b. Abdominal distention and tenderness develop as intestinal obstruction becomes more acute

   c. Fever

   d. Bloody mucus on rectal examination

   e. Shock-like state develops if intussusception not reduced

- Differential Diagnosis

  1. Anaphylactoid purpura

  2. Enterocolitis

  3. Volvulus

  4. Gastroenteritis

  5. Incarcerated hernia

- Diagnostic Tests/Findings: Barium enema diagnostic procedure of choice; also therapeutic

- Management/Treatment: Rapid referral for reduction (medical or surgical)

Pyloric Stenosis

- Definition: Congenital hypertrophy of circular muscle of pyloric sphincter, resulting in an obstructive process

- Etiology/Incidence

  1. Unknown; appears to be genetic basis of inheritance

  2. Affects 1:150 male infants and 1:750 female infants

  3. Slight familial incidence

■ Clinical Findings

1. Not present at birth

2. Vomiting after feedings—progressive, non-bilious, projectile usually 2 to 4 weeks after birth; vomiting progresses in intensity

3. "Hungry" infant

4. Poor weight gain

5. Constipation

6. Eventual dehydration

7. Physical Findings

    a. Visible gastric peristaltic waves from left to right across abdomen

    b. Palpable pyloric "olive"

        (1) A firm, mobile, non-tender mass to right of umbilicus, below liver edge

        (2) Palpated most easily following vomiting

    c. Dehydration—variable

    d. Lethargy and irritability as process continues

■ Differential Diagnosis

1. Food related disorders

    a. Overfeeding

    b. Improper handling

    c. Milk allergy

2. Gastroesophageal reflux

3. Gastroenteritis

4. Adrenal insufficiency

■ Diagnosis Tests/Findings

1. Radiographic studies show elongated, narrow pyloric canal ("string sign"); delayed or no gastric emptying

2. Blood chemistries to R/O electrolyte imbalances

■ Management/Treatment: Refer for surgical evaluation

Colic

- Definition: A complex of symptoms which includes paroxysmal severe crying episodes (may persist for several hours); apparent abdominal pain and irritability in an otherwise healthy infant

- Etiology/Incidence

  1. Cause of colic unknown; no consistent correlation with birth order, race, socioeconomic status, breast/bottle feeding, age or emotional health of parents

  2. Incidence unknown due to lack of agreement on precise definition; usually occurs in infants less than 3 months of age

- Clinical Findings— usually presents by 2 to 4 weeks of age and resolves by 3 to 4 months

  1. Spells of unexplained irritability, fussiness or crying; behaviors differ in degree among infants

  2. Face may be flushed, may have circumoral pallor; abdomen may be distended; legs may be drawn up to abdomen and hands clenched; frequent flatus

  3. Episodes are rhythmic, usually occurring in evening, lasting from 3 to 5 hours or longer

  4. Normal physical examination

- Differential Diagnosis

  1. "Normal crying" in infant whose parents have low tolerance

  2. Intolerance or allergy to formula or substances in diets of breast feeding mothers

  3. Intestinal obstruction

  4. Incarcerated hernia

  5. Otitis media

  6. Peritoneal infection

  7. Pyelonephritis

- Diagnostic Tests: None.

- Management/Treatment

  1. Detailed history of sleep, diet, crying, "typical day," soothing

techniques; parental concerns

2. Parental support/counseling

a. Reassure parents that physical examination is normal

b. Educate parents regarding average amount of time infants of particular age cry

c. Acknowledge the stress and difficulty of caring for infants when they cry more than average

d. Discuss factors which seem to trigger or increase crying

e. Correct any recognized existing problems with feeding techniques. (under/over feeding, sucking, burping, etc.)

f. Changes in formula composition, while frequently tried, are seldom effective unless true allergy or intolerance exist; breastfeeding mothers occasionally can identify particular foods in their diet which appear to increase crying

g. Help parents learn to read and respond to their infant's cues

(1) To gauge readiness for interaction

(2) To recognize fatigue

(3) To avoid over stimulation

h. Discuss effective/soothing techniques—holding baby upright, rocking, position infant in prone position across the lap

i. Medication use is controversial and questionably effective

j. A supportive, sympathetic health professional is important in the treatment process

k. Close follow-up:

(1) Telephone every 1 to 2 days until improvement

(2) Re-evaluate in one week

Malabsorptive Disorders

■ Definition: Includes those congenital and acquired deficiency disease states of absorption and digestion which are characterized by an osmotic diarrhea as a result of inability of intestine to absorb nutrients and electrolytes normally

■ Etiology/Incidence: Malabsorptive disorders are classified according to the phase of digestion affected

1. Abnormalities of the intestinal phase

   a. Secondary lactose malabsorption is most common malabsorption in pediatrics

   b. Infectious—bacterial, viral

   c. Infestations—*Girdia lamblia*

   d. Celiac disease

   e. Selective inborn absorptive defects

2. Intraluminal phase abnormalities—cystic fibrosis

3. Malnutrition

4. Decreased conjugated bile acids

   a. Biliary atresia

   b. Hepatitis

   c. Short bowel syndrome

5. Defective delivery phase—congestive heart failure, diseases of lymphatic circulation

6. Miscellaneous—intractable diarrhea of early infancy

7. Family history may suggest genetic basis

- Clinical Findings

1. Onset of symptoms significant

2. Growth failure is most common presentation

3. Dietary history may distinguish undernutrition from malabsorption

4. Common findings

   a. Chronic diarrhea

   b. Frequent, large, pale, oily and foul smelling stools

   c. Increased flatus

   d. Abdominal distention

5. Disease-specific findings

   a. Lactose malabsorption—persistent diarrhea after infectious diarrhea; bloating; abdominal pain

   b. Cystic fibrosis—recurrent pulmonary infection; decreased muscle mass; "salty" taste; bulky, greasy stools

    c. Celiac disease—irritability, anorexia, protuberant abdomen, pallor

    d. Defects in intestinal phase processes—signs and symptoms of water soluble vitamin and mineral deficiencies

        (1)   Pallor

        (2)   Fatigue

        (3)   Anemia

        (4)   Dermatitis

        (5)   Glossitis

    e. Defects in biliary processes—deficiency of fat-soluble vitamins

        (1)   Hyperkeratosis

        (2)   Ecchymosis

        (3)   Hematuria

        (4)   Rickets

- Differential Diagnosis

    1. Undernutrition

    2. Chronic renal disease

    3. Non-gastrointestinal disease which causes small stature

- Diagnostic Tests/Findings

    1. Stool—inspection; microscopic examination and culture

        a. Occult blood—damage to intestinal mucosa

        b. Polymorphonuclear leukocytes—inflammation

        c. 3 fresh samples for ova and parasites—detect 50 to 80% of giardiasis

        d. pH < 5.5 and reducing substances—sugar malabsorption

    2. Hgb, Hct

    3. Urinalysis

    4. Sweat test > 60 mEg/L chloride—diagnostic for cystic fibrosis

    5. CBC, electrolytes—useful if abnormal

- Management/Treatment

1. Depends upon identified cause

2. Refer to gastroenterologist for further work-up

3. Secondary lactose intolerance—short-term avoidance of lactose containing foods

4. Cystic fibrosis—pancreatic enzyme replacement and fat-soluble vitamin supplements; protein and caloric supplement

5. Celiac disease—gluten-free diet; lactose-free diet until mucosa heals

Gastroesophageal Reflux

- Definition: A retrograde flow of gastric contents into the esophagus
- Etiology/Incidence

   1. Result of a neuromuscular failure of lower esophageal sphincter

   2. Occurs in 1 in 500 live births

   3. Begins in infancy; spontaneous improvement by 6 to 9 months common

   4. Spontaneous resolution believed to be related to more upright posture of older infant

- Clinical Findings—wide range based on severity

   1. Regurgitation; may have poor weight gain

   2. Esophagitis—heartburn, dysphagia

   3. Anemia; occult blood in stool

   4. Irritability

   5. Pulmonary—coughing, choking, wheezing, stridor

   6. May have abnormal posturing of head and neck

- Differential Diagnosis

   1. Gastroenteritis

   2. Milk intolerance, food intolerance

   3. Pyloric stenosis

   4. Improper feeding/handling techniques

   5. Partial intestinal obstruction

   6. Reactive airway disease

7. Neurologic disorders

- Diagnostic Tests/Findings
    1. Mild cases—none
    2. Others
        a. Upper GI series—25% false-positive results
        b. Gastric scintiscan—sensitive in detecting reflux
        c. Flexible endoscopy and esophageal biopsy—to evaluate esophagitis
        d. Prolonged pH monitoring—considered by many to be the "gold standard"; differentiates between pathologic and physiologic reflux

- Management/Treatment
    1. Mild—moderate
        a. Reassurance to parents
        b. Postural elevation one or two hours after eating; prone with head elevated if possible
        c. Small, frequent feedings with careful burping
        d. Careful weight monitoring
        e. Careful observation for signs/symptoms of aspiration
    2. Severe (F.T.T., esophageal stricture, recurrent pneumonia)
        a. Medication—metaclopramide or bethanechol, cimetidine, ranitidine
        b. Surgery—Nissen fundoplication

Acute Infectious Gastroenteritis

- Definition: A group of clinical syndromes pedominantly manifested by GI tract symptoms (anorexia, nausea or vomiting, diarrhea) of various severity

- Etiology/Incidence
    1. May affect up to 10% of infants younger than one (1) year in U.S.
    2. Reported to account for more than 3 million ambulatory pediatric— 20% of visits per year
    3. General incidence has decreased in U.S. over past decades
    4. Incidence varies with causative organism, age, season, geographic

location, and host susceptibility

5. Predisposing factors

    a. Poor sanitation

    b. Improper hand washing

    c. Improper food handling

    d. Day care

    e. Recent travel

    f. Immuno-compromised

    g. Recent antibiotics

6. Viral agents

    a. More common in winter

    b. Rotavirus—most common virus; affects all age groups, predominantly in children 6 to 24 months

    c. Norwalk—affects all ages

    d. Adenovirus—occurs during most of the year

7. Bacterial

    a. More common in summer

    b. *Campylobacter jejuni*—most common cause of bacterial gastroenteritis in children 1 to 5 years in U.S.

    c. Salmonella—may occur at any age; highest incidence in children less than 5 years; peak in first year; often secondary to food poisoning

    d. Shigella—most common in children 1 to 4 years old; prevalent in poor hygiene environments

    e. *E. Coli*—more frequent in winter; most common in newborns

    f. *Yersinia Enterocolitica*—more frequent in winter; occurs more frequently in children less than 3 years

8. Parasitic

    a. *Entamoeba histolytica (amebiasis)*—children under 5 years affected less

    b. *Giardia lambia*—most common intestinal parasite in humans world wide; more frequent in children than adults

    c. *Enterobius vermicularis* (see Pinworms)

■ Clinical Findings

    1. State of hydration

        a. Skin turgor—normal, decreased, markedly decreased

        b. Skin color—normal, pale, gray or mottled

        c. Weight loss—3 to 5%; 8 to 10%; 12 to 15%

        d. Mucous membranes—dry, parched, moist

        e. Tears—decreased, absent

        f. Urine output—mildly decreased, anuria

        g. Fontanel—flat, sunken

        h. Alertness—normal, variable, lethargic

        i. Pulse—normal, tachycardic

    2. Presence of other infectious processes that may be causing diarrhea or vomiting, e.g.,

        a. Otitis media

        b. Pneumonia

        c. Streptococcal pharyngitis

    3. Physical examination may find

        a. Hyperactive bowel sounds

        b. Diffuse abdominal tenderness

        c. Fever

        d. Splenomegaly (bacterial)

FACTORS	VIRUS	SHIGELLA	SALMONELLA	CAMPYLOBACTER	GIARDA LAMBLIA
Age	Any	1-4 yrs	Less than 5 yrs; Peaks in 1st yr	Any. Most common bacterial cause in children 1-5 yrs	Any; most common parasite in U.S.
Respiratory Symptoms	Common	Uncommon	Uncommon	Uncommon	None
Vomiting	Commonly precedes diarrhea	Common	Common	Common	Common; bloating and flatulence
Fever	Commonly precedes diarrhea	Common	Sometimes	Common	Rare
Stools Type	Large volume, less frequent watery	Watery yellow green, bloody, mucoid	Loose, slimy, green, seldom bloody	Profuse watery bloody	Loose, watery, greasy
Blood	Rare	Common	Sometimes	Common	Rarely bloody
Odor	Variable	No change	Spoiled eggs	Variable	Foul smelling
Leukocytes	Rare	Common	Common	Common	None

- ■ Differential Diagnosis
    1. Malabsorption (celiac disease, cystic fibrosis, acquired lactose deficiency)
    2. Inflammatory bowel disease
    3. Food allergy
    4. Metabolic disease
    5. Necrotizing enterocolitis
    6. Pseudomembranous colitis
    7. Reye syndrome
- ■ Diagnostic Tests/Findings
    1. Dehydration status—weight, BUN, specific gravity, electrolytes, pH, HCO_3, acid-base balance especially in infants
    2. Stool culture and sensitivity; stool for ova and parasites; WBC; reducing substances; pH

3. Urine—urinalysis, culture and sensitivity

■ Management/Treatment

1. Most diarrhea and vomiting is benign and self-limiting

2. Most important aspect of management is to assess degree of dehydration; correct existing dehydration, restore and maintain fluid and electrolytes and acid-base balance

3. Infants are particularly at risk for rapid dehydration; concomitant fever accelerates risk of dehydration

4. Approach to management of dehydration is changing from use of intravenous fluids to increasing use of oral rehydration

5. The American Academy of Pediatrics Committee on Nutrition recommends

   a. Oral rehydration fluids to treat mild, moderate or severe dehydration

   b. Rehydration fluid therapy should consist of glucose-electrolyte solutions with 75 to 90 mmol/L of sodium

   c. Maintenance fluid therapy should consist of glucose-electrolyte solutions with 40 to 60 mmol/L of sodium

   d. Carbohydrate-to-sodium ratios should never exceed 2:1 ratio in either type of therapy

   e. Feeding should be reintroduced within 24 hours of onset of diarrhea and may include breast milk, dilute formula, or milk for infants, and rice cereal, potatoes, bananas for older infants and children (Offit, 1993)

6. "Bowel rest" probably not necessary in most cases; advance to normal diet as soon as possible to avoid "starvation" diarrhea

7. Most home remedies (Jello, Gatorade, soft drinks) contain inappropriately high concentrations of carbohydrates and low sodium concentrations

8. Nursing mothers may continue to breast feed

9. Inadequate circulating blood volume necessitates intravenous therapy

10. Hospitalization may be indicated if compliance of caregiver is questionable or if excessive vomiting interferes with rehydration

11. Antimicrobials not generally indicated except for select cases to

shorten clinical course, decrease excretion of causative organism or to prevent complications

  a. Shigella—TMP-SMX

  b. Infants < 3 months with salmonella in whom sepsis is suspected— ampicillin or chloramphenicol or TMP-SMX or cefotaxime

  c. Campylobacter infections identified early in course of illness— erythromycin

  d. *Giardia lamblia*—quinacrine, furazolidone, metronidazole

  e. *Entamoeba histolytica*—iodoquinal, metronidazole

  f. Enterobius Vermicularis (see Pinworms)

12. Use of antidiarrheal agents discouraged

13. Temporary lactose or sucrose intolerance may occur in 20% of infants following infectious diarrhea; formula may be substituted with non-lactose, non-sucrose formula for short period

Pinworms (Enterobiasis)

- Definition: Most common helminth infestation in U.S.
- Etiology/Incidence
  1. *Enterobius vermicularis*
  2. Usually affects children; estimated 20% of children in U.S. harbor this parasite; more common in crowded environments
  3. Transmitted fecal-oral route; food, drink, fomites and inhaled dust also implicated
- Clinical Findings
  1. Nocturnal anal pruritis (hallmark of infection)
  2. Vaginal itching, discharge, vulvar pruritis
  3. Dysuria
  4. Irritibility
  5. Insomnia
  6. Evidence of eczematous dermatitis of perianal and perineal areas
- Differential Diagnosis
  1. Anal fissure

2. Perianal and perineal irritation secondary to urinary tract infections, bubble bath

3. Sexual abuse

4. Vaginal foreign body

- Diagnostic Test/Findings

   1. "Scotch tape" test—tape is pressed against perianal area on 3 to 5 successive mornings prior to bathing and before child defecates; eggs detected on microscopic examination; 3 negative results following treatment, 1 week apart, indicate eradication

   2. Direct use of stool for egg detection unreliable diagnostic method

- Management/Treatment

   1. Medication

      a. Pyrantel pamoate (Antiminth)—11 mg/kg orally for one dose; repeated in 2 weeks

      b. Mebendazole (Vermox)—100 mg orally for one dose (same dose all body weights); repeated in 2 weeks

      c. Piperazine citrate (Vermizine)—65 mg/kg/day for 7 days (maximum 2.5 g/day)

   2. Treatment of entire family simultaneously usually recommended

   3. Prevention directed at good personal hygiene

      a. Careful hand washing before meals and after toilet use

      b. Avoid thumb sucking

      c. Avoid scratching affected areas

      d. Keep nails short and clean

      e. Frequent laundering of linens, undergarments in hot H_2O

      f. Wash toilet seats

   4. Reassurance that pinworms rarely cause serious disease

   5. Prognosis usually excellent, but high carrier rate results in frequent reinfection

Constipation

- Definition: Passage of infrequent hard stools due to defects in either filling or emptying the rectum
- Etiology/Incidence
    1. Functional (inorganic), e.g., dietary factors; voluntary stool withholding
    2. Organic, e.g., Hirschsprung, anal-rectal stenosis, volvulus, strictures
    3. Drugs, e.g., antidepressants, narcotics, psychoactive
    4. Metabolic, e.g., dehydration, hypothyroidism, hypokalemia
    5. Neuromuscular, e.g., spinal cord lesions
    6. Psychiatric, e.g., anorexia nervosa
- Clincial Findings
    1. Organic constipation commonly presents during first months of life
    2. Infants who eliminate only 1 to 2 times per day during first month may be showing a hereditary predisposition toward constipation
    3. In latter part of first year or second year, straining, streaks of blood on hard stool with infrequent defecation may appear
    4. Physical examination frequently reveals a distended abdomen with a palpable round mass in lower left quadrant
    5. Child with functional constipation will generally have normal anal sphincter tone and large rectal vault
    6. Internal rectal examination—used to evaluate presence of impaction
- Differential Diagnosis: Determine differences between organic and nonorganic (functional) as stated previously
- Diagnostic Tests/Findings: None indicated unless organic pathology suspected
- Management/Treatment
    1. Infants younger than 6 months with tendency toward constipation will benefit from introduction of apricots, prunes, pineapple, non-starchy vegetables and an occasional water or juice bottle; rice cereal should be avoided; may be necessary to give dark corn syrup or Maltsupex, 1 to 2 teaspoons 1 to 3 times daily (may aggravate colicky infant);

glycerin suppositories may be used as an alternative

2. In toddlers and young children with voluntary stool withholding due to painful elimination, initial treatment may include 1 to 2 hypertonic phosphate enemas followed by mild laxatives for 1 to 2 weeks to establish painless, regular bowel training

3. Maltsupex; prunes, apricots, raisins, bran products; liberal water and juice intake

Encopresis

■ Definition: Repeated fecal incontinence in the absence of organic defect or illness by a child older than 4 years of age

■ Etiology/Incidence

1. Often associated with constipation

2. Withholding stool results in functional or acquired megacolon with need for progressively larger stools to stimulate defecation

3. Is often a complication of fecal impaction and consists of involuntary seepage of liquid stool beyond fecal bolus

4. Vicious cycle may ensue—constipation → pain → withholding → acquired megacolon → larger stool → constipation

5. Estimated to affect 2 to 3% pre-school and elementary school-aged children

6. Greater incidence in boys than girls

■ Clinical Findings

1. Stool incontinence/"dribbling"

2. Abdominal pain; abdominal distention; anorexia

3. Moodiness

4. Enuresis (30%)

5. Retentive posturing

6. Physical Findings

   a. Physical examination is usually normal

   b. Abdominal examination may be normal, or may reveal soft, non-tender mass in midline or lower left quadrant

   c. Rectal examination may reveal decreased anal tone, large, distended rectal vault and hard, formed or soft, liquid stool

    d. Anal sphincter may show fissure/irritation

- Differential Diagnosis
  1. Hirschsprung's Disease
  2. Irritable bowel disease
  3. Chronic, intermittent diarrhea
  4. Hypothyroidism, hypopituitary, hypercalcemia
  5. Crohn disease, ulcerative colitis
  6. Lead intoxication
  7. Anal stricture/fissure
  8. Neuromuscular, spinal cord lesion, cerebral palsy
  9. Obstructive uropathy

- Diagnostic Tests/Findings
  1. Usually none; occasionally an abdominal radiograph is used to assess volume of impacted stool and rectal/colonic distention
  2. Females—urinalysis, urine culture; for possible concomitant UTI

- Management/Treatment
  1. Goals
     a. Establish regular bowel habits
     b. Lessen stool retention
     c. Restore neuromuscular function
     d. Minimize negative emotional impact of encopresis
  2. Initial management plan
     a. Counseling
        (1) Educate parents/child; should be pointed out that most soiling is an involuntary "overflow" mechanism
        (2) Remove blame
     b. Hypertonic phosphate enemas (3 ml/kg)
        (1) Each morning and evening until return is free of solid stool (not for use in those with medical problems or very young because of side effects)

(2)   Reexamine child within 3 days

c. Other modalities may include medicated suppositories; oral laxatives, e.g., bisacodyl, senna (Dulcolax or Senokot); polyethylene glycol-elecrolyte solutions (Pettei & Davidson, 1993)

3. Prevention of reaccumulation of stool

a. "Force" one or two stools daily with stimulant or osmotic laxatives (senna, cascara, milk of magnesia)

4. Final stage focuses on establishing regular bowel pattern

a. Taper laxatives as tolerated, (e.g., daily for 2 weeks, every other day for 2 to 4 weeks)

b. Bowel training—sit on toilet for 5 to 15 minutes twice daily (same times every day)

c. High fiber diet

d. Increased fluid intake

5. Follow-up

a. Telephone availability as necessary

b. Periodic office visits, depending on severity, need, compliance

(1)   Disorder can be chronic and recurrent

(2)   Treatment should continue for a prolonged period (usual is a minimum of 6 months)

c. Counsel/refer for associated psychosocial issues

6. Treatment resistant—refer to child psychiatrist/pediatric gastroenterologist

Appendicitis

- Definition: An acute inflammation of the vermiform appendix
- Etiology/Incidence—usually due to an obstruction of the appendix by fecal material or foreign body which causes stasis in appendix

1. Rare before 2 years; peak age between 15 and 24 years of age

2. Slightly higher incidence in males

3. Increased incidence in spring and fall

4. Familial tendency

■ Clinical Findings

1. Poorly localized periumbilical or mid-abdominal pain initially; typically pain migrates to right lower quadrant (classic presentation); appendix may be in an abnormal position and produce flank or upper abdominal pain

2. Anorexia

3. Vomiting (variable)—seldom precedes pain

4. Diarrhea or constipation

5. Low-grade fever

6. If appendix ruptures, child may report less pain; as infection spreads, diffuse abdominal pain with tenderness, vomiting and malaise follows

7. Physical findings

   a. Abdominal tenderness/rigidity

      (1) McBurney's Point (in older child); right iliac fossa (younger child)

      (2) Bowel sounds may be depressed or hyperactive

      (3) Peritoneal signs

      (4) Rectal examination—may show tenderness

■ Differential Diagnosis

1. Gastroenteritis

2. Constipation

3. Urinary tract infection

4. Pelvic inflammatory disease

5. Ruptured ectopic pregnancy

6. Ovarian torsion

7. Sickle cell crisis

8. Lower lobe pneumonia

9. Inflammatory bowel disease

10. Intussusception

11. Mesenteric lymphadenitis

12. Diabetic ketoacidosis

■ Diagnostic Tests/Findings

1. CBC—WBC 10,000-20,000/mm^3

2. Urinalysis—to rule out urinary tract infection

3. Radiograms may detect calcified appendicolith, intestinal obstruction

4. Ultrasound—for diagnosis of nonperforated appendicitis

■ Management/Treatment: Immediate referral for surgical consultation

Recurrent Abdominal Pain (Chronic Non-specific Abdominal Pain of Childhood)

■ Definition: Defined as 3 or more episodes of abdominal pain, without organic pathology, that interferes with normal activity over a 3-month period of time

■ Etiology/Incidence

1. Little specific information available concerning pathophysiologic mechanisms

2. Pain sensations presumed to originate from nerve endings in submucosa, musculature, or serosa of abdominal organs

3. No evidence of consistent pattern of psychopathology; stress is sometimes a factor

4. Affects 10 to 15% of school-aged population

5. Problem predominately in preadolescence

6. Increased family prevalence

7. About 5 to 10% of affected children have organic disease

■ Clinical Findings

1. Patient usually looks well

2. Pain episodes usually lasting less than one hour; inconsistent in its relationship to food and activity

3. Bowel dysfunction and vomiting are commonly associated symptoms

4. No symptoms of organic disease

5. Some may report headaches and limb pain at other times

6. Nighttime awakening is usually absent

7. Physical Findings—normal

- Differential Diagnosis
  1. Appendicitis
  2. Mesenteric lymphadenitis
  3. Peptic ulcer
  4. Inflammatory bowel disease
  5. Constipation/chronic stool retention
  6. Malabsorption/lactose intolerance
  7. Parasites
  8. Lead poisoning
  9. Pelvic inflammatory disease
  10. Urinary tract infection
  11. Cholecystitis
  12. Meckel's diverticulum
  13. Sickle cell
  14. Migraine (abdominal expression)
  15. Endometriosis
  16. Malingering
- Diagnostic Test/Findings: Most often a diagnosis of exclusion
- Management/Treatment
  1. Identify significant sources of environmental or interpersonal stress in child or family
  2. Identify impact of recurrent pain on children and family
  3. Assist family/child to recognize existing situations/dynamics which may be associated with the abdominal pain
  4. Encourage development of healthy coping mechanisms in response to stress

Inflammatory Bowel Disease (IBD)

- Definition
  1. Disorder characterized primarily by chronic intestinal inflammation of unknown cause

2. Crohn disease and ulcerative colitis are the two major forms in children; believed to be two separate disorders, they share many clinical features

3. Ulcerative colitis involves only the colon

4. Crohn disease may affect any part of the gastrointestinal tract

- Etiology/Incidence

1. Pathogenesis unknown

2. Theoretically, a genetically determined immunologic response to an environmental trigger

3. No evidence that diet or emotional factors are primary cause

4. Incidence of ulcerative colitis is between 3 and 15/100,000 per year and 5 and 8/100,000 per year for Crohn disease

5. Age of presentation for ulcerative colitis ranges from 15 to 25 years; Crohn disease rarely occurs before age 10 and 25 to 40% begin before 20 years of age

6. Positive family history, usually

- Clinical Findings

1. Abdominal pain

   a. In right lower quadrant related to food intake typical in Crohn disease

   b. Lower abdominal and on left more typical of ulcerative colitis

2. Weight loss

   a. More severe in Crohn disease

   b. 10 to 30% of children with IBD present with short stature

3. Bloody diarrhea — hallmark of ulcerative colitis

4. Related findings are anorexia, fatigue, anemia

5. Extraintestinal signs (more common in ulcerative colitis)

   a. Skin lesions

   b. Arthritis

   c. Fever

   d. Uveitis

   e. Aphthous ulcers

6. Local lymphadenopathy; perianal fistulas, tags, and abscesses common in Crohn disease

7. Abdominal examination may be normal or tender

- Differential Diagnosis: Appendicitis, infectious gastroenteritis, irritable bowel, malabsorption disorders, peptic ulcer disease, rheumatoid arthritis, systemic lupus erythematosus

- Diagnostic Tests

1. No single diagnostic test

2. CBC—leukocytosis; microcytic anemia with low serum iron and elevated total iron-binding capacity

3. Erythrocyte sedimentation rate—often elevated

4. Serum total protein and albumin—low with undernutrition and protein losing enteropathy

5. Stool or blood; rule out bacterial pathogens

6. Radiologic examination of gastrointestinal tract used to define extent of lesions; in Crohn disease, lesions can occur from esophagus to anus with intervening skip (normal) areas

7. Colonoscopic examination—in ulcerative colitis, continuous lesions occur from rectosigmoid up to unaffected area

- Management/Treatment

1. Refer to pediatric gastroenterologist

2. Appropriate therapy requires a specific diagnosis, sites of gastrointestinal tract affected and assessment of disease severity

3. Treatment directed toward decreasing inflammation

   a. Corticosteroids are cornerstone for moderate to severe colitis and with Crohn disease of esophagus, stomach or small intestine

   b. Sulfasalazine for colonic disease—used in treatment of mild to moderate ulcerative colitis and in Crohn disease affecting the large intestine

   c. Immunosuppressive agents for steroid dependent/resistant disease

4. Antibiotics—metronidazole to manage fistulas and perianal complications; effective in treatment of Crohn disease

5. Nutritional rehabilitation—high caloric; high protein; mineral and

vitamin supplement

6. Surgery in treatment failures

    a. Total colectomy is curative of ulcerative colitis

    b. No surgical cure for Crohn disease due to discontinuous lesions

    c. Supportive psychological care

Viral Hepatitis

■ Definition: Infection primarily or exclusively involving the liver.

■ Etiology/Incidence

1. Hepatitis A virus (HAV)—formerly known as "infectious"

    a. Most common form in pediatric population; highly contagious

    b. Incubation period 15 to 45 days

    c. Transmission from person to person by fecal-oral route

    d. Associated with ingestion of raw shellfish, overcrowding, poor sanitation; spreads readily in child care centers

2. Hepatitis B virus (HBV)—formerly known as "serum hepatitis"

    a. Incubation period 45 to 160 days

    b. Transmitted through blood or body fluids such as wound exudates, semen, cervical secretions and saliva; perinatally during delivery or during neonatal period

    c. Children at risk for infection include

        (1) Residents in institutions for developmentally disabled

        (2) Those with clotting disorders and those receiving blood products

        (3) Hemodialysis patients

        (4) Household contacts of HBV carriers

        (5) Most infected persons in U.S. acquire infection during adolescence or as an adult

3. Hepatitis C virus (HCV) (parenterally transmitted non-A, non-B hepatitis)

    a. Incubation period 14 to 170 days

    b. Transmission parenterally and possibly through sexual contact;

role of person to person contact not well defined; most cases in U.S. not associated with blood transfusions

    c. Groups at high risk include parenteral drug users, health care workers with frequent blood exposure, persons with multiple sexual partners

    d. Most frequently found in adults; infrequent in children less than 15 years of age

4. Hepatitis D virus (HDV)

    a. Only occurs with hepatitis B and spread in same manner

    b. Incubation period 45 to 160 days

    c. Endemic in Mediterranean Basin; in U.S. found most frequently in parenteral drug abusers, hemophiliacs and persons immigrating from endemic areas

    d. Transmission from mother to newborn is uncommon

5. Hepatitis E virus (enterically transmitted non-A, non-B hepatitis)

    a. Most recent type of viral hepatitis

    b. Strong association with ingestion of contaminated water in developing countries (fecal-oral route)

    c. Incidence in U.S. is very low

    d. More common in adults than children; high incidence of mortality in pregnant women

6. High-risk persons

    a. Hemodialysis patients

    b. Drug addicts

    c. Homosexual males

    d. Institutionalized patients

    e. Health professionals

■ Clinical Findings

1. Hepatitis A

    a. Produces mildest illness; infection self-limited, usually lasting less than 2 weeks

    b. In infants and preschool children most infections are asymptomatic or cause mild nonspecific symptoms without jaundice

  c. Infants may fail to gain weight

  d. Adolescents and older children may demonstrate more severe symptoms usually seen in adults

  e. Systemic symptoms may include fever, lethargy, nausea/vomiting, abdominal discomfort (may go unnoticed)

  f. Jaundice and dark-colored urine usually follow systemic symptoms, but may also be presenting symptoms

  g. Convalescent period may last several weeks with complete return of appetite, activity level, and well-being; no chronic infection or hepatitis-A carrier state

2. Hepatitis B

  a. Initial signs and symptoms may include arthralgia or macular rashes; many of the systemic manifestations are the same as hepatitis A; may last longer than hepatitis A; spectrum from mild clinical findings to fulminant fatal hepatitis

  b. Anicteric or asymptomatic infection is common in children

  c. Physical examination may show icteric skin and mucous membranes; liver may be enlarged and tender; splenomegaly and lymphadenopathy are fairly common

  d. Can result in chronic hepatitis and chronic carrier state

    (1) Chronic HVB infection with persistence of HB_sAg occurs in 90% of newborns who become infected by perinatal transmission and in 6% to 10% of older children, adolescents and adults

    (2) Occurs more frequently in immunocompromised individuals

    (3) Chronically infected persons—at increased risk for cirrhosis and hepatocellular carcinoma in later life

3. Hepatitis C

  a. Infection is usually mild or asymptomatic; onset is usually insidious with jaundice and malaise

  b. Chronic hepatitis and HCV carrier states occur in 50% of infected individuals

4. Hepatitis D

    a. Infection is clinically evident and may be severe

    b. Fulminant hepatitis may occur in chronic HBV individuals

    c. Should be suspected in those patients with severe episode of acute viral or very severe chronic hepatitis

  5. Hepatitis E

    a. Acute illness with malaise, anorexia, fever

    b. Jaundice

    c. Abdominal pain and arthralgia

- Differential Diagnosis
  1. Biliary atresia
  2. Infectious mononucleosis
  3. Leptospirosis
  4. Toxoplasmosis
  5. Choledochal cysts
  6. Hemolytic-uremic syndrome
  7. Reye syndrome
  8. Lupus erythematosus
  9. Juvenile rheumatoid arthritis
  10. Inflammatory bowel disease
  11. Sickle cell liver disease
  12. Liver dysfunction secondary to drug exposure
  13. Wilson disease
  14. Cystic Fibrosis

- Diagnostic Tests/Findings
  1. Hepatitis A

    a. Serologic tests for anti-HAV and IgM

    b. Presence of IgM anti-HAV antibodies usually indicates recent infection

    c. These antibodies are replaced with IgG anti-HAV antibodies and are indicative of prior infection

2. Hepatitis B
   a. Serologic tests available to detect HBV antigens, HBsAg and HBeAg, and detection of antibodies to HBsAg (anti-HBs), antibody to hepatitis B core antigen (anti-HBc), IgM antibody to core antigen, IgM anti-HBc, and antibody to HBeAg (anti-HBe)
   b. HBsAg—identifies acutely infected persons except during "window" phase
   c. IgM anti-HBc is highly specific in establishing acute infection during early infection as well as "window phase" in older children and adults; not present, usually, in perinatal infection
   d. Chronic hepatitis B shows HBsAg and anti-HBC in serum
   e. Anti-HBc and anti-HBs—identifies individuals who have had HBV infection; persists indefinitely
   f. Anti-Hbs alone—present in persons immunized with hepatitis B vaccine

3. Hepatitis C
   a. Serologic test for anti-HCV positive in most patients
   b. False positives may be seen in other kinds of liver disease

4. Hepatitis D
   a. Presence of anti-HD in serum

5. Hepatitis E—no serologic test commercially available; diagnosis by exclusion

6. Additional diagnostic tests may be abnormal
   a. Direct and indirect serum bilirubin levels—elevated
   b. Serum transaminase—elevated
   c. WBC—leukopenia, lymphocytosis in early phase of illness
   d. IgM values—elevated, especially in hepatitis A
   e. Sedimentation rate—elevated, especially in hepatitis A; often used to monitor course of the disease

■ Management/Treatment
   1. Hepatitis A
      a. Treatment is supportive as it is for all other types of viral hepatitis;

decreased activity, nutritious diet and multivitamins are the usual recommendations

b. Hospitalization may be required for profound weakness and/or dehydration

c. Prevention

    (1) Scrupulous hand washing and thorough cleaning of eating utensils is effective in controlling spread of hepatitis A in households and child care centers

    (2) Immune globulin (IG)—highly effective in prevention or in decreasing course of disease if given early enough after exposure or before exposure; also, recommended for susceptible individuals traveling to or working where hepatitis A is endemic

    (3) Licensed HAV vaccine not available

2. Hepatitis B

a. Treatment is supportive as described for hepatitis A

b. Prevention

    (1) Since blood is common source of HBV risk of transmission is directed at identification of infected carriers

    (2) Hepatitis B vaccine

        (a) Recommended for all infants as part of routine childhood immunization schedule. See Health Maintenance/Promotion chapter

        (b) Immunization of all children during or before adolescence is necessary and recommended (see Health Maintenance/Promotion chapter)

        (c) Also recommended for health care professionals; both patients and staff in institutions; hemodialysis staff and patients; recipients of frequent blood transfusions; household and sexual contacts of HBV carriers plus a number of other specific groups and individuals (AAP, 1994)

    (3) Post-exposure prophylaxis

        (a) Percutaneous (e.g., needle stick) or permucosal (sexual exposure)—hyperimmune B, immune globulin (HBIG) and hepatitis B vaccine recommended

    (b) Newborns of mothers who are HBsAg-positive—both HBIG and hepatitis B vaccine is recommended (see Health Maintenance/Promotion chapter)

3. Hepatitis C

    a. Interferon has been approved by the Food and Drug Administration for the treatment of chronic hepatitis C; beneficial in small proportion of cases

    b. No official prophylaxis for hepatitis C; results of studies on IG have been equivocal (AAP, 1994)

4. Hepatitis D

    a. No treatment effective; supportive therapy

    b. Since HDV is always associated with an HBV infection, prevention of HBV will likewise prevent HDV

5. Hepatitis E

    a. Treatment directed at supportive therapy

    b. IG as a preventive measure has not been demonstrated

Questions

Select the best answer

1. Typical pathognominic clinical features of pyloric stenosis include all of the following, except

   a. Average age of clinical presentation is 3 weeks
   b. Progression of bile free vomiting that increases in amount and frequency
   c. Presence of a sausage-shaped mass palpated in upper right quadrant
   d. A firm, small (olive) mobile mass palpated in upper right quadrant

2. A healthy, thriving, 4-month-old boy suddenly has episodes of drawing knees to chest and screaming as if in acute abdominal pain. These episodes are separated by intervals in which baby appears normal and comfortable. This history is classic with

   a. Gastroenteritis
   b. Intussusception
   c. Pyloric stenosis
   d. Hirschbrung's Disease

3. Which of the following statements about appendicitis is untrue?

   a. Appendicitis is the most common reason for abdominal surgery in childhood
   b. Appendicitis is the most common cause of severe abdominal pain in all age groups in pediatrics
   c. Colicky abdominal pain, tenderness and fever are common signs and symptoms
   d. The most intense site of pain may be at McBurney point which is located midway between the anterior superior iliac crest and the umbilicus

4. Which of the following is not consistent with a diagnosis of nonorganic recurrent abdominal pain?

   a. May have aggravation of symptoms during times of stress and tension
   b. Nighttime awakening is usually absent
   c. Predominant in preadolescence
   d. Absence of vomiting

5. This common cause of diarrhea in children under 2 years is often seen in day care outbreaks. Stools are watery without blood or mucus.

   a. Shigella
   b. Norwalk virus
   c. Salmonella

d. Virus

6. This organism is a frequent cause of gastroenteritis in children with Sickle Cell disease. Stools are loose, slimy and may be bloody.

   a. *Campylobacter jejuni*
   b. Shigella
   c. Enterotoxigenic *E. coli*
   d. Salmonella

7. All of the following statements about gastroesophageal reflux are true, except

   a. It reflects incompetence or relaxation of the lower esophageal sphincter
   b. Usually requires surgical intervention
   c. It is sometimes associated with anemia
   d. It predisposes patient to respiratory problems

8. Although controversy exists regarding treatment of acute gastroenteritis of less than 48 hours duration, which of the following management suggestions could normally be included for a 10-month-old without evidence of dehydration

   a. Limit all foods except Gatorade or tea as tolerated until stools return to normal
   b. Discontinue breast feeding for 24 to 48 hours
   c. Stool culture x 3
   d. Continue normal diet as tolerated

9. Colic is most commonly caused by

   a. Milk allergy
   b. Poor maternal-infant attachment
   c. Intolerance to food in diet of breast feeding mother
   d. None of above

10. An ideal oral solution recommended for the acute phase of rehydration will contain

   a. 75 to 90 mmol/L of sodium
   b. 20 to 30 mmol/L of sodium
   c. 10% glucose
   d. carbohydrate to sodium ratio of 4:1

11. The most common cause of bacterial acute gastroenteritis in children between 1 and 5 years of age in the U.S. is

   a. Salmonella
   b. Norwalk agent
   c. Enterotoxigenic *E. coli*
   d. *Campylobacter jejuni*

12. The most common parasitic cause of acute gastroenteritis in children in the U.S. is

    a. *Entamoeba histolytica*
    b. *Giardia lamblia*
    c. Amebiasis
    d. *Enterobius vermicularis*

13. A child who contracts this parasite (see above) is likely to present with

    a. Loose, watery, greasy stools
    b. A brief prodrome of respiratory symptoms prior to vomiting and diarrhea
    c. Fever of > 101 degrees
    d. Bloody, non-odorous stools

14. An 11-year-old girl presents with a history of intermittent abdominal pain for the past 6 months. The finding which would be least likely to support a diagnosis of IBD is

    a. A normal abdominal examination
    b. Aphthous uclers
    c. Negative family history
    d. Weight gain of four pounds in past 6 months

15. The finding which would likely support a possible diagnosis of recurrent abdominal pain is

    a. Weight loss of 3 to 5 pounds since last visit one year ago
    b. Pain does not awaken child
    c. Infrequent headaches
    d. History of pain interfering with normal activities

16. While there is no single diagnostic test for IBD, the diagnosis could be supported by the following laboratory finding

    a. Elevated erythrocyte sedimentation rate
    b. Elevated serum total protein and albumin
    c. Leukopenia
    d. Low serum iron and low total iron-binding capacity

17. Eventually a diagnosis of IBD is made. Findings which are more common in Crohn disease than in ulcerative colitis include

    a. Bloody diarrhea and abdominal pain
    b. Fever and weight loss
    c. Perianal fistulas and abscesses
    d. Rectal bleeding and skin lesions

18. Which of the following statements reflects current understanding of IBD?

    a. Current research supports the theory that emotional stress is a primary cause of

IBD
b. Children with IBD commonly present between 7 to 10 years
c. If other treatments fail, surgery is curative for Crohn disease
d. While disease-free discontinuous areas are common in Crohn disease, the distribution of lesions in ulcerative colitis is continuous

19. The most common cause of malabsorption in pediatrics in the U.S. is

a. Cystic fibrosis
b. Secondary lactose intolerance
c. *Giardia lamblia*
d. Celiac disease

20. Stools which are described as slimy, green and smell like spoiled eggs are typical of

a. Campylobacter
b. Shigella
c. Salmonella
d. *E. coli*

21. Which of the following statements regarding encopresis is false?

a. Physical examination is usually normal
b. Soft, liquid stool in rectal vault
c. A child may present with a complaint of diarrhea
d. There is a greater incidence in girls

22. A newborn with Hirschsprung disease is likely to present with

a. Respiratory distress and scaphoid abdomen
b. Vomiting and diarrhea
c. Poor feeding and distended abdomen
d. Lethargy and tachypnea

23. The following statements regarding gastroesophageal reflux are true, except

a. Feeding adjustments such as small, frequent feedings may be sufficient treatment
b. Placing infant in a left lateral position after meals is sound advice
c. The use of medications should be reserved for more severe, unresponsive cases
d. Spontaneous improvement common, by 6 to 9 months

24. The most common cause of intestinal obstruction in children under 3 years is

a. Pyloric stenosis
b. Intussusception
c. Appendicitis
d. Volvulus

25. The most common organism causing gastroenteritis in newborns is

    a. Yersinia
    b. Rota virus
    c. Norwalk agent
    d. *E. coli*

26. Pharmacologic treatment recommendations for enterobiasis includes

    a. Mebendazole — 100 mg x 1
    b. Sulfasalazine — 50 mg/k/d x 1
    c. Azathioprine — 1.5 to 2 mg/k/d x 1
    d. Metronidazole — 15 mg/k/d x 1

27. Which of the following statements regarding colic is untrue?

    a. Colic usually presents by 1 month of age and resolves by 4 months
    b. Changing the formula or diet of the breast feeding mother usually helps
    c. Physical descriptions of an infant with distended abdomen and knees drawn to chest are consistent with colic
    d. The use of medication is controversial

28. The single most helpful test to order for a toddler with a history of poor growth, recurrent respiratory infections and bulky, greasy stools is

    a. Erythrocyte sedimentation rate
    b. Colonoscopy
    c. Stool for reducing substances, culture and O&P
    d. Sweat test

29. Nutritional management of the toddler with celiac disease includes

    a. Pancreatic enzyme replacement
    b. Gluten-free diet
    c. Fat-soluble vitamin supplements
    d. Sucrose-free diet

30. The incubation period of hepatitis B virus (HBV) is believed to last from

    a. 45 to 160 days
    b. 14 days to indefinitely
    c. 60 to 180 days
    d. 15 to 45 days

Answer Key

1.	c	16.	a
2.	b	17.	c
3.	b	18.	d
4.	d	19.	b
5.	d	20.	c
6.	d	21.	d
7.	b	22.	c
8.	d	23.	b
9.	d	24.	b
10.	a	25.	d
11.	d	26.	a
12.	b	27.	b
13.	a	28.	d
14.	d	29.	b
15.	b	30.	a

Bibliography

American Academy of Pediatrics (1994). *Report of the committee on infectious diseases* (23rd ed.). Elk Grove Village, IL: American Academy of Pediatrics.

DeWitt, T. (1989). Acute diarrhea in children. *Pediatrics in Review, 11*(1), 6-13.

DiPalma, J., & Colon, A. (1991). Gastroesophageal reflux in infants. *American Journal of Family Practice, 43*(3), 857-864.

Finberg, L. (1990). Assessing the clinical clues to dehydration. *Contemporary Pediatrics, 7*(4), 45-57.

Garcia, V., & Randolph, J. (1990). Pyloric stenosis: Diagnosis and management. *Pediatrics in Review, 11*(10) 292-295.

Israel, E. J. (1993). Inflammatory bowel disease. In R. Dershewitz (Ed.). *Ambulatory pediatric care* (2nd ed.). (pp. 415-418). Philadelphia: J. B. Lippincott.

Jackson, D. & Grand, R. (1991). Crohn's disease. In *Pediatric gastrointestinal disease*. Philadelphia: B. C. Decker.

Kirscher, B. S. (1988). Inflammatory bowel disease in children. *Pediatric Clinics of North America, 35*(2), 189-208.

Krugman, S. (1992). Viral hepatitis- A, B, C, D, and E infection. *Pediatrics in Review, 13*, 203-212.

Menveille, E., & Walsh, T. (1992). "Problems in elimination." In J. Weiner (Ed.), *Textbook of child and adolescent psychiatry*. Washington, DC: American Academy of Child Psychiatry.

Mezoff, A. & Balisteri, W. (1990). New GI therapies: Any better than antacids? *Contemporary Pediatrics, 7*(4) 101-126.

Murphy, M. S., & Walker, W. A. (1991). Celiac disease. *Pediatrics in Review, 12*, 325-330.

Nowicki, M. J., & Balisteri, W. (1992). Hepatitis A to E. *Contemporary Pediatrics, 9*(11), 118-128.

Offit, P. A. (1993). Rotavirus. In F. D. Burg, J. R. Ingelfinger, & E. R. Wald (Eds.), *Gellis & Kagan's current pediatric therapy* (14th ed.). (pp. 652-653). Philadelphia: W. B. Saunders.

Perman, J. A. & Schwartz, K. G. (1992). Hepatitis. In R. A. Hoekelman (Ed.), *Primary pediatric care* (2nd ed.). (pp. 1278-1279). St. Louis: Mosby Yearbook.

Pettei, M. J., & Davidson, M. (1993). Constipation and encopresis. In F. D. Burg,

J. R. Ingelfinger & E. R. Wald (Eds.). *Gellis & Kagan's current pediatric therapy* (14th ed.). (pp. 198-200). Philadelphia: W. B. Saunders.

Sondheimer, J., & Silverman, A. (1993). Acute infectious diarrhea. In Hathaway, Hay, Groothuis & Paisley (Eds.), *Current pediatric diagnosis & treatment* (11th ed.). (pp. 591-593). Norwalk CT: Appleton & Lange.

Trends, Professional Issues, Health Policy

Marilyn W. Edmunds
Debra Hardy Havens

Health Policy

Improvement in health is a major policy emphasis in both national goal statements (Healthy People 2000 Objectives) and international policy statements (WHO "Health for All")

■ Purpose

1. Overall objective—all persons to obtain a level of health by the year 2000 that will permit them to lead socially and economically productive lives

2. Specific objectives focus on equal access, acceptability, availability, continuity, cost and quality of care

    a. To achieve equal access to all, focus on

       (1) Establishment of community-based primary health care systems

       (2) Redistribution of health and specialty services to overcome regional inequalities

       (3) Emphasis on self-reliance and participation by the individual and community members in health matters

       (4) Increased emphasis on provision of services to specific target groups

       (5) Increased involvement of existing health organizations and groups

       (6) Expanded education of health professionals

       (7) Expansion of traditional roles

       (8) New focus by government on health rather than cure and on the roles that transportation, housing, and industry can play in bringing about a healthy society (Healthy People 2000, 1990)

    b. Acceptability

       (1) Individuals receive care that they want

       (2) Individuals receive care that is appropriate

    c. Availability

       (1) Individuals have access to health care services and facilities

       (2) Individuals have access to choice of providers

     d. Continuity

        (1) Individuals have access to primary care providers

        (2) Individuals have access to follow-up care

     e. Cost

        (1) Individuals are not denied health care because of lack of money

        (2) Cost is reasonable for services provided

        (3) Investment of money in health care leads to improved health

     f. Quality of care

        (1) Care leads to symptoms reduction or sense of well-being

        (2) Patients are satisfied with care received

        (3) Mortality-morbidity indicators show improvement

■ Primary health care delivery

  1. First contact with the health care system; implies continuity and coordination of care

  2. Currently in the U.S., health care is fragmented, costly, unavailable to many, with an emphasis on specialty care not primary care.

  3. Nursing has submitted an "Agenda for Health Care Reform" which contains three major parts

     a. A restructured health care system that will focus on the consumers and their health, with services to be delivered in familiar, convenient sites

     b. Basic core of essential health care services to be available to everyone

     c. A shift from the predominant focus on illness and cure to an orientation toward wellness and care (National Leadership Coalition for Health Care Reform, 1991)

■ Resource utilization

  1. Attempts to reduce duplication

  2. Attempts to reduce under-utilization/over-utilization

■ Policy research utilization/application

  1. Major research trend is in outcome studies. Agency for Health Care

Policy and Research, NIH are funding research with clinical applications

2. National Institute for Nursing Research funds major nursing research

- International health care trends

1. WHO "Healthy People" objectives unite the world

2. Major shift to emphasis on primary care

3. Trend toward earlier preventive efforts

4. Stress on improvements in sanitation, housing, nutrition, and immunization

5. Attention focused on promotion of individual measures to promote health and prevent disease

Nurse Practitioner Role Development

- History of the Role

1. In the early 1960s the Millis Report indicated that because of a physician shortage, many children were receiving inadequate medical care

2. A survey of the American Academy of Pediatrics (AAP) found that most physicians were willing to delegate certain patient care tasks

3. As a result of this response a plan to expand the role of the nurse was developed

    a. In 1964, Dr. Loretta C. Ford and Dr. Henry K. Silver started the first pediatric nurse practitioner program at the University of Colorado Health Sciences Center in Denver, Colorado

    (1) Length of initial program was 4 months of study and 18 months of clinical practice

    (2) Susan Stearly was the first nurse and only student in the Colorado program

    b. Also in 1964 across the country, Priscilla Andrews and Dr. John Connelly began a Pediatric Nurse Practitioner program at Massachusetts General Hospital in Boston, Massachusetts. This class was composed of public health nurses (Murphy, 1990)

4. In 1969 the American Academy of Pediatrics passed a statement saying, ". . . a physician may delegate to a properly trained individual, working under his direct supervision, the responsibility of providing

appropriate portions of health examinations and health care of infants . . ." (MacQueen, 1979, p. 31). The American Academy of Pediatrics also developed training and certificate guidelines for PNPs

5. In 1971 the American Nurses Association and the American Academy of Pediatrics jointly published "Guidelines on Short-term Continuing Education Program for PNP/As." This was one of the more formal attempts at developing standards for the multiple programs that were developing around the country

6. By 1980 there were almost 300 programs across the country (Bullough, Sultz, Henry & Fiedler, 1984)

7. Pediatric nurse practitioners, as the first nurse practitioners, served as the model for the inception of other nurse practitioners, e.g., school nurse practitioners, family nurse practitioners, adult nurse practitioners, gerontological nurse practitioners, ob-gyn nurse practitioners

■ Preparation of Nurse Practitioners

1. Most of the early nurse practitioners were graduated from certificate programs offered both within and outside of university settings. By 1989, 85% of all federally funded nurse practitioner programs were at the master's level and only 15% were certificate programs (Mezey, 1993)

2. Most evidence now clearly supports master's level preparation for nurse practitioners although initially, the appropriate educational model was not clear

3. The evolution from certificate programs to well integrated knowledge and skills in master's programs has been fairly consistent across the country

■ Role of Nurse Practitioner Movement and Professional Organizations

1. In 1973 a group of pediatric nurse practitioners representing six states organized the National Association of Pediatric Nurse Associates and Practitioners (NAPNAP)

   a. To set standardized guidelines for PNP practice, NAPNAP and the AAP published a "Scope of Pactice Statement" in 1974. This statement later resulted in "The Standards of Practice for PNP/As" issued jointly by NAPNAP and the Association of Faculties of PNP/A Programs (Murphy, 1990)

   b. American Nurses Association was also setting up a PNP Council under the Maternal-Child-Health division the very same year

2. Purpose of Professional Organizations

   a. Benefits

      (1) Provides collective voice for promoting nursing and quality health care

      (2) Monitors and influences laws and regulations

      (3) Communicates information

      (4) Public relations

   b. Relationship to practice

      (1) Study practice issues

      (2) Establish standards for practice

      (3) Act as collective bargaining agent for nurses

      (4) Provides visible presence in the community because of its legitimacy in representing nursing perspectives

■ Changes in the role

1. Originally when the role was in its formative stages it was viewed as

   a. A means to improve the image and stature of nurses within the healthcare and consumer community

   b. A quick solution to the shortage of physician services and access to primary care

2. Originally there was both support and resistance for the nurse practitioner role; research focused on the need to prove the impact of the role

3. Research also originally focused on the need to prove the existence of the role; quality, cost effectiveness, productivity, clinical decision making skills and job satisfaction (McGivern, 1993)

4. Policymakers originally saw nurse practitioners as physician substitutes

5. Nurse practitioners saw the physician maldistribution of the 1960s as an opportunity to increase the availability of primary care services

6. During the 1980s a change took place in the health care environment; the physician shortage of the 60s gave way to a physician glut; nurse practitioners were abandoned in favor of physicians

7. Now, in the 90s, with increased emphasis on primary care and

decreased need for physician specialists and sub-specialists, the nurse practitioner is being looked at as a viable, cost effective member of the health care delivery system

- Types of Roles
    1. Collaborator—establishes communication with other health care professionals to influence care
    2. Researcher
        a. Uses the knowledge of the research process to create knowledge and apply it to practice by sharing it with others
        b. Masters prepared nurse obligated to participate "in activities that contribute to the ongoing development of the profession's body of knowledge" (ANA, 1985, p. 1. Code of Ethics)
    3. Educator—teaches other professionals, family or patients. Requires
        a. Knowledge of the teaching/learning process
        b. Assessment of the learner
        c. Development of teaching plan
        d. Selection of teaching mode
        e. Implementation of plan
        f. Evaluation of teaching and learning effectiveness
        g. See (Teaching and learning in Creasia & Parker, 1991) for a succinct summary
        h. Learning theories
    4. Consultant
        a. Informal—individual draws from personal expertise to advise others, validate current practice, or provide specialized knowledge to help others
        b. Formal—contractual services on a wide variety of health care topics and for a variety of reasons
    5. Clinician—provides direct care or provides clinical information to others
        a. Has expert knowledge
        b. Maintains skills
        c. Evaluates practice

6. Administrator—manages others in the delivery of health care or may case manage the care of a group of patients

   a. Requires knowledge of organizational structures

   b. Requires management styles/strategies

   c. Requires leadership styles/strategies

   d. May require case management skills—administers the care of patients but may not provide the care

7. Independent practice

   a. Legal considerations

      (1) State nurse practice act must be broad and flexible enough to allow for full scope of practice

      (2) Obtain legal assistance in establishing practice

         (a) Small Business Administration Service Corp of Retired Executives (SBA-SCORE) provide free consultation

         (b) Evaluate best legal structure for practice, e.g., corporation, partnership, etc.

      (3) Establish cadre of health professionals to collaborate with

   b. Fiscal

      (1) Consider need for funds to cover 6 to 12 months of operation

      (2) Contact Small Business Administration regarding loan opportunities

      (3) Develop relationshps with your local banker and merchants

      (4) Negotiate directly with major third party payers

         (a) Describe who you are and your credentials

         (b) Describe what you are prepared to do

         (c) Describe the contract you would like to establish

         (d) Discuss fees and terms

   c. Accountability

      (1) Provide for self audit

      (2) Work with local nurse practitioner professional organizations to make certain local standards of practice are met

      (3) Examine quality of clinical documentation

   (4)   Establish open relationship with other nurse practitioners, physicians and health care providers

8. Other role functions

   a. Advocacy—promotes what is best for the client, ensuring that the clients needs are met, and protects the client's rights (Kozier, Erb, & Blais, 1992)

      (1)   Children/families

      (2)   Nursing profession

      (3)   World health/public health

   b. Ethical actions

      (1)   Ethical decision-making models applied to practice

      (2)   Advocacy, accountability, and loyalty are moral concepts (Fry, 1990)

      (3)   Care/caring, compassion, human dignity also important

      (4)   A discussion of nursing's policy on ethics may be found in Ethics in Nursing: Position Statements and Guidelines (ANA, 1988, Pub. No. G-175)

9. Marketing the role

   a. Always identify yourself as a nurse practitioner

   b. Use professional cards with your title, credentials

   c. Use brochures, educational materials for descriptions and functions of the role

   d. Take opportunities with radio, television, newspapers to identify yourself as a nurse practitioner and provide information

   e. Volunteer your nurse practitioner service at health fairs, neighborhood center, community functions

   f. List services in the telephone directory under "Nurse Practitioner"

   g. Work with local nurse practitioner organizations to focus media attention upon nurse practitioners

   h. Work with other health care providers on volunteer committees

   i. Donate time to a political campaign

   j. Send announcements of your practice to local medical societies, hospitals, pharmacists, physical therapists, etc. as relevant in your area

    k. Establish referral systems with other nurse practitioners and health professionals

- Legal ramifications

    1. The use of malpractice claims for regulating the quality of health care, escalating costs of providing medical care, maldistribution of primary care physicians and growing consumer demand for affordable quality care have created pressure on the health care system to provide low cost alternatives for the delivery of health care services

    2. These trends have led to increased use of nonphysician providers (many of whom are nurse practitioners) and new statuatory recognition of these providers (Eccard & Gainor, 1993)

    3. Problems arise from the legal perspective when nurses are defined under the nonphysician provider "umbrella" since nurses are separately licensed, contrary to some nonphysician providers, and practice their profession separate from medicine

    4. Most states have expanded or amended their nurse practice acts to cover nurse practitioners while others have given physicians more delegative powers

    5. Some states have a separate level of licensure for advanced practitioners

    6. Individual certification of nurse specialists is the best approach to legal coverage because it makes practitioners accountable for their own practice (Bullough, 1993, p. 274)

    7. Legal regulations vary widely from state to state

Knowledge Base

- Scientific content

    1. Medicine

    2. Physical assessment

    3. Statistics and research

    4. Physiology

    5. Anatomy

    6. Microbiology

7. Psychology

8. Sociology

9. Nutrition

10. Pharmacology

- Elements of theory

    1. Development of theory

        a. Relatively specific and concrete set of concepts and propositions that purports to account for or characterize phenomena of interest to the discipline of nursing

    2. Application

        a. Theories allow the nurse to assess, plan, implement and evaluate care

    3. Evaluation

        a. Use of theories allows the nurse to determine the relevance of the theory to actual practice

        b. Data should be provided to allow the nurse to modify practice

- Applicable psychosocial theories: The strength of the nurse practitioner is their unique preparation which integrates psychosocial theory into clinical practice

    1. Nursing theories

        a. Nightingale's environmental theory

        b. Henderson's complementary-supplementary model

        c. Johnson's behavioral system model

        d. Rogers' science of unitary human beings

        e. King's theory of goal attainment

        f. Neuman's systems model

        g. Orem's theory of self-care

        h. Roy's adaptation model

        i. Leininger's theory of transcultural nursing

        j. Watson's science of caring

        k. Parse's theory of man-living-health

2. For a succinct summary of each of these theories see Creasia & Parker, 1991, pp. 5-18

3. Other theories

    a. Change theory—ability to initiate change or to assist others in making modification in themselves or in the system

        (1) Change theory focuses on how to make change

        (2) Examples of change theorists: Lewis, K.—unfreezing, moving, refreezing; Lippitt, R.—diagnose, assess, select progressive change objectives, terminate; Havelock, R.—build relationships, acquire resources, choose solution, stabilize; Rogers, E.—knowledge, persuasion, decision, decision-implementation, confirmation

        (3) For a concise summary of change theory see Kozier, Erb & Blais, 1992, p. 211

    b. Developmental theory

        (1) Development is patterned, orderly, and predictable with purpose and direction

        (2) Development is continuous throughout life, although the degree of change in many areas decreases after adolescence

        (3) Can occur simultaneously in several areas, e.g., physical and social, but rate of change in each area varies

        (4) Proceeds from simple to complex

        (5) Pace varies among individuals

        (6) Physical and mental stress during periods of critical developmental change, such as puberty, make a person particularly susceptible to outside stressors (Morton, 1989 p. 47)

■ Health behavior

Becker Health Belief Model intends to predict which individuals would or would not use preventive measures based upon perceived susceptibility; perceived seriousness; perceived threat. Health risk appraisal includes a variety of questions about health behavior and attempts to evaluate the patient's risk in a variety of areas. Focus is on decreasing statistical risk by changing behavior through knowledge of risk.

■ Stress

General theory of behavior and response first described by Selye in which the body adapts, as long as possible, to stress. Some degree of stress can be healthy

1. Stress as a stimulus

2. Stress as a response

3. Stress reaction (adaptive response)

4. Stress reaction (sustained response)

5. Stress exhaustion

- Education

    1. Most early programs were certificate programs

    2. In the early 1970s, baccalaureate level preparation was considered

    3. Seems there is now a general consensus that the nurse practitioner role requires specialized knowledge and skills, which is best acquired in a master's degree program (Mezey, 1993)

    4. Continuing education is the obligation of the professional

        a. Participant—many states require continuing education as a condition of continuous licensure

        b. Provider—must meet predetermined criteria to award continuing education credit

- Credentialing

    1. Accreditation—"The process by which a voluntary, non-governmental agency or organization appraises and grants accreditation status to institutions and/or programs or services which meet predetermined structure, process and outcome criteria" (ANA, 1979)

        a. Purpose of accreditation—protects public, by recognizing practitioners who have successfuly completed an approved course of study

        b. Can serve as a mechanism to identify providers who can be reimbursed for services

        c. Accrediting bodies

            (1) National League for Nursing (NLN)—accredits schools of nursing

            (2) Joint Commission on Accreditation of Health Care Organizations (JCAHO)—accredits hospitals and health care organizations and agencies

    d. Establishes standards for the profession

      (1) Designed initially to improve quality

      (2) Designed to protect public safety

      (3) Designed to standardize services and facilities by being explicit about what is expected

2.   Licensure: "A process by which an agency of state government grants permission to individuals accountable for the practice of a profession to engage in the practice of that profession and prohibits all others from legally doing so. It permits use of a particular title. Its purpose is to protect the public by ensuring a minimum level of professional competence." (ANA, 1979)

    a. Reciprocity—acknowledgement and acceptance by one state of another state's licensure of a nurse

    b. Registration—individual has met certain criteria and is therefore "registered" within the state and entitled to practice within that state

3.   Certification—"A process by which a non-governmental agency or association certifies that an individual licensed to practice as a professional has met certain predetermined standards specified by that profession for specialty practice. Its purpose is to assure the public that an individual has mastered a body of knowledge and acquired skills in a particular specialty." (ANA, 1979)

    a. As of 1991, all but five states recognized National Certification as a means for certifying nurse practitioners and/or nurse midwives. The mechanisms for achieving certification vary by state and include various types of criteria, e.g., treatment protocols, collaborative agreements in addition to national certification requirements

    b. Conditions for certification maintenance or recertification must be met, often involving clinical practice, continuing education, re-examination, periodic self-assessment examinations and peer review

4.   Certifying bodies

    a. American Nurses Credentialing Center (ANCC)—specialty examinations in nursing fields, plus adult, pediatric, gerontological, family, and school nurse practitioners

    b. National Certification Board of Pediatric Nurse Practitioners and

Nurses (NCBPNP/N)—specialty examinations for pediatric nurse practitioners and pediatric nurses

c. National Certification Corporation for the Obstetric, Gynecologic and Neonatal Nursing Specialties (NCC)—specialty examinations for Ob/Gyn nurse practitioners, and other maternal, infant and women's health specialties

Professional Issues

■ Standards of Practice

1. The development of standards has focused on setting minimum levels of acceptable performance and has attempted to provide the consumer with a means of measuring the quality of nursing care they receive (Eccard & Gainer, 1993)

   a. The ANA defines a standard as an "authoritative statement by which the quality of practice, service or education can be judged"

   b. Standards were developed in 1966 following an organizational revision of the ANA which resulted in the creation of five divisions of practice that corresponded to distinct specialty areas

   c. Both generic standards applicable to all nurses in all areas of practice have been developed in addition to specialty areas

3. Various specialty groups have also developed standards, e.g., National Association of Pediatric Nurse Associates and Practitioners (NAPNAP); Nurses Association of the American College of Obstetricians and Gynecologists (NAACOG) now known as Association of Womens' Health, Obstetric, and Neonatal Nurses (AWHONN); American College of Critical-Care Nurses; American Association of Nurse Anesthetists are but a few of the several specialty nurses organizations with their own Standards of Practice. (Eccard & Gainor, 1993)

4. Legal implications and parameters

   a. Former protocols or standards provide legal protection if nurse practitioner challenged about specific tasks, actions, knowledge

   b. Protocols should be a simple series of steps that will always apply to certain problems or presenting symptoms

   c. Protocols should be the minimum requirements for safe care

   d. Protocols should be updated as scientific knowledge changes

   e. Protocols should be realistic depending on the practice setting in which they will be utilized

    f. Protocols must be followed without fail. A deviation from the protocol should be documented in the chart (Moniz, 1992).

    g. Informal practice may provide some legal protection if it can be documented that this is the standard of practice within a community or state

■ Evaluation of practice

  1. Peer review

    a. Provides evaluation which recognizes and rewards nursing contribution

    b. Leads to higher standards of practice within a community and discourages practice beyond the scope of legal authority

  2. Quality assurance—a system to evaluate and monitor the quality of patient care and the quality of facility management (JCAHO, 1988)

    a. Provides for accountability and responsibility of individual practitioner in delivering high quality care

    b. Can be used as a means of evaluating and improving patient care

    c. Can serve as a model by which individual nurse practitioners can ensure quality care within their own practice through an organized approach to problem solving

    d. Provides a framework for systematic, continuous evaluation of individual clinical practice

    e. Can reduce exposure to liability

    f. Can identify educational needs of nurse practitioners

    g. Can improve documentation of care provided

    h. Components of quality assurance

      (1) Structure—focuses on organization of client care system

      (2) Process—focuses on activities and performance of care givers in relation to client's needs

        (a) Identifies the person(s) responsible for quality assurance activity

        (b) Delineates the scope of care provided

        (c) Identifies the important aspects of care

        (d)   Evaluates the appropriateness of identified quality indicators

        (e)   Collection and analysis of data

   (3)   Outcome

        (a)   Evaluation of care

        (b)   Client's health care status, welfare and satisfaction

        (c)   Results of care in terms of change in the client

        (d)   Resolution of problem(s)

        (e)   Evaluation of whether general patient care has improved as a result of the evaluation process

        (f)   Communicate process results to appropriate individuals in the institution

   (4)   Effectiveness

        (a)   Are expectations reasonable?

        (b)   Are changes made?

   (1)   Efficiency

        (a)   Are outcomes possible with reasonable effort?

        (b)   Are tasks selected reasonable?

   (6)   Client and provider interactions

        (a)   Is there a mechanism for evaluating patient satisfaction?

        (b)   Is there a mechanism for patient participation in policy development and implementation?

 i. Additional methods

   (1)   Auditing—examining records to see how well they meet established criteria

   (2)   Selected studies—detailed evaluation of information related to a specific disease or process

   (3)   Patient satisfaction—evaluation of subjective response

   (4)   Utilization review—evaluation in which extent of services described or resources used is measured against a standard

   (5)   Peer review—evaluation of care given by similar providers. Focus is on reasonableness of care, what is commonly

expected as care in that setting for that problem

- Risk management

  Includes systems and activities which are designed to recognize and intervene to reduce the risk of injury to patients and consequent claims against health care providers. It is based on the assumption that many injuries to patients are preventable

  1. Management liability

      a. Evaluation of sources of legal risk in a practice

          (1) Patients

          (2) Procedures

          (3) Quality of record keeping

      b. Educational or procedural activities in order to reduce risk in identified risk areas

  2. Malpractice—any professional misconduct, unreasonable lack of skill, or infidelity in professional or fiduciary duties, or illegal or immoral conduct. Negligence is the failure of an individual to do something that a reasonable person would do, that results in injury to another. Malpractice is the alleged failure on the part of a professional to render services with the degree of care, diligence, and precaution that another member of the same profession in similar circumstances would render to prevent injury to someone else. In order to recover for negligent malpractice, it must be established:

      a. A duty to care by provider to the patient violated the applicable standard of care

      b. Patient suffered a compensable injury that such injury was caused in fact and proximately caused by the substandard conduct (King, 1986)

      c. Safety (client, staff, and volunteers) was compromised

  3. Malpractice insurance

      a. Mistakes do happen, despite the best intentions

      b. Malpractice insurance will not protect a nurse practitioner from charges of practicing medicine without a license if they are practicing outside the legal scope of practice within the state

      c. It is universally recommended that all nurse practitioners carry their own insurance

    d. The National Practitioner Data Bank collects information on adverse actions against health care practitioners, including nurses. All hospitals must query the data bank every two years regarding health care providers on their medical staffs, those to whom they have granted clinical privileges, or new appointments

4. Personal/professional liability

    a. Many nurse practitioners are covered under a professional liability insurance policy purchased by their employers

    b. This type of insurance covers problems which are of a more general nature; malpractice insurance may be a component of this type of policy

5. General types of liability policies

    a. An insurance contract or agreement between insurer and insured. Two major policy options

        (1) Occurrence coverage—covers events of alleged malpractice which occurred during the policy period, regardless of the date of discovery or when the claim was filed

        (2) Claims made coverage—covers only those claims filed during the policy coverage period, regardless of when they occurred, optional tail coverage contract extends the coverage of a claims made policy into the future to cover all claims filed after the basic claims made coverage period

■ Prescriptive Authority

1. Important to ensure adequacy of therapeutic regimens

2. Addressed state by state

3. To date, over 35 boards provide for some degree of prescriptive authority; the degree of authority varies. (Pearson, 1994)

4. Depending on the full scope of the state law a nurse practitioner may obtain a federal DEA registration number

■ Testimony as an expert witness in a court of law

1. Standards of care in professional nursing negligence action must be established by expert testimony

2. Nurses are the best people to give testimony on standards of care for nurses

3. Competency of an expert witness is tested by the sufficiency of the

witness's knowledge of the subject matter

4. The degree or depth of the expert's knowledge affects how much weight or credence the jury should give the testimony

5. How to prepare testimony if you are the expert witness or are defending yourself

   a. Prepare thoroughly, with concise, well supported and well documented materials

   b. Know the State Nurse Practice Act and how to apply it to situations

   c. Be aware of existing regulations and how promulgated

   d. Be aware of any Standards of Care written by American Nurses' Association or other professional organizations

   e. Be knowledgeable about reasonable, acceptable, and proper existing practice

   f. Present with confidence, authority and conviction

   g. A professional appearance and demeanor is critical

6. How to deliver and respond to questions

   a. Communicate directly with questioners, directing answers toward the judge and jury

   b. Maintain composure; be relaxed

   c. State opinion and do not change it; do not overtly react to other witnesses that may disagree

   d. Avoid vague imprecise expressions such as "I think" or "I believe;" avoid superlatives such as "always" and "never."

   e. When you know the answer, give it concisely and precisely, but do not answer more than you are asked

   f. When it comes to giving your opinion, it is not always necessary to answer only "yes" or "no." It is often appropriate to say a few more words to explain your opinion.

   g. Take time to allow the question to register and to prepare your answer. This allows the attorney to make appropriate objections before you answer. If an objection is made and overruled, you must answer the question

   h. If you do not understand a question, ask to have it repeated or clarified

i. If you do not remember or know an answer, it is better to acknowledge this than make a mistake. If the answer involves exact time or number and you know the appropriate answer, state your recollection as an approximation (Northrup & Kelly, 1987, p. 531)

■ Interaction with the legal system

1. Evaluate your legal requirements by talking to an attorney or other health care professional

2. Utilize tools available to identify prospective legal counsel

   a. See *Martindale-Hubbell Directory of Attorneys*

   b. Check with friends, colleagues, professional associations

   c. Use Bar Associations and other attorney referral services

3. Interview prospects

   a. Develop rapport between yourself and attorney

   b. Discuss what services the attorney feels may be necessary and services they are willing to perform

   c. Establish the fee structure, payment terms, and estmated total cost. (Northrup & Kelly, 1987)

■ Political activism: Mandatory if nurse practitioners are to remain a viable role. Many policies have the potential to impact on nurse practitioners

1. Analyze health/public/social policy

   a. Determine objective of policy

      (1) What is the problem?

      (2) Problem definition affects policy structure

   b. What are the social dimensions of the policy?

      (1) Who will be affected?

      (2) Examine issues of race, gender, economic class, education, etc.

   c. What are the political dimensions of the policy?

      (1) Is specific legislation required?

      (2) Is it politically feasible to pass legislation?

      (3) How will this policy be implemented?

    d. What are the economic dimensions of the policy?

        (1) Who will pay for policy implementation?

        (2) What are the costs involved?

        (3) What will be accomplished by the money invested?

    e. Who are the opponents and proponents of the policy?

    f. What are other social, political or economic alternatives to the policy?

2.   How to recommend and contribute to development of policy

    a. The process of recommending policy (political process)

        (1) Provide information or research to legislators who are interested in submitting legislation; they are looking for good ideas

        (2) Initiate meetings with policy makers to inform them

    b. Formation of community interest groups

        (1) Numbers of people create visibility for the problem

        (2) Numbers of people provide more resources in addressing the problem

        (3) Attract media attention to put issue on the policy agenda

    c. How to form a coalition

        (1) Define your problem broadly

        (2) Examine all constituent groups affected by the problem

        (3) Initiate meetings between members of different constituent groups

        (4) Determine areas where interests are similar and where interests are different

        (5) Agree to work together on problems where interests or goals are the same; not work against each other where interests are not the same; work together on interests which are of great importance to some group members but not highly important to others

3.   Advocacy for the establishment and implementation of public policy

    a. Always represent yourself as a nurse practitioner

  b. Take the initiative to approach policy makers

  c. Coordinate efforts with national associations and other interested parties when appropriate

 4. Formal legislative process (usual process)

  a. Federal level

   (1) Issue may be placed on public agenda by interested groups or other means may be used

   (2) Bill introduced into Congress

   (3) Referred to committee for hearings

   (4) Referred to House and Senate for debate and vote

   (5) If both Houses concur, bill goes to President; if they do not, it goes to conference committee

   (6) Conference committee debate and vote

   (7) Legislation either dies or is sent back to both houses

   (8) To President for signature or veto

   (9) If signed by President, bill becomes law. If vetoed, Congress can vote to overturn veto

   (10) After bill becomes law, appropriate agency drafts rules and regulations to implement law

   (11) Draft Regulations published in *Federal Register* for public comment

   (12) After public comment period, final regulations are promulgated and published

   (13) Law is implemented via regulations

  b. State and Local Level

   (1) Basic process is similar although not so complex

   (2) (See Dye, 1992)

  c. Role of Lobbyist

   (1) Professional workers whose job is to get information to policy makers to help influence policy formation

   (2) Assist with developing plan and implementation of achieving goals and objectives

(3) Expertise is often in knowing who to influence and how to do so

d. Policy often influenced by informal process

(1) Influence of friends and family

(2) Associations with church or social clubs

Types of health care delivery systems

■ Managed Care

1. Broad term which describes networks of providers who contractually agree to provide services for particular patient groups

2. Major dimensions include reviewing and intervening in decisions about health services to be provided—either prospectively or retrospectively; limiting or influencing patient's choice of providers; and negotiating different payment terms or levels with providers

3. Types of managed care systems

a. Health Maintenance Organization (HMO)—An organized system of health care that provides, directly or through contracts with others, a specified range of comprehensive health services to a voluntarily enrolled population for prepaid per capita payments. They are both insurers and providers of health care

(1) Emphasizes health promotion and health maintenance

(2) Patient's choice of health care providers and hospitals, services is limited

b. Preferred Provider Organization (PPO)—A preferred provider organization is an entity through which a partnership is established between a group of "preferred providers"—doctors, hospitals and others—and an insurance company, self-limited employer or its intermediary to provide specified medical and hospital care and sometimes related services at a negotiated price. Providers negotiate lower fees in anticipation of a greater volume of patients and agree to basic managed care principles such as utilization review, accompanying guidelines for hospital admissions, and limited use of facilities and resources

(1) Marketed to purchasers as opposed to consumers

(2) Physicians are paid per person or capitated payment depending upon the number of individuals enrolled with

them as primary providers, and patients pay a small co-payment at time of service

- Private practice: Physicians who accept fee for service, third party reimbursement from private insurance plans, Medicare and Medicaid. They are unaffiliated with other physician or organizational groups and charges are based on current market rates

- Home health care: Care provided by a public agency or private organization primarily engaged in providing skilled nursing services and other therapeutic services

  1. Has policies established by a group of professional personnel to govern the services which it provides

  2. Provides for supervision of services

  3. Maintains clinical records on every patient

  4. Has in effect an overall plan and budget

  5. Meets applicable federal, state and local law

- Health centers

  1. Federally funded centers designed to meet specific population needs, e.g., pregnant women, low birth weight babies, the elderly

  2. Provides provision for direct reimbursement to nurse practitioners in rural areas

  3. Examples include Community Health Centers, Federal Qualified Health Centers, Federal Qualified Health Center Look-A-Likes, Rural Health Clinics, Migrant Health Clinics, Indian Health Clinics, National Health Service Corps

- University teaching hospitals

  1. Service and research institutions

  2. Educational training system for health professionals

  3. Quality of care usually high; continuity of care may be decreased

- Hospitals

  1. Clinical service-based facilities of varying size

  2. Often meet special community needs

  3. May develop care specialty for a geographic area

Reimbursement

Types of reimbursement (Provider reimbursement mechanisms). Top agenda item for nurse practitioners. Traditionally, nurse practitioners have not been paid directly for services performed unless authorized by a physician or performed under the supervision of a physician. Nurse practitioners argue that reimbursement should be provided directly to provider and at rate determined for service provided, not by type of provider

■ Direct reimbursement

1. Advantages of direct reimbursement include

    a. Increases the availability and improves accessibility of health care to the consumer

    b. Increases consumer choice of health care providers

    c. Provides for comprehensive or full service health care for the consumer

    d. Provides for cost-effective health care through improved utilization of nurse practitioners

    e. Legitimizes the nurse practitioner role

    f. Decreases restrictions on practice imposed by limited reimbursement mechanisms

2. Impact of restrictions on direct reimbursement for nurse practitioner services

    a. Reinforces dominance of physicians

    b. Reduces collegial relationships

    c. Limits professional autonomy in nursing

    d. Limits consumer choice

    e. Limits access to services, particularly in underserved areas or with underserved population groups (Labar, 1983)

3. Government opinion has been that direct payment to nurse practitioners would be inflationary, increasing utilization and fee-inflation. If nurse practitioners provide complimentary rather than substitutive services, both physicians and nurse practitioners could bill for patient services, thus increasing overall health care utilization and costs

■ Fee-For-Service

1. Traditional form of payment made to physicians and health care providers. The provider gets paid a fee for each service that is provided

■ Medicare

1. Provides health insurance protection for over 33 million aged and disabled individuals. The program covers hospital service, physician services, and other medical services for those eligible, regardless of income

2. Medicare is administered by the Health Care Financing Administration (HCFA) in the Department of Health and Human Services. Many of the day-to-day operations, including the reviewing and paying for claims, are performed by organizations such as Blue Cross/Blue Shield plans or private insurers under contract to HCFA. These organizations are referred to as Part A intermediaries and Part B carriers

3. The program has two parts: Hospital insurance (Part A) that covers inpatient hospital and related institutional care; Supplementary Medical Insurance (Part B) covers physician services and other related medical services and supplies

   a. Part A covers inpatient hospital care. In some cases, it also covers short-term skilled nursing facility care after a hospital stay, home health agency visits, and hospice care

   Medicare pays for inpatient hospital services according to a prospective payment system (PPS). Under this system, each Medicare patient is classified according to his or her medical condition into diagnosis-related groups (DRGs). Hospitals are paid a predetermined rate for each patient treated within a given DRG. Hospitals with costs below the payment rates are allowed to keep the surplus, while hospitals with costs above the payment rates must absorb the cost

   b. Part B, the Supplementary Medical Insurance (SMI) program, is a voluntary program; individuals must enroll and pay a premium to receive benefits. All persons are entitled to Part A and all persons over age 65 are eligible to enroll. The program covers the services of physicians, outpatient hospital care, laboratory and x-ray services and other related medical services and supplies. In certain instances, the services of nonphysician providers, like nurse practitioners, are covered

      (1) The program is financed by beneficiary premiums and general revenues. Medicare generally pays 80% of the reasonable charges for covered services, after the beneficiary has met the annual deductible. The beneficiary is liable for

> 20% of the reasonable charge, an amount that is known as coinsurance

> (2) Medicare pays for most Part B services including physician services, on the basis of a reasonable charge. The reasonable charge is the lesser of the actual charge, the physician or supplier's customary charges for the service, and the prevailing charge for the service in the community

> (3) By accepting "assignment" on a claim, a provider, (i.e., nurse practitioner, physician, supplier) agrees to accept Medicare's reasonable charge as payment in full. There are incentives for providers to enter into agreements to accept assignment on all Medicare claims. Persons who enter into such agreements are known as "participating" providers

> If physician or provider does not accept assignment, the patient is liable for the 20% and difference between what is paid by Medicare and the actual charge

> (4) The Omnibus Budget Reconciliation Act of 1989 (OBRA 89), Public Law 101-239, enacted a new payment system for physician's services. Instead of a reasonable charge basis, physician's services will be paid on a fee schedule that uses a resource-based-relative-value-scale (RBRVS). Under RBRVS, physician payments are determined according to the resources and effort (including the physician's time) needed to perform a service. In general terms, the fee schedule will reduce payments for most surgical services, while increasing payments for primary care services such as office visits. Beginning in 1992, the fee schedule is being phased in over a 5-year period

4. Nurse Practitioners: For a Nurse Practitioner's (NP) services to be covered under Medicare, an NP must:

   a. Be a registered professional nurse who is currently licensed to practice in the State in which the services are furnished

   b. Satisfy the applicable requirements for qualification as NP in the State in which the services are furnished

   c. Meet at least one of the following requirements:

      (1) Be currently certified as a primary care nurse practitioner by the American Nurses' Credentialing Center or by the National Certification Board of Pediatric Nurse Practitioners

and Nurses

(2) Have satisfactorily completed a formal educational program of at least one academic year that prepares registered nurses to perform an expanded role in the delivery of primary care and that includes at least four months (in the aggregate) of classroom instruction, and awards a degree, diploma, or certificate for successful completion of the program; *or*

(3) Have successfully completed a formal education program (that does not qualify under the immediately preceding requirement) that prepares registered nurses to perform an expanded role in the delivery of primary care and have been performing that expanded role for at least 12 months during the 18-month period immediately preceding February 8, 1988, the effective date for the provision of the services of nurse practitioners as reflected in the conditions for certification for rural health clinics (Medicare handbook 1991)

5. Medicare Covered Services

Coverage is limited to the services an NP is legally authorized to perform in accordance with State Law (or State regulatory mechanism established by State Law). The NP must meet training, education, and experience requirements prescribed by the Secretary of Health and Human Services

The services of an NP may be covered under Part B if all of the following conditions are met:

a. They are the type that are considered physician's services if furnished by a doctor of medicine or osteopathy (MD/DO)

b. They are performed by a person who meets the definition of an NP (See above)

c. The NP is legally authorized to perform the services in the State in which they are performed

d. They are performed in collaboration with an MD/DO. The term "collaboration" means a process whereby an NP works with a physician to deliver health care services within the scope of the NP's professional expertise with medical direction and appropriate supervision as provided for in jointly developed guidelines or other mechanisms defined by Federal regulations and the law of the State in which the services are performed; and

    e. They are not otherwise precluded from coverage because of one of the statutory exclusions

6. Medicare Reimbursement for NP Services

Under certain conditions, Medicare will reimburse for services of an NP in the following ways

    a. Incident to:

        (1) Services of nonphysician personnel, (i.e., nurse practitioners) furnished "incident-to" physician services in private practice is limited to situations in which there is direct physician supervision. Direct personal supervision in the office setting does not mean that the physician must be present in the same room with his or her assistant. However, the physician must be present in the office suite and immediately available to provide assistance and direction throughout the time the assistant is performing services. Such services must be an integral, although incidental, part of the physician's personal professional services, and they must be performed under the physician's direct supervision

        (2) Services performed by nurse practitioners "incident-to" a physician's professional services include not only service ordinarily rendered by a physician's office staff person, (e.g., medical services such as taking blood pressures and temperatures, giving injections, and changing dressings), but also services ordinarily performed by the physician himself or herself such as physical examinations, minor surgery, setting casts for simple fractures, interpreting radiographs, and other activities that involve an independent evaluation or treatment of the patient's condition

        (3) Services Excluded from coverage:

        NP services may not be covered if they are otherwise excluded from coverage even though an NP may be authorized by State law to perform them. For example, the Medicare law excludes from coverage routine foot and dental care, routine physical checkups, examinations prescribing or fitting eyeglasses (except after cataract surgery) or hearing aids, cosmetic surgery and services that are not reasonable and necessary for the diagnosis or treatment of an illness or injury or to improve the functioning of a malformed body member

    (4)   Billing and payment under "incident-to":

When an NP performs an "incident-to" service in a physician's office/clinic, the service must be submitted to Medicare by the employing physician, under his/her name, provider number, and the most accurate Current Procedural Terminology (CPT) code that describes the treatment being furnished. The payment is made at the full physician rate and paid to the employer

  b. Billing and Payment in other circumstances:

Billing and payment for NP services is available only in limited circumstances as follows:

    (1)   Skilled Nursing Facilities (SNFs): Payment for services furnished in Skilled Nursing Facilities or Nursing Facilities in urban areas, as defined by law. Under the Social Security Act, a SNF must meet certain "conditions of participation" that concern the quality of care provided, proper training for employees, residents' rights, and safety code requirements. Other requirements include that the facility is primarily engaged in providing residents:

        (a)   Skilled nursing care and related services for residents who require medical or nursing care

        (b)   Rehabilitation services for the rehabilitation of injured, disabled, or sick persons, and not primarily for the care and treatment of mental diseases.

It is also possible that part of another institution is treated as a SNF

    (2)   Medicare pays for nurse practitioner and clinical nurse specialist services in SNFs in non-rural areas on a reasonable charge basis. This amount, however, may not exceed the physician fee schedule amount for the service. The payment is made to the NP's employer

  c. Rural Health Clinics: Nurse practitioners can own rural health clinics where reimbursement is covered under the Medicare program. In addition, services of NPs and CNSs in rural health clinics are paid to the clinic on a reasonable cost basis. Payment is made to the clinic

    d. Rural Areas:

        (1) A rural area is defined as any area outside of an urban area for which an urban area is defined as a "Metropolitan Statistical Area" (MSA) or New England County Metropolitan Area (NECMA) as defined by the Executive Office of Management and Budget or otherwise defined by law

        (2) Rural Inpatient Settings: The payment amount for the services provided by a nurse practitioner is limited to 75% of the physician Fee Schedule amount when they are performed in a hospital setting. In this case, the payment is made only under assignment and made to the hospital

        (3) Rural Outpatient Settings: For all other services, (outpatient), an 85% limit is applicable. Payment is made only under assignment. Also, payment can be made directly to an NP providing services in a rural area or to his or her employer or contractor

■ Medicaid

    1. Program is authorized by Title XIX of the Social Security Act, which is a Federal-State matching program providing medical assistance to approximately 25 million low income persons who are aged, blind, disabled, or members of families with dependent children

    2. Federal funds account for 56% of total program expenditures

    3. Each state designs and administers its own Medicaid program, setting eligibility and coverage standards within broad federal guidelines. There is substantial variation among the states in terms of eligibility requirements, range of services offered, limitations placed on those services, reimbursement policies

    4. Every state except Arizona participates, as well as District of Columbia, American Samoa, Guam, Puerto Rico, the Virgin Islands, and the Northern Mariana Islands

    5. At the state level, Medicaid is administered by a designated state agency

    6. Federal oversight of the Medicaid program is the responsibility of the Health Care Financing Administration (HCFA)

    7. There are proposals to increase provider participation, improve coordination between Medicaid and other programs, and provide

outreach, education, and social services to pregnant women and children

8. Reimbursement regulations

a. Providers must accept Medicaid payment as payment in full and may not collect from beneficiaries

b. Medicaid pays only after any other insurance or third party payment sources available to the beneficiary have been exhausted

c. Payments must be sufficient to enlist enough providers so that covered services will be available to Medicaid beneficiaries to the extent they are available to the general population in a geographic area

d. Payments are either prospective or retrospective for institutional care; payments are usually the lesser of the provider's actual charge for the service and maximum allowable charges established by the state for physician services. Some states have a flat fee schedule and payments may be unrelated to actual provider charges

9. Medicaid reimbursement to nurse practitioners

a. Budget Reconciliation Act of 1989 (H.R. 3299) required states to cover the services of certified pediatric and family nurse practitioners beginning July 1, 1990 when practicing within the scope of state law and regardless of whether they are under the supervision of, or associated with a physician or other provider (*Congressional Record*, 1989)

b. Level of payment determined by state Medicaid Agency. Current reimbursement at 60 to 100% of physicians' rate (Pearson, 1993)

c. Pediatric and Family nurse practitioners may directly bill Medicaid for their services and may apply for a provider number from their state

d. States may pass regulations for direct payment for Medicaid to other nurse practitioners not identified in the federal statutes. Currently, 42 states pay nurse practitioners (Pearson, 1993)

■ Prospective Reimbursement to Hospitals

1. Payment mechanism based upon the projected costs of caring for a patient with a particular problem. Under this system, each Medicare patient admitted to a hospital is classified according to his or her medical condition into a diagnosis-related group (DRG). Hospitals are paid a predetermined rate for each patient treated with a given DRG.

Hospitals with costs below the payment rate are allowed to keep a percentage of the surplus, while hospitals with costs above the payment rate must absorb the loss

2. Nurse practitioners not paid directly for services delivered in hospital

- Third-party payers

    1. Two-thirds of total health care revenue comes from third party agencies—private insurance companies or government

        a. Public sources (federal, state, local) pay for 40% costs

        b. Private sources pay for 60%

            (1) Includes direct out-of-pocket expenses

            (2) Includes amount paid for insurance

- Other third party payers

    1. Civilian Health and Medical Program of the United Services (CHAMPUS)

        a. Federal health plan that provides coverage to the military personnel and their families

        b. Program is a means of cost sharing authorized health care services and benefits for dependents of active duty personnel and retirees, dependents and surviving dependents of service members

        c. Program utilizes a variety of health personnel and reimburses them for their services

        d. Nurse practitioners are reimbursed for services

    2. Federal Employees Health Benefit Programs

        a. FEHBP is the largest employer-sponsored group health insurance program in the world, serving 10 million participants and offering over 250 insurance plans

        b. Offers wide variety of plans

        c. Nurse practitioners are recognized as designated health care providers under the system

Questions

Select the best answer

1. Healthy People 2000 is

   a. A report on the health status of 2000 people in the U.S.A.
   b. An international health policy paper
   c. A statement of national health policy goals to help all people live socially and economically productive lives
   d. A research analysis of what makes people healthy

2. WHO "Health for All" is

   a. A report on who is healthy in the world
   b. A general policy statement on improving the world's health care
   c. A research study on the components of health in all countries
   d. A discussion of who is healthy

3. Nursing has submitted an "Agenda for Health Care Reform" which includes

   a. A restructured health care system that will focus on the consumers and their health, with services to be delivered in familiar, convenient sites
   b. A predominant focus on illness and acute care
   c. The insistence on more specialty training for physicians
   d. A two-tiered system of health care for the wealthy and the poor

4. The major trend in health policy research is now

   a. Outcome studies
   b. Process studies
   c. Structure studies
   d. Primary care studies

5. Which of the following is not considered in the overall cost reduction strategy in the delivery of health care services

   a. Individuals are not denied health care because of lack of money
   b. All individuals may have free care
   c. Cost is reasonable for services provided
   d. Investment of money in health care leads to improved health

6. The process of quality assurance focuses on

   a. Activities and performance of care given in relation to client's needs
   b. Accessibility of care

    c. Organization of client care
    d. Outcome of care

7. Which of the following methods is not appropriate in evaluating care?

    a. Examining records to see how well they meet established criteria
    b. Detailed evaluation of information related to a specific disease or process
    c. Evaluation of patient satisfaction
    d. Evaluation of care given by other institutions for the same disease process

8. The predominant component of malpractice is

    a. Negligence in providing professional care
    b. Overcharging fees
    c. Provider uses acceptable standards of care
    d. Patient suffers no injury

9. In preparing to give testimony as an expert witness you should

    a. Be aware of existing regulations and how promulgated and implemented within the state
    b. Be aware of all other relevant legal cases
    c. Give as much information as possible each time a question is asked
    d. Make certain the judge understands what you are saying, even if you have to repeat it

10. The trend for nurse practitioner prescriptive authority is

    a. The majority of states allow nurse practitioners to write prescriptions for controlled substances
    b. There is a large degree of variability among states regarding the prescribing authority of nurse practitioners
    c. The majority of states have not drafted legislation or regulations which deal with NP prescribing
    d. To use presigned prescription pads

11. The most important major components which should be considered in examining health/public/social policy include

    a. Political, social, economic and professional components of the policy
    b. How powerful are the opponents of the policy
    c. How to sell the policy to the media
    d. What kind of supporters exist for the policy

12. In working to form a coalition

    a. Keep policy focus very narrow
    b. Include all groups remotely involved in the problem

   c. Do not work with groups who do not totally agree on every issue of the problem

   d. Agree to not work against each other where interests are not the same

13. The federal legislative process includes

   a. The President refers the Bill to committees for hearings

   b. Bill becomes law when passed by Congress

   c. President may sign or veto Bill submitted to him

   d. Draft regulations are published in *Congressional Record* for public comment

14. The legislative process

   a. Does not follow a formal legislative path

   b. Is often influenced by informal processes

   c. Makes it illegal for paid, professional workers to give information to policy makers to help influence policy formation

   d. Is ended if President vetoes the Bill

15. Managed care is a broad term which describes

   a. The manager in a health maintenance organization

   b. The type of care provided in a Preferred Provider Organization

   c. Networks of providers who contractually agree to provide services for particular patient groups

   d. Networks of hospitals who provide patient care for acutely ill patients

16. A Health Maintenance Organization is an organized system of

   a. Health care facilities

   b. Health care that provides through contracts, a specified range of comprehensive health services to a voluntarily enrolled population for prepaid per capita payments

   c. Health care which must provide health care to all clients in a geographic area

   d. Health care providers who provide specialty services on an out-patient basis

17. A Preferred Provider Organization is an entity through which

   a. Providers negotiate lower fees with insurance companies in anticipation of a greater volume of patients

   b. Providers all work in the same clinic and admit to the same hospital

   c. The providers work on a "fee-for-service" basis

   d. Services are marketed to consumers

18. Characteristics of University Teaching Hospitals include

   a. Focus on hospital is clinical services

   b. Cost of care is lower because provider services are given by individuals in educational training curricula

   c. Quality of care is often low because of inexperienced clinicians

   d. Continuity of care may be a problem because of staff rotation and turnover

19. The term accreditation means

   a. The process by which a voluntary, non-governmental agency or organization appraises and grants accreditation status to institutions and/or programs or services which meet predetermined structure, process and outcome criteria

   b. The process by which a governmental agency appraises and grants accreditation status to institutions and/or programs or services which meet predetermined structure, process and outcome criteria

   c. Professional regulations which oversee the conduct and function of a profession's affairs

   d. A process by which an agency of state government grants permission to individuals accountable for the practice of a profession to engage in the practice of that profession and prohibits all others from legally doing so

20. The term licensure means

   a. The process by which a voluntary, non-governmental agency or organization appraises and grants accreditation status to institutions and/or programs or services which meet predetermined structure, process and outcome criteria

   b. The process by which a governmental agency appraises and grants accreditation status to institutions and/or programs or services which meet predetermined structure, process and outcome criteria

   c. Professional regulations which oversee the conduct and function of a profession's affairs

   d. A process by which an agency of state government grants permission to individuals accountable for the practice of a profession to engage in the practice of that profession and prohibits all others from legally doing so

21. The purpose of licensure is to

   a. Standardize programs or facilities

   b. Protect the public by ensuring a minimum level of professional competence

   c. List programs or facilities which meet certain standards

   d. Designate professional standards of practice

22. Certification is

   a. Process by which a non-governmental agency or association certifies that an individual licensed to practice as a professional has met certain predetermined standards specified by that profession for specialty practice

   b. Process by which an agency of state government grants permission to individuals accountable for the practice of a profession to engage in the practice of that profession and prohibits all others from doing so

c. The process by which a voluntary, non-governmental agency or organization appraises and grants accreditation status to institutions and/or programs or services which meet predetermined structure, process and outcome criteria

d. The process by which a governmental agency appraises and grants accreditation status to institutions and/or programs or services which meet predetermined structure, process and outcome criteria

23. The purpose of certification is to

a. Assure the public that an individual has mastered a body of knowledge and acquired skills in a particular study
b. Improve quality of programs
c. Have a list of qualified candidates
d. Recognize outstanding performance

24. Standards of practice are

a. The prevailing set of professional knowledge and skills established by an informal evaluation of practice within a community
b. Authoritative statements by which the quality of practice, service or education can be judged
c. Composed of informal discussions among health care providers within a community
d. A scientifically documented "gold standard" against which all practice is measured

25. Quality assurance programs can

a. Provide for accountability and responsibility of individual practitioners in delivering high quality care
b. Be tied to revenue generation
c. Increase exposure of practitioner to liability
d. Only evaluate the quality of records kept

26. Malpractice insurance

a. Will not protect a nurse practitioner from charges of practicing medicine without a license if they are practicing outside the state legal scope of practice
b. Will protect against entries into the National Practitioner Data Bank
c. Will protect a nurse practitioner from making a clinical mistake
d. Will pay for legal defense in the alleged failure on the part of a professional to render services with the degree of care, diligence, and precaution that another member of the same profession in similar circumstances would render

27. Personal/professional liability insurance covers

a. Liability issues of a more general nature

   b. Items such as homes, automobiles in addition to malpractice insurance
   c. Areas not covered by employer insurance
   d. Malpractice incidents exclusively

28. You are an Ob/Gyn nurse practitioner and you care for a baby whose parents sue you 10 years later because they claim your care damaged their child. You would want to have

   a. Malpractice insurance
   b. Occurrence coverage
   c. Claims made coverage
   d. Personal liability insurance

29. Advantages of direct reimbursement to nurse practitioners include

   a. Reinforces dominance of physicians
   b. Limits professional autonomy in nursing
   c. Limits consumer choice
   d. Provides for cost-effective health care through improved utilization of nurse practitioners

30. Medicare is

   a. Legislation from Social Security Act, Title 19
   b. Provides health insurance to low income persons
   c. Administered by Health Care Financing Administration
   d. Administered by a designated state agency

31. Medicare Part A provides for

   a. Inpatient hospital care, short-term skilled nursing facility care
   b. Outpatient physician services
   c. Laboratory and radiography services
   d. 80% of reasonable charges for covered services

32. Medicare Part B provides for

   a. Inpatient hospital care according to a prospective payment system
   b. Short-term skilled nursing facility care following hospitalization
   c. Home health agency visits and hospice care
   d. Services of physicians, outpatient hospital care, laboratory and radiography services

33. Which of the following services of nurse practitioners are covered by Medicare, part B

   a. All services delivered to Medicare patients
   b. Only those provided with a physician physically present at all times

c. Only routine physical examinations performed for prevention of illness and wellness promotion

d. "Incident to" physician services in private practice with physician supervision and with physician consultation immediately available

34. Medicaid is

a. Authorized through Social Security Act, Title 18
b. A Federal-State matching program providing medical assistance to low income persons
c. A program designed primarily to assist patients who are elderly
d. Administered by insurance company or organization

35. Medicaid reimbursement to nurse practitioners

a. Covers the services of gerontological and adult nurse practitioners
b. Level of coverage determined by state Medicaid Agency with considerable variation among states
c. Payment is always directly to agency and not to provider
d. Payment is based on usual and customary charge

36. Nationally nurse practitioners are reimbursed through which of the following programs?

a. DRGs
b. Private insurance companies
c. CHAMPUS and FEHBP
d. Blue Cross-Blue Shield

37. The nurse practitioner role originally began

a. In Colorado in 1975
b. As an experimental program in an Internal Medicine Clinic
c. With the pediatric nurse practitioner movement in an effort to expand traditional nursing functions to overlap those traditionally performed by physicians
d. As a Ph.D. program in human development

38. The nurse practitioner role has focused on

a. Provision of care to ambulatory patients with an emphasis on primary health care
b. Diagnosis and management of unstable acutely ill patients
c. Diagnosis and treatment of major acute illnesses
d. Specialty role development

39. Legal authority for nurse practitioner is granted by

a. State law and regulations (usually Nurse Practice Act)

    b. Federal law
    c. Health Care Financing Agency
    d. Medical and Pharmacy Practice Acts

40. Knowledge base of nurse practitioners is composed of

    a. Scientific content
    b. Applicable theory
    c. Scientific content and Theory
    d. Nursing Theory and Psychosocial Theory

41. Developmental theory is an example of a theory which

    a. Proceeds from the simple to the complex
    b. Theory which is in the early phase of developing
    c. Nursing theory which has developed to guide the practice of nurses
    d. Scientific content which is taught in all nursing schools

Answers

1.	c		22.	a
2.	b		23.	a
3.	a		24.	b
4.	a		25.	a
5.	b		26.	a
6.	a		27.	a
7.	d		28.	b
8.	a		29.	d
9.	a		30.	c
10.	b		31.	a
11.	a		32.	d
12.	d		33.	d
13.	c		34.	b
14.	b		35.	b
15.	c		36.	c
16.	b		37.	c
17.	a		38.	a
18.	d		39.	a
19.	a		40.	c
20.	d		41.	a
21.	b			

Bibliography

1992 Medicare Explained. Commerce Clearing House: Chicago, IL.

American Nurses Association. (1979). *The study of credentialing in nursing: A new approach*, Staff working papers, (pp. 2, 28). Kansas City: ANA.

American Nurses Association. (1985). *Code of ethics*. Kansas City: ANA.

American Nurses Association. (1988). *Ethics in nursing: Position statements and guidelines*. Pub. No. G-175. Kansas City: ANA.

Bullough, B. (1993). State nurse practice acts. In M. D. Mezey & D. O. McGivern (Eds). *Nurses, nurse practitioners: Evolution to advanced practice* (pp 267-280). NY: Springer Publishing.

Bullough, B., Sultz, H., Henry O. M., & Fiedler, R. (1984). Trends in pediatric nurse practitioner education and employment. *Pediatric Nursing, 10,* 193-196.

Congressional Record. (1989).

Creasia, J. L., & Parker, B. (1991). *Conceptual foundations of professional nursing practice*. St. Louis: Mosby Yearbook.

Dye, T. R. (1992). *Understanding public policy* (7th ed.). Englewood Cliffs, NJ: Prentice Hall.

Eccard, W. T., & Gainor, E. E. (1993). Legal ramifications for advanced practice. In M. D. Mezey & D. O. McGivern (Eds.), *Nurses, nurse practitioners: Evolution to advanced practice* (pp. 281-321). NY: Springer Publishing.

Edmunds, M. W. (1991). NPs who replace physicians: Role expansion or exploitation? *Nurse Practitioner, 16*(9), 46, 49.

Fry, S. T. (1990). Measurement of moral answerability in nursing practice. In C. F. Waltz and O. I. Strickland (Eds.). *Measurement of clinical and educational nursing outcomes*. Vol IV. New York: Springer Publishing.

Health Law. (1990). Committee on Energy and Commerce. U.S. Government Printing Office. Washington, D.C. Committee Print 101-104. 101st Congress 2nd Session.

Joint Commission on Accreditation of Healthcare Organizations. (1988). *Overview of quality assurance and monitoring and evaluation*. Chicago: JCAHCO

King, J. H. (1986). *The law of medical malpractice* (2nd ed.). St. Paul: West Publishing Co.

Kozier, B., Erb, G., & Blais, K. (1992). *Advocacy and change in concepts and issues in nursing practice* (2nd ed.). Redwood City CA: Addison-Wesley.

Labar, D. (1983). *Third party reimbursement for services of nurses.* Kansas City, MO: American Nurses Association.

MacQueen, J. C. (1979). The challenges of the PNP/A movement. *Pediatric Nursing, 5,* 31-35.

McGivern, D. O. (1993). The evolution of advanced nursing practice. In M. D. Mezey and D. O. McGivern (Eds.). *Nurses, nurse practitioners: Evolution to advanced practice* (pp. 3-30). NY: Springer Publishing.

Medicare Carriers Manual Part 3—*Claims Process* issued by Department of Health and Human Services, Health Care Financing Administration, Transmittal No. 1463, HCFA Pub. 14-3.

Mezey, M. (1993). Preparation for advanced practice. In M. D. Mezey & D. O. McGivern (Eds.), *Nurses, nurse practitioners: Evolution to advanced practice* (pp. 31-58). NY: Springer Publishing

Mittelstadt, P. M. (1993). Federal reimbursement of advanced practice nurses' services empowers the profession. *Nurse Practitioner, 18*(1), 43-49.

Moniz, D. (1992). The legal danger of written protocols and standards of practice. *Nurse Practitioner,* 17(9), 58-60.

Morton, P. G. (1989) *Health assessment in nursing.* Springhouse, PA: Springhouse Corporation.

Murphy, M. A. (1990). A brief history of pediatric nurse practitioners and NAPNAP 1964-1990. *Journal of Pediatric Health Care, 4,* 332-337.

National Leadership Coalition for Health Care Reform. (1991). *A comprehensive reform plan for the health care system.*

Northrup, C., & Kelly, M. (1987). *Legal issues in nursing,* St. Louis: Mosby Year Book.

Pearson, L. (1994). 1993-1994 Update: How each state stands on legislative issues affecting advanced nursing practice. *Nurse Practitioner, 19*(1), 16-25.

Pearson, L. (1993). 1992-1993 Update: How each state stands on legislative issues affecting advanced nursing practice. *Nurse Practitioner, 18*(1), pp. 23-28

Public Health Service. (1990). *Healthy People 2000.* (DHHS Publication No. PHS 91-50212). Washington, DC: U.S. Government Printing Office.

The Medicare 1991 Handbook, U. S. Department of Health and Human Services, Health Care Financing Administration. Publication No. HCFA 10050, SSA ICN-461250.

Wilkinson, M. G. (1991). Teaching and learning. In J. L. Creasia and B. Parker, (Eds). *Conceptual foundations of professional nursing practice.* (pp. 263-266). St. Louis: Mosby Yearbook.

INDEX

For information on Certification Review Courses, Home Study Programs and Review Books contact:

Health Leadership Associates, Inc.
Post Office Box 59153
Potomac, Maryland 20859

1-800-435-4775

REVIEW BOOK/AUDIO CASSETTE ORDER FORM
HEALTH LEADERSHIP ASSOCIATES, INC.

PLEASE PRINT OR TYPE

NAME: _____

ADDRESS: Street _____ Apt. # _____ City _____ State _____ Zip Code _____

TELEPHONE: _____ (HOME) _____ (WORK)

Section 1: AUDIO CASSETTES

Professional "live" audio recordings of Review Courses are approximately 15 hours in length unless otherwise noted and include detailed course handouts. Continuing Education contact hours are available for these audio cassette Home Study Programs.

QTY	REVIEW COURSE TITLE	PRICE	
____	Adult Nurse Practitioner	$150.00	_____
____	Ambulatory Women's Health Care Nursing	$150.00	_____
____	Clinical Specialist in Adult Psychiatric and Mental Health Nursing	$150.00	_____
____	Family Nurse Practitioner	$330.00	_____
	(Consists of ANP, PNP & Childbearing Management courses)		
____	* Generalist Gerontological Nurse	$ 75.00	_____
____	Generalist Medical-Surgical Nurse	$150.00	_____
____	* Generalist Pediatric Nurse	$ 75.00	_____
____	* Generalist Psychiatric and Mental Health Nurse	$ 75.00	_____
____	Gerontological Nurse Practitioner	$150.00	_____
____	Home Health Nurse	$150.00	_____
____	Inpatient Obstetric/Maternal Newborn/Low Risk Neonatal/Perinatal Nurse	$150.00	_____
____	** Childbearing Management	$ 45.00	_____
____	Pediatric Nurse Practitioner	$150.00	_____
____	** Test Taking Strategies and Techniques	$ 30.00	_____
____	Women's Health Care Nurse Practitioner	$150.00	_____
	(Formerly Ob/Gyn Nurse Practitioner)		

* 8 Hour Course, ** 2-4 Hour Course

SUB TOTAL: _____

Maryland Residents add 5% sales tax: _____

CEU FEE ($10/course): _____

Shipping: 2-4 Hour Course $ 4.00   _____

All other Courses $10.00   _____

TOTAL: _____

PAYMENT DUE METHOD OF PAYMENT

☐ Check or money order (US funds, payable to Health Leadership Associates, Inc.) A $25 fee will be charged on returned checks.

☐ Purchase Order is attached. P.O. # _____

☐ Please charge my ☐ MasterCard ☐ Visa

Credit Card# _____ Exp. date _____

Signature _____

Print Name _____

REVIEW GUIDES & AUDIO CASSETTES

1) Section 1 Total $ _____

2) Section 2 Total $ _____

3) Section 3 Total $ _____

TOTAL PAYMENT DUE $ _____

Section 2: REVIEW BOOKS

QTY	BOOK TITLE	PRICE	
____	Adult Nurse Practitioner Certification Review Guide (second edition)	$ 47.75	_____
____	Family Nurse Practitioner Certification Review Guide Set (Includes ANP, PNP, and Women's Health Care NP Guides)	$123.25	_____
____	Generalist Pediatric Nurse Certification Review Guide (second edition)	$ 47.75	
____	Gerontological Nursing Certification Review Guide for the Generalist, Clinical Specialist, and Nurse Practitioner (revised edition)	$ 47.75	
____	Pediatric Nurse Practitioner Certification Review Guide (second edition)	$ 47.75	
____	Psychiatric Certification Review Guide for the Generalist and Clinical Specialist in Adult, Child, and Adolescent Psychiatric and Mental Health Nursing	$ 47.75	
____	Women's Health Care Nurse Practitioner Certification Review Guide (Formerly Ob/Gyn Nurse Practitioner)	$ 47.75	

SPECIAL OFFERING

____	TODAY and TOMORROW'S WOMAN - MENOPAUSE: BEFORE AND AFTER (Girls of 16 to Women of 99) (Author: Virginia Layng Millonig)	$ 19.95	

SUB TOTAL: _____

Maryland Residents add 5% sales tax: _____

CEU FEE ($10.00) _____

Shipping $5.00 for one book: _____

$2.00 for each additional book: _____
(Except $1.00 for each add'l. *Today and Tomorrow's Woman*)

TOTAL: _____

For orders of 10 or greater call 1-800-435-4775.
(All prices subject to change without notice)

Section 3: REVIEW BOOK/AUDIO CASSETTE DISCOUNT PACKAGES

A discounted rate is available when purchasing Review Book(s) and Audio Cassettes together. When purchasing packages, indicate Book/Audio Cassette selections in sections 1 and 2. Calculate amount due in this section.

QTY	PACKAGE SELECTION	PRICE	
____	8 Hour Course / 1 Review Guide	$120.00	_____
____	15 Hour Course / 1 Review Guide	$190.00	_____
____	FNP Package	$415.00	_____

FNP Package consists of Adult NP, Pediatric NP, Women's Health Care NP Guides & Audio Cassettes of the ANP, PNP, and Childbearing Management Courses.

SUB TOTAL: _____

Maryland Residents add 5% sales tax: _____

CEU Fee ($10) _____

TOTAL: _____
(Shipping charge included in package rate)

RETURN POLICY

Due to the nature of the material contained in the review books and audio cassettes, returns on books ONLY will be accepted one week post delivery. No returns on audio cassettes except for defective audio cassettes which will be replaced.

MAIL TO: Health Leadership Associates, Inc.
P.O. Box 59153 Potomac, MD 20859

OR PHONE: (800) 435-4775; (301) 983-2405

OR FAX: (301) 983-2693